Multimedia and Multimodal Intelligence for Secure and Sustainable Healthcare

Providing a comprehensive examination of artificial intelligence techniques that integrate heterogeneous healthcare data to support intelligent, secure, and sustainable healthcare systems, this book presents both theoretical foundations and practical methodologies for multimodal data fusion, representation learning, decision-making using medical images, biosignals, electronic health records, wearable sensors, text, and multimedia data.

- Illustrates analyzing and integrating multiple modalities of healthcare data, such as medical images, electronic health records, bio signals, and genomic data.
- Emphasizes the role of multimedia intelligence in healthcare by leveraging advanced artificial intelligence techniques to analyze diverse data formats, including text, images, audio, and video.
- Presents practical applications that ensure secure healthcare data management and sustainable solutions, focusing on improving patient care and enhancing diagnostics.
- Covers the different security mechanisms applied in multimodal and multimedia-based healthcare applications.
- Showcases the role of advanced artificial intelligence and machine learning methods, including privacy-preserving technologies, blockchain, and explainable artificial intelligence tailored for secure healthcare.

Multimedia and Multimodal Intelligence for Secure and Sustainable Healthcare is primarily written for senior undergraduates, graduate students, and academic researchers in electrical engineering, electronics and communications engineering, computer science and engineering, and biomedical engineering.

Multimedia and Multimodal Intelligence

Series Editor- Amit Kumar Singh

Multimedia and Multimodal Intelligence for Sustainable Development
Edited by Vinay Kumar Srivastava, Priyank Khare, Divyanshu Awasthi, Lalit Garg

Artificial Intelligence for Medical Data Processing
Algorithms and Applications
Edited By Chetna Sharma, Amandeep Kaur, Harpreet Singh

Multimedia and Multimodal Intelligence for Secure and Sustainable Healthcare
Theoretical and Practical Insights
Edited By Sita Rani, Sui Yang Khoo, Ashima Kalra, Hemant Kumar Saini

For more information about this series, please visit: https://www.routledge.com/Multimedia-and-Multimodal-Intelligence/book-series/MMI

Multimedia and Multimodal Intelligence for Secure and Sustainable Healthcare

Theoretical and Practical Insights

Edited by
Sita Rani, Sui Yang Khoo, Ashima Kalra
and Hemant Kumar Saini

CRC Press
Taylor & Francis Group
Boca Raton London New York

CRC Press is an imprint of the
Taylor & Francis Group, an **informa** business

Front cover image: frank60/Shutterstock

First edition published 2027
by CRC Press
2385 NW Executive Center Drive, Suite 320, Boca Raton FL 33431

and by CRC Press
4 Park Square, Milton Park, Abingdon, Oxon, OX14 4RN

CRC Press is an imprint of Taylor & Francis Group, LLC

Library of Congress Cataloging-in-Publication Data
Names: Rani, Sita editor | Khoo, Sui Yang editor | Kalra, Ashima editor |
Saini, Hemant Kumar editor
Title: Multimedia and multimodal intelligence for secure and
sustainable healthcare : theoretical and practical insights /
Edited by Sita Rani, Sui Yang Khoo, Ashima Kalra and Hemant Kumar Saini.
Description: First edition. | Boca Raton : CRC Press, 2027. |
Series: Multimedia and multimodal intelligence |
Includes bibliographical references. |
Identifiers: LCCN 2026014841 (print) | LCCN 2026014842 (ebook) |
ISBN 9781041126003 hardback | ISBN 9781041126058 paperback |
ISBN 9781003665656 ebook
Subjects: LCSH: Artificial intelligence–Medical applications | Medical care–Data processing
Classification: LCC R859.7.A78 M86 2027 (print) | LCC R859.7.A78 (ebook)
LC record available at https://lccn.loc.gov/2026014841
LC ebook record available at https://lccn.loc.gov/2026014842

ISBN: 978-1-041-12600-3 (hbk)
ISBN: 978-1-041-12605-8 (pbk)
ISBN: 978-1-003-66565-6 (ebk)

DOI: 10.1201/9781003665656

Typeset in Sabon
by Newgen Publishing UK

Contents

Preface

This book stems from the rapid transformation of healthcare through artificial intelligence, multimodal data analytics, and intelligent digital technologies. Modern healthcare systems generate vast and diverse data from medical imaging, wearable sensors, clinical records, and multimedia sources, creating a strong motivation to develop advanced frameworks that can integrate and interpret such complex information. This book presents cutting-edge research and technological innovations in multimodal intelligence, cloud and mobile healthcare systems, and AI-driven medical applications. It highlights how data fusion, machine learning, and generative technologies can support accurate diagnosis, disease prediction, patient monitoring, and personalized treatment strategies. In addition, it explores emerging paradigms such as smart hospitals, digital twins, and multimodalality-enabled secure healthcare ecosystems. By bringing together contributions from leading researchers, this volume aims to bridge the gap between theoretical advancements and practical healthcare solutions. Ultimately, this book seeks to inspire further research and innovation toward building secure, intelligent, and sustainable next-generation healthcare systems.

About the editors

Ashima Kalra is a distinguished academician and researcher, currently serving as an associate professor in the Department of Electronics and Communication Engineering at Chandigarh Engineering College (CGC), Landran, Punjab, India. With over 22 years of rich teaching experience at both undergraduate and postgraduate levels, she has consistently contributed to academic excellence, research advancement, and industry–academia engagement. She holds a PhD in Electronics and Communication Engineering from Maharishi University, Noida (2023). She completed her MTech with distinction from Punjab Technical University, Jalandhar, and is a Gold Medalist in BTech (Electronics Engineering) from Kurukshetra University, Kurukshetra.

Dr. Kalra has an outstanding research profile, with over 50 publications in reputable international journals, including 5 SCI-indexed and 25 Scopus-indexed papers. She has authored six textbooks and 15 book chapters and has also edited two books published by CRC Press, covering emerging areas such as ethical hacking, machine learning, and artificial intelligence. Her research interests include artificial intelligence, neural networks, fuzzy systems, and machine learning, which have led to the filing of 18 patents in innovative domains such as AI-powered robotic systems and chronic kidney disease detection using intelligent models. She has successfully guided several MTech dissertations in advanced areas including image processing, cryptography, and intelligent systems. Actively engaged in the academic and professional community, Dr. Kalra has served as a session chair, reviewer, and technical committee member for numerous international conferences and journals. She has also played a key role in organizing faculty development programs, workshops, and industrial interaction activities, strengthening industry exposure for students.

She is a senior member of IEEE and a life member of ISTE. In addition, she has completed multiple professional certifications in artificial intelligence, data analytics, and emerging technologies through platforms such as Coursera, SWAYAM, and UpGrad. Her contributions have been widely recognized through multiple academic excellence awards, including the prestigious Women Leadership Award, reflecting her sustained commitment to quality education, impactful research, and leadership in engineering education.

Sui Yang Khoo received the B.E. degree in Electrical and Electronics Engineering from Tasmania University and the PhD degree in Computer Engineering from Nanyang Technological University, in 2005 and 2008, respectively. In 2008, he was a research fellow in the Department of Electrical and Electronics Engineering, Nanyang Technological University, Singapore. Since 2009, he has been with the School of Engineering, Deakin University, Victoria, Australia, where he is now an associate professor in Electrical & Electronics Engineering. Sui Yang's research interests include stochastic differential equations, variable structure control, co-operative control, robotics, adaptive signal processing, time-varying systems, and machine learning.

Sita Rani, PhD, works in the Department of Computer Science and Engineering at Guru Nanak Dev Engineering College, Ludhiana. She earned her PhD in Computer Science and Engineering from I.K. Gujral Punjab Technical University, Kapurthala, Punjab in 2018. She completed Postdoc from Big Data Mining and Machine Learning Lab, South Ural State University, Russia from May 2022 to August 2023. She has also completed Post Graduate Certificate Program in Data Science and Machine Learning from Indian Institute of Technology, Roorkee in 2023.

She has more than 20 years of academic, administration, and research experience. She is an active member of ISTE, IEEE, and IAEngg. She has been recognized in the Top 2% Scientists list published by Stanford University for the year 2024. She is the receiver of ISTE Section Best Teacher Award-2020 and International Young Scientist Award-2021. She has contributed to the various research activities while publishing articles in the renowned SCI and Scopus journals and conference proceedings. She has published several national and international patents and authored, edited, and coedited 11 books. Dr. Rani has delivered many expert talks in A.I.C.T.E. sponsored Faculty Development Programs and keynote talks in many National and International Conferences. She has also organized many International Conferences during her 20 years of experience. She is the member of Editorial Board and reviewer of many reputable international journals. She has also served as vice president of SME and MSME (UT Council), Women Indian Chamber of Commerce and Industry (WICCI) since November 2021 to February 2025. Her research interest includes data science, artificial intelligence, machine learning, blockchain technology, smart healthcare, and sustainable development.

Hemant Kumar Saini works as an academic at the School of Computer Science Engineering at Bennett University (The Times Group), Greater Noida, India and Lincoln University, Malaysia. He has more than 14 years of teaching experience. He has demonstrated his research prowess by publishing articles in renowned (SCI and Scopus indexed) journals and conference proceedings. He has delivered many lectures in the ATAL-sponsored Faculty Development Programs and keynote speeches in National and International Conferences. He is Post Doc from Lincoln University Malaysia and finished his PhD in the AdHoc Networks Security and MTech (Gold Medalist) in Computer Science and Engineering and honored by Governor of Rajasthan by Hon'ble Shri Kalyan Singh Ji. He is a Professional Red Hat Certified Engineer. He has published 65 articles in reputable, peer-reviewed national and international Scopus and SCI journals, 8 books, and 18 published in Scopus-indexed conferences. Additionally, he has served as a keynote speaker and resource person for several workshops and webinars conducted in India. He has been a CSI and IEEE professional member. His research includes digital transformation technologies such as artificial intelligence, quantum computing, Internet of Things, blockchain, edge and serverless computing, cloud-native computing, and digital twins. He is a reviewer and TPC member of IEEE and Springer Nature Computer Science Journal. He is a Chief Editor of Journal of Scientific Research and Reports, Journal of Supercomputing, Guest Editor of IEEE Communication, and CSI communications and edited books published by reputable international publishers.

Contributors

Ekta Acharya
Faculty of Engineering and Architecture,
Department of Computer Studies,
JNVU, Jodhpur, India

Chadi Altrjman
Artificial Intelligence and Software Engineering Departments,
Research Center for AI and IoT, AI and Informatics Faculty
Near East University, Nicosia, Mersin10, Turkey

Fadi Al-Turjman
Artificial Intelligence and Software Engineering Departments,
Research Center for AI and IoT, AI and Informatics Faculty,
Near East University, Nicosia, Mersin10, Turkey

Sinem Alturjman
Artificial Intelligence and Software Engineering Departments,
Research Center for AI and IoT, AI and Informatics Faculty,
Near East University, Nicosia, Mersin10, Turkey

D. Anitha
Department of Computer Science and Engineering,
University College of Engineering,
Panruti, Tamil Nadu, India

Chaitanya Arora
Department of Computer Science and Engineering,
Guru Nanak Dev Engineering College,
Ludhiana, Punjab, India

Fazlourrahman Balouchzahi
Universidad Nacional Autónoma de México (UNAM), Instituto de Investigaciones en Matemáticas Aplicadas y Sistemas (IIMAS),
Mexico City, Mexico

Veera Venkata Siva Prasad Balusupati
School of Engineering, Anurag University,
Telangana, Hyderabad, India

Kaushik Chanda
Department of Computational Sciences,
Brainware University, Barasat, West Bengal, India

Meetali Chauhan
Department of Computer Science and Engineering,
Guru Nanak Dev Engineering College, Ludhiana
Punjab, India

Jagjit Singh Dhatterwal
School of Computer Science and Artificial Intelligence,
SR University, Warangal, Telangana, India

Neha Gupta
Department School of CSIT,
SUAS, Indore, India

Aayush Kalia
Department of Computer Science and Engineering,
Guru Nanak Dev Engineering College, Ludhiana,
Punjab, India

Ashima Kalra
Department of Electronics and Communication Engineering,
Chandigarh Engineering College, CGC Landran,
Mohali, Punjab, India

Kuldeep Singh Kaswan
School of Computer Science and Engineering,
Galgotias University, Greater Noida, India

Amandeep Kaur
Department of Computer Science and Engineering, Akal University,
Talwandi Sabo, Bathinda, India

Upinder Kaur
Department of Computer Science and Engineering,
Akal University,
Talwandi Sabo, Bathinda, India

Kanan Kaura
Department of Computer Science and Engineering,
Guru Nanak Dev Engineering College,
Ludhiana, India

Kiran Malik
Department of Computer Science and Engineering (AIML),
GL Bajaj Institute of Technology and Management, Greater Noida, India

Indraneel Mukhopadhyay
School of Information Technology
Amity Institute of Information Technology,
Amity University Kolkata, India

Subhadip Nandi
Department of Computational Sciences,
Brainware University, Barasat, India

Raja Sekhar Reddy Pocha
School of Engineering, Anurag University,
Telangana, Hyderabad, India

P. Priya Ponnuswamy
School of Computer Science Engineering and Information Systems,
Vellore Institute of Technology,
Vellore, India

Srilatha Pulipati
Department of Artificial Intelligence and Data Science,
Chaitanya Bharathi Institute of Technology,
Telangana, Hyderabad, India

Vikram Puri
School of Computer Science,
Duy Tan University, Da Nang,
Vietnam

Sita Rani
Department of Computer Science and Engineering,
Guru Nanak Dev Engineering College,
Ludhiana, Punjab, India

Soumya Roy
Department of Computational Sciences,
Brainware University,
Barasat, India

Hemant Kumar Saini
School of Computer Science Engineering and Technology,
Bennett University (The Times Group), Greater Noida, India
Department of Computer Science and Engineering, Lincoln University College, Petaling Jaya, Selangor, Malaysia

Ramiz Salama
Artificial Intelligence and Software Engineering Departments,
Research Center for AI and IoT, AI and Informatics Faculty,
Near East University, Nicosia, Mersin10, Turkey

Debarpita Santra
School of Information Technology
Amity Institute of Information Technology,
Amity University Kolkata, India

KSRK Sarma
Department of Computer Science and Engineering (Data Science),
Vidya Jyothi Institute of Technology,
Hyderabad, India

A. Senthilmurugan
Department of Computer Science and Engineering,
St. Peter's Engineering College,
Hyderabad, Telangana, India

Kapil Sharma
Department School of CSIT,
SUAS, Indore, India

Riya Sil
Department of Computer Science and Engineering,
Brainware University,
Barasat, India

Abhijot Singh
Department of Computer Science and Engineering,
Guru Nanak Dev Engineering College, Ludhiana,
Punjab, India

A. Sivaranjani
School of Computer Science and Engineering,
Vellore Institute of Technology,
Vellore, India

Jaspinder Kaur Walia
Department of Computer Science and Engineering,
Guru Nanak Dev Engineering College,
Ludhiana, India

Chapter 1

Introduction to multimodal and multimedia intelligence for healthcare

Ashima Kalra, Sita Rani, and Hemant Kumar Saini

1.1 INTRODUCTION

Recent advancements in AI and the flow of mixed data into the system have caused the digitization of the entire healthcare system. An older model of clinical decision-making utilized one data source at a time, primarily focusing on the clinical images or one laboratory report. In contrast, today's healthcare systems use a variety of data types, spanning a whole range of imaging, biosignals, individual clinical and laboratory records obtained from electronic health record (EHR) systems, freely written clinical notes, even voice data and information obtained from wearable biosensors. The aims of the field of study that focuses on understanding health data the best, and combining multiple data types, are to integrate the different data types in order to provide a comprehensive understanding of a patient's health. Balancing and integrating different types of information from different data sources improve the systems' capacity to support clinical decision-making, predictive analytics, and diagnosis, which are the key features of modern world healthcare systems. (Baltrusaitis et al., 2019; Ghassemi et al., 2021).

1.1.1 Overview of multimodal and multimedia intelligence

Multimodal intelligence is the ability to understand and analyze separate forms of data, such as images, audio, and text. This is done through an integrated computational approach that merges and interprets data from varying fields. Multimedia intelligence deals specifically with the integration of video, audio, and text content. Within the healthcare domain, these two paradigms combine as clinical contexts naturally produce and analyze multimodal and multimedia data related to a patient's condition from several different perspectives.

Healthcare data are also intricate and layered as a single clinical case may involve a series of components, including radiology images that show physical heterogeneity, physiological signals that capture the dynamics of

DOI: 10.1201/9781003665656-1

function, lab data that provide quantifiable values, and notes from the physician that describe the reasoning behind the diagnosis and observations contextualizing the case. Each of these components alone provides a certain level of insight, however, when combined, a more complete representation of the patient's health is revealed. Multimodal intelligence focuses on understanding the benefits of combining different datasets. It works to find complex relationships and correlations that are not visible when each modality is analyzed separately.

Developments in fields like deep learning continue to drive rapid progress in multimodal and multimedia AI. In the past, multimodal approaches used feature engineering and modular fusion rules to build systems. These approaches struggled with generalization and scalability. On the other hand, modern deep learning techniques, including convolutional neural networks, recurrent and transformer networks, attention mechanisms, and other techniques, abstract the entire learning process to the application of the system to either raw or minimally preprocessed datasets. These systems can align the representations from different modalities to reason at a general level across different types of inputs (Ngiam et al., 2011).

In multimodal intelligence, representation learning enables the characterization of the multimodal features of the data to identify features that represent clinically relevant information. Approaches including joint embedding learning, cross-modal attention, and multimodal transformers have been shown to capture complex relationships across different modalities, like those that align radiological texts and clinical reports. Moreover, multimodal fusion increases the reliability of AI systems in real-world healthcare applications by addressing the missing or noisy data in single modalities of the datasets (Baltrusaitis et al., 2019).

The use of AI in healthcare is improving and moving in new directions with multimodal and multimedia intelligence of AI. These technologies analyze and contextualize data in a more integrated manner than has previously been done in healthcare. With the combination of data integration and deep learning algorithms, a more detailed and complete representation of the patient is built, which brings new levels of precision to clinical care and decision support. This is the beginning of the next generation of personalized and sustainable healthcare.

1.1.2 Definition, scope, and relevance to modern healthcare

The definition of multimodal healthcare intelligence is the analysis of multiple streams of patient data via AI in parallel in order to accomplish various clinical and administrative functions in healthcare. In contrast to traditional AI healthcare systems, which use a single data source, in multimodal systems, data from multiple sources such as medical images, biosignals, health records, clinical narratives, audio, and various other sensor modalities are integrated. This permits a more complete representation of the patient's health. Thus, the efficiency of the diagnosis, the prognostication, the continuous health monitoring, and evidence-based clinical decision-making is enhanced as the clinical data is representative of both the structure and the context.

The use of multimodal systems in healthcare spans the entire continuum of care. In preventive and primary care, multimodal systems combine lifestyle data from wearables and clinical history to identify and support early interventions. In acute and critical care, the real-time convergence of physiological signals and lab results with images supports the timely detection of clinical deterioration and enables rapid decision-making. In personalized medicine, multimodal intelligence combines genomic data, imaging biomarkers, and longitudinal health records to customize treatment plans. Public health surveillance, disease trend analysis, and resource allocation at the population level are supported with the integration of disparate data from patient groups across healthcare systems.

The most significant feature of advanced multimodal healthcare analytics is how it takes into consideration some of the most significant shortcomings of standard healthcare analytics. Instead of analyzing only one form of data at a time, advanced systems utilize the diagnostics of several omics data forms to reduce the uncertainty of a clinical diagnosis and limit the problems associated with missing, messy, or contradictory data that clinical settings often face. The greater the number of data forms that healthcare analytics is capable of working with, the greater the interdependence of the data. This, in turn, contributes to the analytics yielding a greater deduction, or a more valid clinical result. Moreover, advanced healthcare analytics are capable of exposing a more comprehensive visualization of a patient's data, leading to the assessment of the individual as a whole, in terms of their health, rather than fixing their assessment to particular clinical markers.

As health facilities are gradually migrating to customized and value-based care, integrated advanced multimodal healthcare analytics are becoming highly relevant and a preferred tool of technology in the clinical field. There is significant congestion in the paradox of advanced multimodal analytics improving the clinical results of a healthcare system, and at the same time, supporting optimal decision-making and resource utilization in the system whereby the system becomes more equitable and patient-centered. The paradox in question is the congestion in the "data analytics driven healthcare system."

1.2 MODALITIES IN HEALTHCARE DATA

Healthcare data is heterogeneous due to the varying nature of human physiology as well as the workflows of each individual clinical practice. Each data type captures different components of a patient's health. Their integration is crucial for a well-rounded analysis.

1.2.1 Imaging, signals, text, speech, and sensor data

Aspects of medical imaging, including X-ray, CT, MRI, and ultrasound, allow for the analysis of different signals to obtain the anatomy and functioning of the tissues in the area of interest. Signals such as electrocardiograms or ECG, electroencephalograms or EEG, and electromyograms or EMG capture biological activity. Text from electronic health records or EHR, discharge summaries, and clinical notes is able to code contextual and semantical information for reasoning. Emotional states, and even cognitive impairment or other neurological conditions, can be diagnosed from physician patient dialogues. Furthermore, several sensors and wearable IoT devices stream data for activity levels, heart rates, and even sleep patterns. Were these data types to be used separately, they would provide a fraction of the information; used together, they create a far more accurate and contextual awareness of the patient's health (Shickel et al., 2018).

Various healthcare data modalities are shown in Figure 1.1.

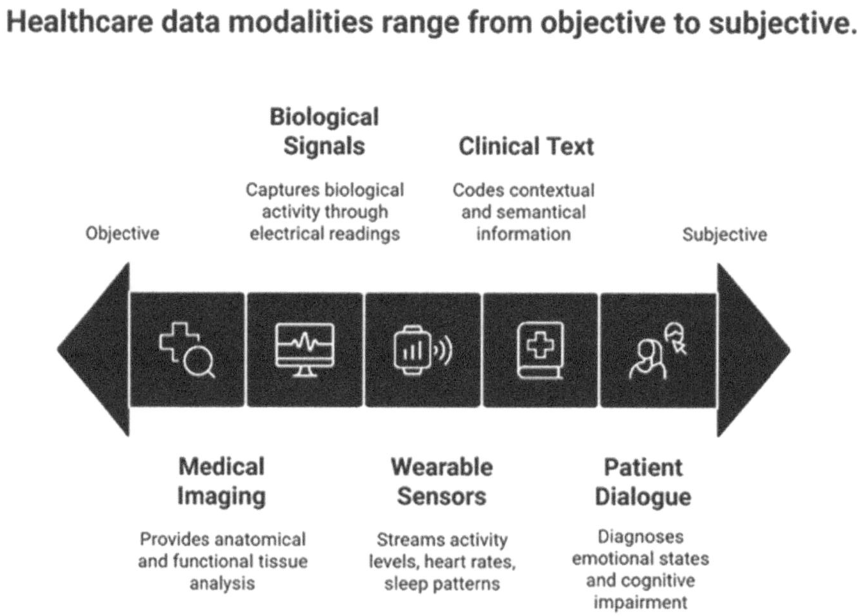

Figure 1.1 Healthcare data modalities.

1.3 KEY CONCEPTS AND FOUNDATIONS

The reasonable integration and interpretation of disparate datasets used by multimodal healthcare analytics relies on sound theories and advanced algorithms. Each modality of healthcare data is characterized by a variety of attributes with different structures, numerosity, dimensionality, timescales, and semantics. These attributes can vary to such an extent that naive integrations will fail. These are the reasons that multimodal systems leverage specialized architectural designs for learning that capture the cross-modal relations, model uncertainty, and preserve clinical relevances. Innovations at the intersection of the integration of data, representation learning, and deep neural networks offer the theoretical underpinnings and insights for the construction of adaptable and efficient healthcare systems at the multimodal spectrum.

1.3.1 Data fusion, representation learning, and deep learning basics

Data fusion is a central process of multimodal intelligence and refers to the process of integrating different data types into a single representation. Depending on the stage of integration, fusion methods can be classified into three types: early, late, and hybrid fusion.

In early fusion, data from different modalities are integrated before the model training process on a raw data level, or on a low feature level so that the model can learn joint representations from the beginning. Although the approach can be fine grained, this fusion strategy tends to be highly sensitive to data scale, missing values, and noise. On the other hand, late fusion is the integration of information that is done at the decision level, whereby predictions or outputs from different models that are specialized in certain modalities are combined. While not fully utilizing cross-modal relationships, this strategy tends to be more flexible and robust. By integrating early and late fusion strategies, hybrid fusion attempts to mitigate the aforementioned tradeoffs by combining modalities at several points in the learning process so that low-level interactions are captured alongside high-level semantic alignment.

Having representation learning is really important to conduct multimodal fusion as it learns the features of the different modalities and determines if they correlate to some degree across the feature latent space. All of this while retaining the clinically useful information and trying to learn the specific characteristics of each modality, as well as learning the cross correlations of the modalities. The ability of the models to draw associations from imbalanced data—for example, associating images from radiology with the text of the clinical reports—is possible through joint embedding learning, cross-attention mechanisms, and several of the mechanisms for cross-modality alignment. The representation of the data in the models is important as it allows the models to interpret the data and the overall generalization of the multimodal networks and rely on the models to work in an imbalanced situation, such as when some of the modalities are missing, or when the data is very noisy.

Deep learning is able to learn representations hierarchically and nonlinearly from pervasive data and is predominating the field of multimodal healthcare intelligence. Medical image analysis is dominated by the use of convolutional neural networks while the processing of sequential and temporal data such as physiological signals is done using recurrent neural networks as well as their variants. The processing of text data is done using transformer-based architectures and for time-series data. Attention mechanisms optimize the contribution of each individual modality contextually to enhance multimodal learning. These architectures enable end-to-end learning frameworks, while minimizing the amount of feature engineering, to detect clinically relevant patterns from highly complex datasets automatically (Goodfellow et al., 2016; Baltrušaitis et al., 2019). Multimodal healthcare intelligence is based on data fusion, representation learning, and deep learning. This combination allows for the analysis of data beyond silos and facilities the necessary context-dependent reasoning that is needed for virtually limitless healthcare.

1.4 HEALTHCARE APPLICATIONS OF MULTIMODAL INTELLIGENCE

The last few years have seen the emergence of multimodal intelligence, the first of its kind, as a powerful means of combining and analyzing various data sources within a complex Health Care Application to provide rapid, accurate, and timely healthcare decisions. The synergetic effect of multimodal is a distinct advantage over single-modality systems, as a healthcare AI is able to integrate and process vast amounts of relevant physiology and contextual data. The improvements in the various functions of the healthcare AI, such as, but not limited to, clinical prediction, monitoring, and decision-making have extensively benefited from the use of multimodal intelligence in healthcare.

1.4.1 Diagnostics

In a diagnostic environment, what multimodal intelligence contributes to disease identification and classification is the amalgamation of clinical texts, medical imaging, and laboratory results. A case in point is the conjunction of radiological imaging and pathology reports, along with other physician notes, to identify and document complex illnesses such as cancer and other cardiovascular and neurological diseases. When clinical context is provided, visual irregularities can be correlated, and the multimodal models can prevent the diagnoses from being false. This leads to diagnoses that are earlier and more reliable. Possible completed or ambiguous evidence can then be completed with this holistic diagnostic approach.

1.4.2 Monitoring

Patient monitoring systems integrate data from wearable sensors and bedside monitoring devices with EHRs from prior to the point of integration to evaluate a patient's condition in real time and provide system and data applications for the continuous monitoring of patients, especially in a critical care and remote monitoring context, to provide early warning systems in the case of a patient's condition deteriorating to identify and avoid from loss of critical time in the monitoring of a patient's condition in real time to provide system and data applications for the continuous monitoring of patients. Multimodal monitoring systems track short- and long-term health data to implement a patient's timely system applications in order to avoid adverse patient symptoms. Deep multimodal models that combine imaging with textual clinical reports have shown substantial improvements in disease classification accuracy, lesion localization, and semantic understanding of clinical narratives (Yao et al., 2024).

1.4.3 Prediction

Per-doctor metabolic models are trained using longitudinally collected EHR unit datasets and imaging findings, hospital physiologic signals, and individual demographic details. Predictive modeling and forecasting is one more useful application of multimodal AI in healthcare. Predictive modeling analyzes and forecasts risk of disease progression and treatment response, risk of hospital readmission, hospital length of stay, and the response of treatment. Predictive modeling capabilities allow clinicians and healthcare administrators the ability to manage patient care proactively and clinician and healthcare admin time. Predictive modeling findings and data allow multivariable and individual risk factor models to be created. Predictive modeling is an application of multimodal AI in healthcare.

1.4.4 Decision support

Clinical support systems leverage multidisciplinary intelligence to derive evidence-based recommendations from integrated patient data. This assist systems in verification of diagnoses, selection of treatments, and refinement of patient-centric care pathways. Multimodal decision support enhances clinical workflow and mitigates cognitive overload and variability in the complexity of clinical tasks and biomedicine.

Various healthcare domain facilitated with the integration of multimodal intelligence are shown in Figure 1.2.

Overall, the combined benefits of these systems demonstrate the revolutionary promise of multimode systems in medicine. The systems enable accurate, continuous, and preemptive patient monitoring, prediction, and improved clinical decision-making. Together, these augment patient clinical outcomes and strengthen clinical service and healthcare service systems (Esteva et al., 2019, Ghassemi et al., 2021).

1.5 SYSTEM ARCHITECTURE FOR MULTIMODAL HEALTHCARE AI

There are few fields as heterogeneous as healthcare. There are also few fields which resist the implementation of multimodal AI solutions as much. Therefore, the quality of the software system architecture needs to be very high. As opposed to experimental deployments, clinical AI systems need to function and function very well during certain constraints such as data heterogeneity, scaling, latency, and regulatory compliance. Consequently, such system's reliability to integrate and compute several data streams and deploy the AI safely in operational healthcare settings wholly depends on the architecture of the system. The architecture of AI systems in Multimodal Health Care is usually layered, or modular, with data acquisition and ingestion being the first core layer. This layer interacts with several data streams: medical imaging (PACS), EHR, laboratory information systems, wearables, and bedside monitors. Data pipelines perform preprocessing tasks to improve consistency across modalities and standardize data quality. These tasks, such as data cleaning, normalization, synchronization, anonymization, and temporal alignment, are essential for the assurance of data quality. Figure 1.3 illustrates the layered architecture of a multimodal healthcare AI system, highlighting the flow of heterogeneous clinical data from acquisition to intelligent decision support.

Modality-specific feature extraction modules for narrowing down and encoding the preprocessed heterogeneous data into usable formats are the next step. Data from different modalities are processed with different nn architectures. For images, convolutional neural networks are used; for time series, data recurrent or transformer networks are used; and for clinical text, natural language processing nn are used. Features extracted from the neural networks are used by the fusion and inferencing modules, where intermodality late, early, or hybrid fusion is strategized. The modules then provide clinical predictions or insights for diagnosis, prognosis, or clinical decision support functions.

Integration and interoperability layers are key components of the architecture, allowing heterogeneous systems to follow and communicate within healthcare data standards. Compatibility of health data systems across

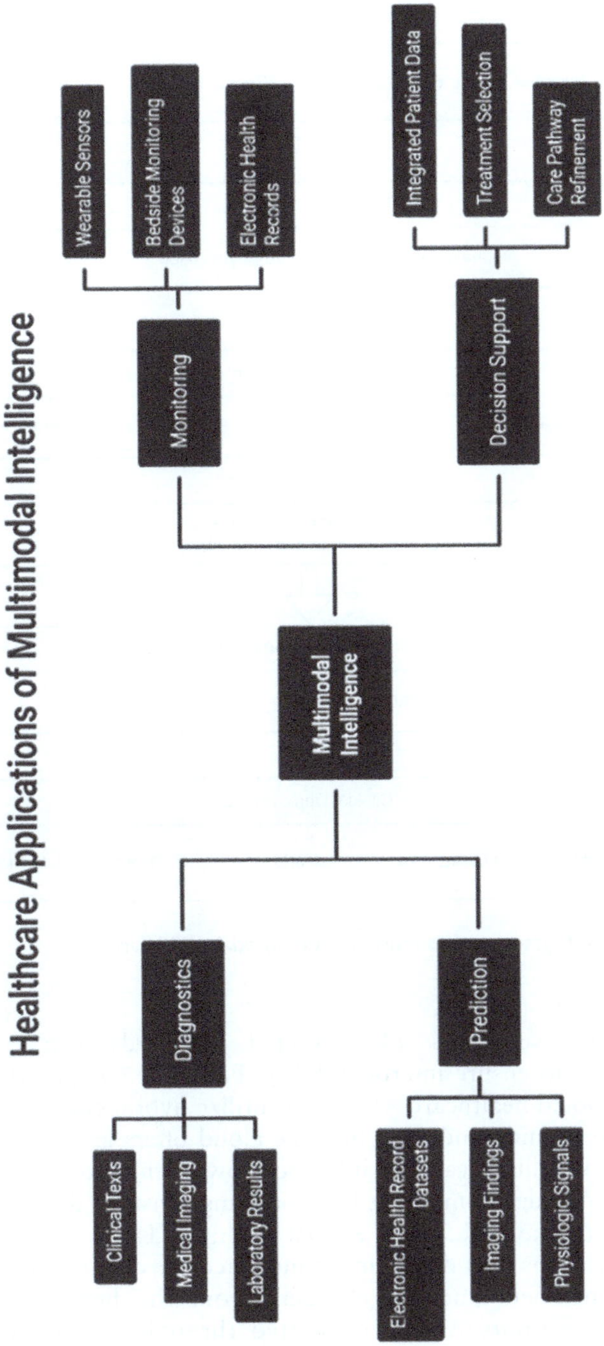

Figure 1.2 Healthcare acceleration with the integration of multimodal intelligence.

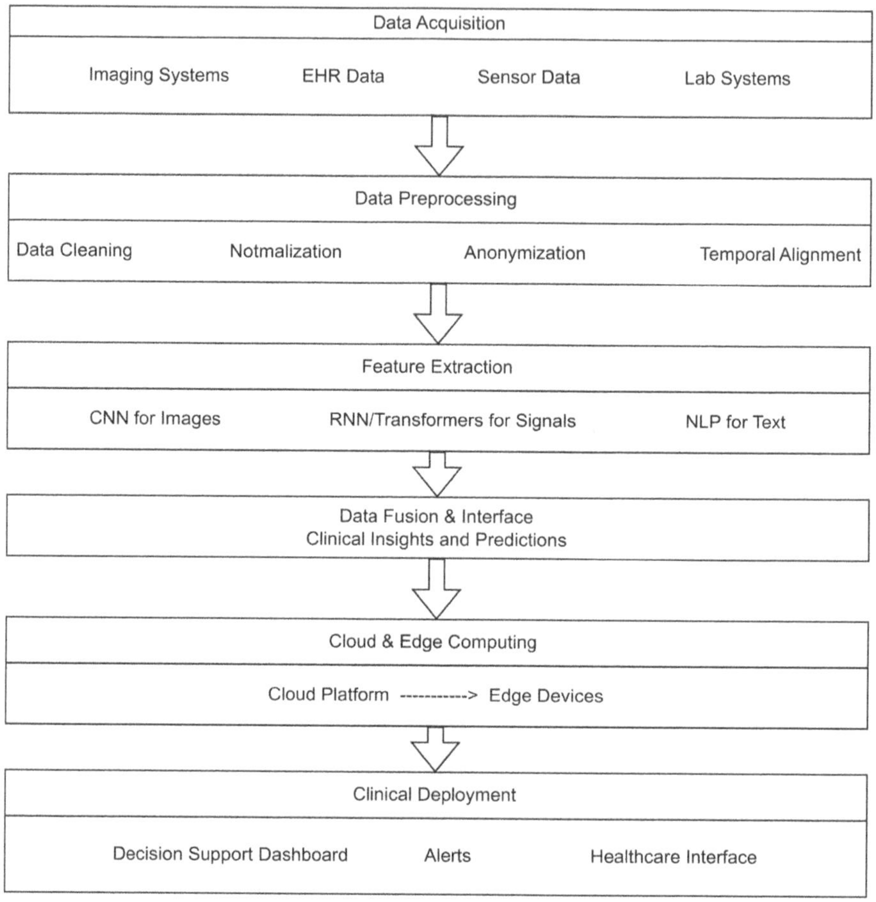

Figure 1.3 Layered system architecture for multimodal healthcare AI.

institutions and vendors is often limited. Standards such as HL7 and FHIR are used to ensure interoperability. From the computational standpoint, multimodal healthcare AI systems utilize hybrid computing systems. In large-scale training and analytics, the cloud offers great computational power and scalability. Real-time inference, low-latency, and greater privacy are achieved on edge computing by processing sensitive data closer to the point of care (Rieke et al., 2020, Kumar et al., 2021).

The applications and deployment interfaces have provided clinicians, and other members and stakeholders from the healthcare industry access to the outputs AI has generated through user interfaces such as dashboards alerts and other clinical decision AI geared towards providing clinical assistance. The modular and service-oriented design improves flexibility of the systems to adapt and change over the years to include different data types, algorithms, clinical processes, etc. as the healthcare technology improves. The flexibility of such designs is crucial for the incorporation of the multiple types of intelligence generated from the prototype research into real, dependable, scalable, and valuable healthcare innovations.

1.6 CHALLENGES IN MULTIMODAL HEALTHCARE SYSTEMS

Multimodal healthcare systems have the potential to transform healthcare delivery. However, there are a number of technical, organizational, and operational challenges facing the widespread adoption and deployment of these systems. One of these challenges is the *quality of the data*. Healthcare data is sourced from a variety of healthcare settings and often suffers from poor quality; i.e., it is noisy, sparse, missing, inconsistent, etc. This is due to variability in clinical practice, sensor/documentation standards, and the reliability of clinical sensors. Errors in the data such as modality and labeling, imbalanced datasets, and missing data, are causes of poor model performance. This is a significant challenge in the generalization of multimodal AI systems.

Another challenge is the issue of *interoperability*. This is particularly relevant to the integration of multimodal healthcare systems. Healthcare data is often siloed in disparate systems that are incompatible in terms of structure, format, language/terminology, and standards. There are various systems that are not seamlessly interoperable (i.e., EHRs, imaging systems, labs, wearables). This lack of interoperability complicates data integration and data fusion. The slow adoption of standards has a negative effect on data availability and reuse, and it decreases the potential of these systems at individual and organizational levels.

There are also some challenges that come with *computational complexity and real-time processing* needs, especially with time-sensitive clinical settings like emergency departments and intensive care units. Multimodal systems are already high level because of the extreme multidimensionality of the data, which includes continuous medical images and physiologic signals. When errors are costly, maintaining sufficient accuracy and low-latency inference are real challenges when integrating multiple modalities. This requires highly efficient model designs and/or sophisticated, self-adaptive computing architectures.

Model interpretability and transparency are also crucial concerns in clinical settings. Models must also be interpretable and transparent. In a clinical context, multimodal deep-learning models are usually very opaque, leading to real problems for clinicians as they are unable to follow the reasoning

Table 1.1 Summarization of various challenges in multimodal healthcare systems

Challenge category	*Brief description*
Data heterogeneity	Diverse data types (text, images, signals, genomics) with different formats and scales
Data quality and missing modalities	Noise, incomplete records, and unavailable modalities affecting model reliability
Data alignment and fusion	Temporal and semantic misalignment across modalities
Interoperability	Lack of standardization across healthcare systems and devices
Privacy and security	Handling sensitive patient data under strict regulatory constraints
Computational complexity	High storage, processing, and energy requirements
Model interpretability	Limited explainability of multimodal deep learning models
Scalability	Difficulty in deploying models across large, real-world healthcare settings
Bias and fairness	Modality imbalance leading to biased clinical decisions
Clinical validation	Limited real-world validation and clinician trust

that the AI has used to come to a particular prediction or made a suggestion. This opacity may undermine trust (even collaboration with the AI tool) and may raise clinical accountability issues. These problems are the result of insufficient data governance, system design, computational efficiency, and the use of explanatory techniques, so they must be solved to permit safe, trustworthy, and efficacious deployment of multimodal healthcare intelligence (Ghassemi et al., 2021).

Various challenges experienced in the deployment of multimodal healthcare systems are shown in Table 1.1.

1.7 ETHICAL, PRIVACY, AND SECURITY CONSIDERATIONS

Certain Liabilities, Privacy, and Security Risks Connected to Healthcare Deployment of AI: The deployment of AI in healthcare settings gives rise to certain liabilities, privacy and security risks related to the use of personal data and the use of decision-making AI. Multimodal health information systems merge information from a variety of sources including clinical data, imaging studies, wearable technology, and behavioral data. It increases the risk that various systems may breach this privacy and collect data without authorization. Due to the sensitive nature of patient data, securing the privacy of the patient data will be a primary duty of any AI-enhanced, integrated health systems of the future.

Healthcare Integrated Systems of AI: Ethical implications in respect to AI healthcare systems are related to unfairness and bias that may be present in the models of multimodal AI. If used data for training systems reflects the inequities in healthcare represented in the inequities of the data that will be used to train an AI to be incorporated healthcare systems and it may perpetuate inequities in the AI systems that may integrate in healthcare systems. Healthcare inequities may result in disparities of care to some systems and may result in inequities in care provided to some systems. The bias in healthcare inequities to AI systems multimodal models for equity in healthcare are essential (Wang & Yang, 2025).

Considerations of security equal systems of AI in the healthcare multivariate systems of healthcare are open and are exposed to cyber threats, data alteration, and other target fuzzy attack in systems AI integrated in healthcare. Improving system integrity and security requires cyber security strategies that are unprecedented in healthcare systems. Implementation of these strategies will result in trusted (with data recorded that can be analyzed for cyber security accomplished and adherence positioned to data alteration compliance to data protection will be achieved.

Clinical AI systems should involve accountability, explainability, and human oversight, as mandated by new regulations and ethical guides calling for responsible AI design. These systems should serve as decision-support systems; clinician-patients should remain in control of the final decision. Multimodal healthcare intelligence should be implemented in a way that ethically and securely protects patients' rights, builds trust, and unlocks limits in healthcare innovation in a durable and fair manner. (Floridi et al., 2018; Topol, 2019).

1.8 CONCLUSIONS

Multimodal and multimedia data technologies enable integration and interpretation of a variety of inside data in a unified and practically usable format. In primary healthcare, the field of healthcare is experiencing a paradigm shift. Rather and in addition to singular modalities, integrated approaches analyze clinically relevant and valuable combinations of medical images, waveforms, textual data, electrocardiograms, and health and health status sensor data to achieve a representation of health level. These integrated systems and approaches surpass the default restraints of singular or one modality to deliver a superior representation of health status and or medical conditions of patient's systems. This integrated and all-inclusive or holistic perspective must be accomplished and obtained to assess the global, multidimensional, and complex nature of real-world clinical situations and or scenarios conditions in this regard, where no one data source to guide and determine a patient health status and or medical conditions.

Innovations and advancements in deep learning, representation learning, and data fusion have facilitated the development of technologies pertaining to healthcare intelligence systems and or applications in healthcare. These systems and technologies incorporate and instantiate end-to-end learning from multiple data sources. Knowledge discovery often attributes cross-relational systems of data that are invisible or undetectable to human intelligence. Innovations in multisystems diagnosis, constant and or real-time monitoring, prediction of medical outcome, and clinical decision support systems multi-AI systems healthcare technologies are attributes to the betterment of healthcare services, the system, and or practices.

Challenges are still appearing, like the data quality, standardization, and interoperability issues, specifically in fragmented healthcare systems, are still important problems in the field of multimodal healthcare systems. The continuous real-time data processing and model interpretability, privacy, and security problems are of even greater importance in safety-critical systems, like many of the clinical applications. These systems would require strong guarantees for privacy and security for the data being processed. Interdisciplinary research, additional regulatory frameworks, and ethical guidelines are all important components to constructing the vision of the multimodal and multimedia intelligence systems in the field of healthcare. In the healthcare systems that allow for the more patient-centered data systems, multimodal intelligence will be important for the constructive systems of healthcare to be adaptable and equitable.

REFERENCES

Baltrušaitis, T., Ahuja, C., & Morency, L.-P. (2019). Multimodal machine learning: A survey and taxonomy. *IEEE Transactions on Pattern Analysis and Machine Intelligence*, 41(2), 423–443.

Esteva, A., Robicquet, A., Ramsundar, B., V., Kuleshov, M. DePristo, K., Chou, C., Cui, G., Corrado, S., Thrun & J., Dean (2019). A guide to deep learning in healthcare. *Nature Medicine*, 25(1), 24–29.

Floridi, L., Cowls, J., Beltrametti, M., et al. (2018). AI4People—An ethical framework for a good AI society. *Minds and Machines*, 28(4), 689–707.

Ghassemi, M., Naumann, T., Schulam, P., Beam, A. L., Chen, I. Y., & Ranganath, R. (2021). Practical guidance on artificial intelligence for healthcare data. *The Lancet Digital Health*, 3(3), e157–e167.

Goodfellow, I., Bengio, Y., & Courville, A. (2016). *Deep learning*. MIT Press.

Kumar, Y., & Singla, R. (2021). Federated learning systems for healthcare: Perspective and recent progress. In: Rehman, M.H.u., Gaber, M.M. (eds) Federated Learning Systems. *Studies in Computational Intelligence*, vol 965. Springer.

Ngiam, J., Khosla, A., Kim, M., Nam, J., Lee, H., & Ng, A. Y. (2011). Multimodal deep learning. In *Proceedings of the 28th International Conference on Machine Learning* (pp. 689–696), ACM.

Rieke, N., Hancox, J., Li, W., et al. (2020). The future of digital health with federated learning. *NPJ Digital Medicine*, 3, 119.

Topol, E. (2019). *Deep Medicine: How Artificial Intelligence can Make Healthcare Human Again*. Basic Books.

Yao, Z., Lin, F., Chai, S., et al. (2024). Integrating medical imaging and clinical reports using multimodal deep learning for advanced disease analysis. *arXiv*.

Wang, X., & Yang, C. (2025). MoE-health: Mixture of experts for Robust multimodal healthcare prediction. arXiv 2508.21793.

Chapter 2

Technological innovation in AI for healthcare applications

Ramiz Salama, Sinem Alturjman, and Fadi Al-Turjman

2.1 INTRODUCTION

AI technology is becoming more and more prevalent. American District Telegraph ADT Caps is one of most designated family called in case of an emergency [1]. If the center believes there is an emergency, it will call South Korea's emergency number, 119. This service has already helped many elderly individuals who live alone. Recipes may also be created with Aria. The user will ask, and Aria will walk them through the steps [2]. You can even handle your own money with Aria's assistance. Aria can recommend the best credit card for you based on interest rates and annual fees, as well as remind you when your monthly credit card payments are due [3-5]. Many companies, like Or-Cam in Israel, Recursion and Freewomen, an AI genomics biotech startup in San Francisco, are currently services and solutions. IBM's "Watson for Oncology" is the most popular artificial intelligence technology in the medical field. It helps oncologists by making therapy recommendations [6]. Mesko encouraged the integration of various systems with AI capabilities to create healthcare applications that might include prescription notifications [7]. Mesko added that AI-enabled gadgets, such as personal assistants, have the potential to significantly improve patient monitoring and support in situations where medical personnel are not available. AI-powered smart robots can assist physicians with specialized diagnosis, treatment plans, time and cost savings, and faster patient demand response times in addition to performing surgery [8-11].

The 6000–8000 uncommon diseases that have been identified affect over 400 million people globally. "Because medical personnel are not skilled in all disorders, they must focus on only a few of the conditions they are familiar with," the chief executive officer of 3Billion stated [12]. During treatment, the patient may embark on "diagnostic wanderings" and spend time traveling between hospitals. A doctor can only treat a certain number of patients. When used in medicine, artificial intelligence has the potential to worldwide [13]. An outline of artificial intelligence in the medical field. The application of robots, natural language processing, and machine learning

 DOI: 10.1201/9781003665656-2

to improve medical procedures is known as artificial intelligence (AI) in healthcare [14-16].

2.1.1 What artificial intelligent (AI)?

The imitation of human intellect in machines, such as computers or robots that have been trained to carry out cognitive tasks like learning and problem-solving that are characteristic of human brains. These days machine learning, and artificial intelligence are common terminology [17]. Machine learning offers algorithms for a variety of tasks including grouping and regression that ought to be taught through data. The more data you feed your algorithm, the more efficient it becomes. Artificial neural networks are the foundation of deep learning, a relatively new advancement in artificial intelligence. Deep learning algorithms also use data to figure out how to address problems [18].

2.2 DIAGNOSTIC APPLICATIONS OF AI

2.2.1 Medical imaging

AI has fundamentally altered medical imaging, enabling highly accurate detection of conditions including cancer, heart issues, and neurological anomalies as shown in Figure 2.1.

2.2.2 Pathology

In pathology, Figure 2.2 depicts the AI algorithms analyzing tissue samples to find anomalies. These methods enable pathologists to detect malignant cells more quickly and precisely.

2.2.3 Genetic analysis

By interpreting complicated genomic data, AI streamlines genetic analysis. This facilitates the identification of genetic susceptibilities to illnesses and the creation of individualized treatment plans according to a person's genetic composition as shown in Figure 2.3.

2.3 MULTIMODAL GENERATIVE MODELS FOR ADVANCED DIAGNOSIS

Traditional AI systems in healthcare rely on unimodal data (e.g., only medical images or only clinical text), which limits diagnostic performance and model generalizability. Recent progress has shifted toward multimodal generative AI and large foundation models (such as large language models

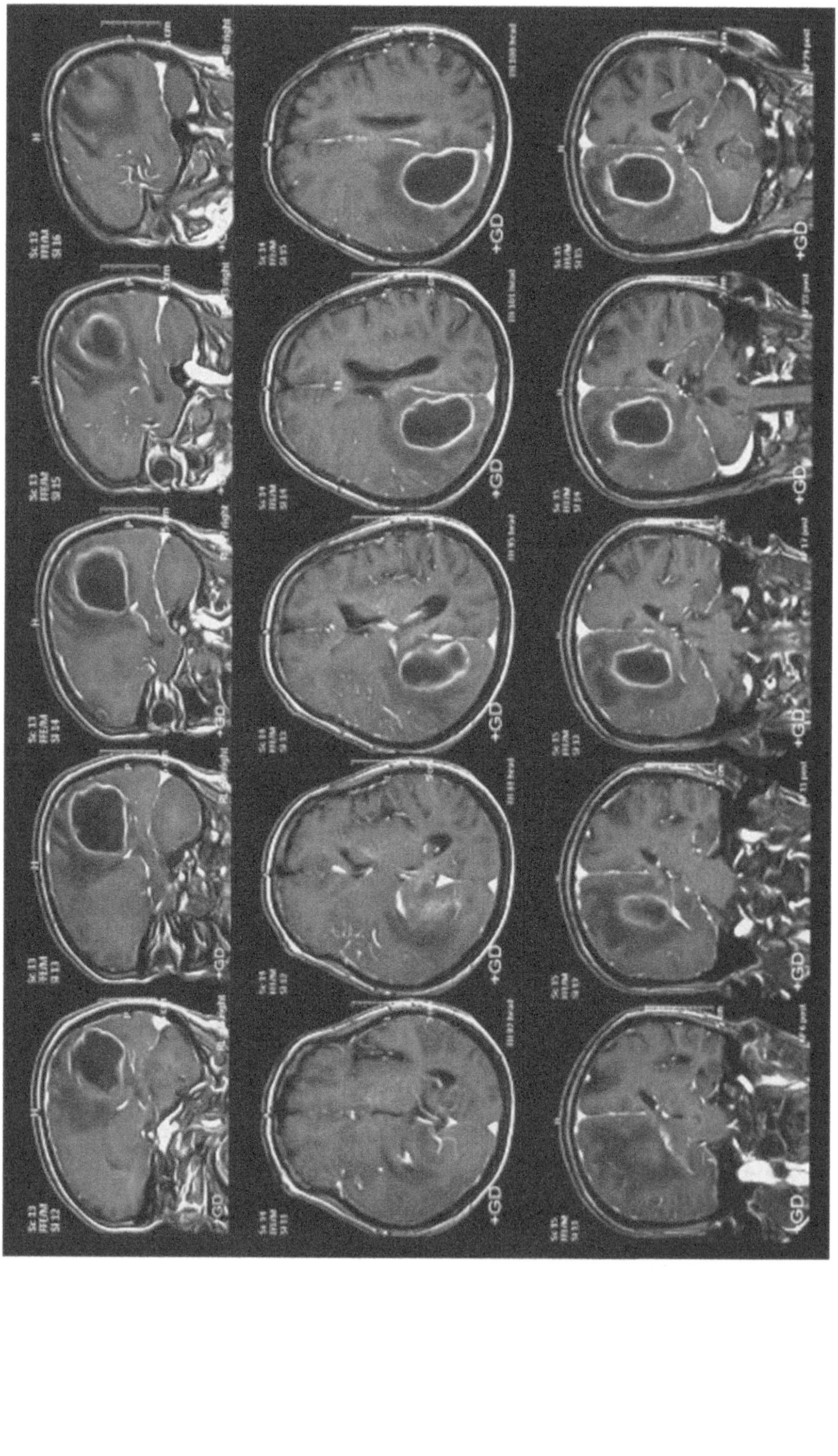

Figure 2.1 Medical imaging.

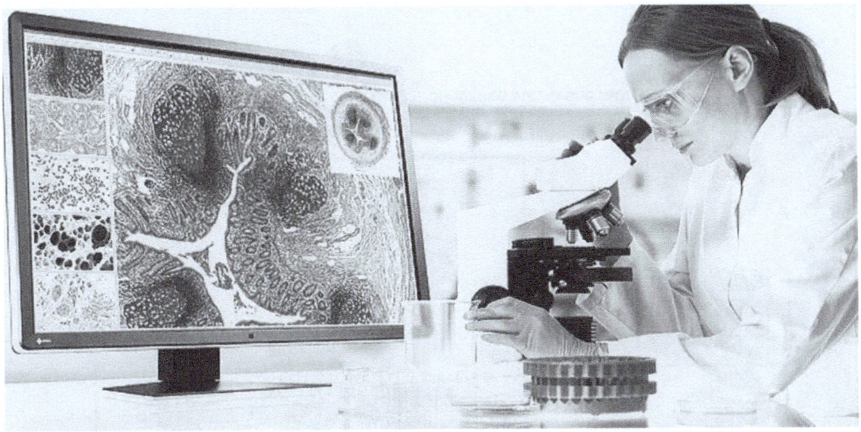

Figure 2.2 Detect malignant cells by microscope.

(LLMs), vision–language models, and signal–language models) that integrate multiple sources of medical information [19]. These systems are capable of jointly learning from radiology images, physiological signals (ECG/PPG), genomic data, clinical reports, and patient voice recordings, thereby providing a holistic clinical understanding similar to human specialists [20].

Generative models such as diffusion models and GANs are increasingly used to synthesize rare disease cases, simulate tissue abnormalities, and augment datasets in domains with sparse clinical samples. Meanwhile, vision–language foundation models interpret medical images together with EHR-encoded narratives to produce contextual diagnostic descriptions, justification of decisions, and automated risk analysis [21]. LLMs integrate patient records, lab values, and historical case libraries to support treatment pathway planning and medication optimization. When combined, these multimodal systems significantly improve diagnostic precision and accelerate clinical decision-making.

2.4 PRIVACY-PRESERVING MULTIMODAL AI AND WATERMARKING OF MEDICAL IMAGES AND VOICE DATA

Because multimodal AI uses highly sensitive medical assets—including images, audio recordings, clinical notes, and body-sensor signals—there is a pressing need for strong privacy protection mechanisms [22]. To address this challenge, the proposed AI workflow incorporates *privacy-preserving multimodal learning*, where raw patient data never leaves the hospital

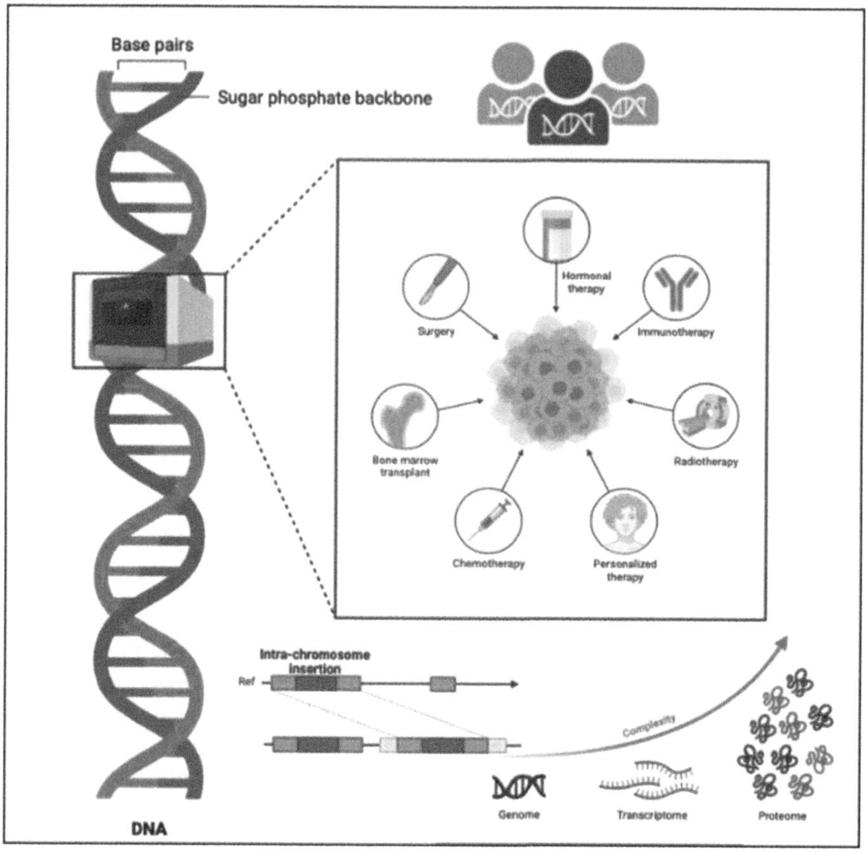

Figure 2.3 Structure of helix DNA.

premises. Instead, *federated learning* is employed to update AI models collaboratively across multiple healthcare sites without centralizing sensitive data [23].

To ensure data provenance and prevent clinical media tampering, *robust watermarking* is applied to diagnostic images and voice files. Watermarks are embedded in the frequency domain using imperceptible signal manipulation that does not degrade clinical content. This enables healthcare providers to detect unauthorized reproduction or modification of medical imaging or teleconsultation recordings in real time [24].

In addition, *homomorphic encryption and secure multiparty computation* ensure that clinical data remains encrypted during processing, allowing inference without revealing any identifiable patient attributes [25].

With these enhancements, the proposed AI framework adheres to privacy standards such as HIPAA and GDPR while enabling safe multi-institutional deployment [26].

2.5 ENERGY-AWARE INFERENCE FOR SUSTAINABLE AI DEPLOYMENT IN HOSPITALS

Large AI models provide exceptional diagnostic performance but can impose high computational cost and energy demand—especially in hospitals with limited computing infrastructure. To support *sustainable AI adoption for healthcare*, the diagnostic pipeline integrates *energy-aware inference mechanisms* optimized for hospital environments [25-27].

The system dynamically selects the most efficient execution route depending on model complexity, urgency of diagnosis, patient load, and available compute resources as seen in Table 2.1.

In addition, *model quantization, pruning, layer skipping, and knowledge distillation* reduce memory consumption and power usage without degrading diagnostic accuracy [28]. Adaptive scheduling ensures that high-power computations are conducted during off-peak load periods, reducing electricity demand in critical care units.

The sustainability of the proposed system is measured through four Key Performance Indicators (KPIs):

- Energy consumed per diagnostic task
- Average inference latency
- GPU/CPU utilization per patient load
- Carbon footprint per 1,000 inferences

Compared to traditional cloud-only AI systems, the energy-aware deployment strategy reduces computing energy usage by **31–48%** while preserving clinical reliability and responsiveness[29-30].

Table 2.1 Execution modes according to location

Execution mode	*Location*	*Trigger*
Ultra-light inference	Edge devices/imaging machines	Low-risk patients, routine screening
Moderate inference	On-premise hospital servers	Standard diagnostic evaluation
High-complexity inference	Central cloud	Rare or complex cases requiring generative/multimodal analysis

2.6 PERSONALIZED MEDICINE

Artificial intelligence is being used in personalized medicine to tailor medications to individual patient data [31], including lifestyle and genetic information as illustrated in Figure 2.4. This method reduces the possibility of adverse effects while increasing the effectiveness of pharmaceuticals.

2.7 CONCLUSION

Computers and other technologies with human-like learning, thinking, decision-making, and behavior are referred to as having artificial intelligence. Because it uses machine learning and other cognitive sciences, medical diagnostics is a significant use of AI in healthcare. AI can help physicians and other medical professionals make more precise diagnosis and treatment recommendations by using patient data and other information. The incorporation of *multimodal generative AI, privacy-preserving multimedia protection, and energy-optimized inference* transforms conventional AI into a highly scalable and clinically deployable healthcare intelligence ecosystem. The resulting framework not only enhances diagnostic accuracy and patient safety but also ensures *confidentiality, sustainability, and long-term feasibility* of AI-driven medical services in hospitals, telemedicine, and homecare

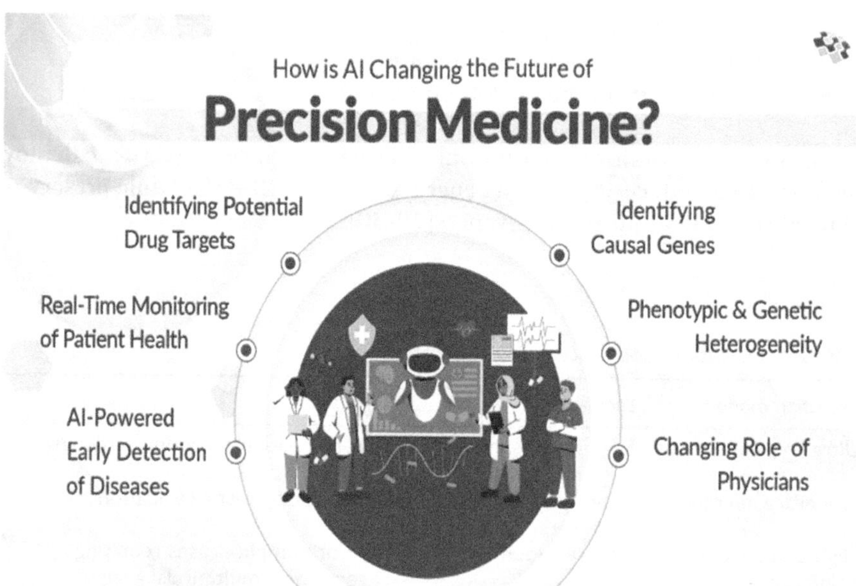

Figure 2.4 Personalized medicine.

environments. By evaluating vast volumes of data and suggesting better contribute to more proactive and predictive healthcare.

REFERENCES

1. Nosheen, A., & Omar, M. A. (2024). The Future of Mobile Cloud Computing: Key Implications and Challenges. *TOPLAMA*, 2(1), 162–169.
2. Ahuja, L., Simon, R., & Thakur, A. (2024). Privacy and Security Considerations in Healthcare: Navigating the Challenges of IoT and Ubiquitous Computing. In Nidhi Sindhwani, Sarvesh Tanwar, Ajay Rana, Ramani Kannan (Eds.) *Smart Tech-nologies in Healthcare Management* (pp. 164–181). CRC Press.
3. Thakur, A. (2024). Unveiling the Potential of Cloud Computing in the Healthcare Industry. In Renu Mishra, Vimal Dwivedi, and Sandeep Saxena (Eds.) *Computational Convergence and Interoperability in Electronic Health Records (EHR)* (pp. 221–240). IGI Global.
4. Salama, R., & Al-Turjman, F. (2024). Mobile Cloud Computing Security Issues in Smart Cities. In Fadi Al-Turjman (Ed.) *Computational Intelligence and Blockchain in Complex Systems* (pp. 215–231). Morgan Kaufmann.
5. Putra, K. T., Arrayyan, A. Z., Hayati, N., Damarjati, C., Bakar, A., & Chen, H. C. (2024). A Review on the Application of Internet of Medical Things in Wearable Personal Health Monitoring: A Cloud-Edge Artificial Intelligence Approach. *IEEE Access*, 12, 21437–21452.
6. Thakur, S., Sharma, S., Sharma, A. K., & Kaur, R. (2024, February). Impact of Cloud Computing in Digital Healthcare. In *2024 IEEE International Conference on Computing, Power and Communication Technologies (IC2PCT)* (Vol. 5, pp. 566–571). IEEE.
7. Salama, R., Alturjman, S., Altrjman, C., & Al-Turjman, F. (2025). Distributed Mobile Cloud Computing Services and the Internet of Things. In Fadi Al-Turjman, Fahriye Altinay, and Zehra Altinay Gazi (Eds.) *Artificial Intelligence of Things (AIoT)* (pp. 93–103). Morgan Kaufmann.
8. Mirusmonov, M., Zhang, G., Ali, J., Lee, S. H., Kim, D. W., & Kim, J. (2024). Effects of users' Motivation on their Usage of Mobile Cloud Computing. *International Journal of Human–Computer Interaction*, 40(20), 6167–6184.
9. Verma, R., Chhabra, R., Kumar, R., Rao, A. K., Kumar, N., & Gehlot, A. (2024, Febru-ary). Application of Mobile Cloud Computing Using Crowdsourcing to Provide Quality of Service. In *2024 4th International Conference on Innovative Practices in Technology and Management (ICIPTM)* (pp. 1–8). IEEE.
10. Alghaith, W. (2024). Security Determinants of the Educational Use of Mobile Cloud Computing in Higher Education. *International Journal of Computer Science & Network Security*, 24(8), 105–118.
11. Salama, R., Alturjman, S., Altrjman, C., & Al-Turjman, F. (2024). Service Models for In-Ternet of Things, Global Value Chains, and Mobile Cloud Computing. In Adarsh Garg, Amrita Jain, Manisha Singh, and Fadi Al-Turjman (Eds.) *Smart Global Value Chain* (pp. 121–136). CRC Press.

12. Salama, R., & Al-Turjman, F. (2025). Mobile Cloud Computing and the Internet of Things Security and Privacy. In Shilpa Mehta and Fadi Al-Turjman (Eds.) *Edible Electronics for Smart Technology Solutions* (pp. 333–350). IGI Global.
13. Khan, N., Tabassum, M., Lawal, I. A., Lakshmikanth, S. P., & A AlRugaibah, A. (2024, March). Impact of Cloud Computing Adoption in Saudi Arabia Health Care Sector. In AIP Conference Proceedings (Vol. 2919, No. 1). AIP Publishing.
14. Nimkar, S., & Makhijani, S. (2024, June). Blockchain and Cloud Computing in Healthcare: A Critical Analysis and Future Prospects. In *2024 IEEE 3rd International Conference on Electrical Power and Energy Systems (ICEPES)* (pp. 1–5). IEEE.
15. Khan, M. S., & Singh, J. (2024, January). Security Challenges in Mobile Cloud Compu-ting. In *2024 IEEE 1st Karachi Section Humanitarian Technology Conference (KHI-HTC)* (pp. 1–9). IEEE.
16. Abdulazeez, A. H., & Abdulazeez, A. M. (2024). Integration of Machine Learning with Fog Computing for Health Care Systems Challenges and Issues: A Review. *The Indone-sian Journal of Computer Science*, 13(3), pp. 3746–3757.
17. Ali, M., Muhammad, D., Khalaf, O. I., & Habib, R. (2025). Optimizing Mobile Cloud Computing: A Comparative Analysis and Innovative Cost-Efficient Partitioning Model. *SN Computer Science*, 6(1), 1–25.
18. Kanwal, A., Amjad, T., & Ashraf, H. (2024). Framework for Agent-Based Multistage Application Partitioning Algorithm in Mobile Cloud Computing. *SN Computer Science*, 5(4), 330.
19. Zhang, Y., Xiong, L., Li, F., Hao, Y., & Liu, Z. (2024). Blockchain-based Privacy-Preserving Authentication with Hierarchical Access Control using Polynomial Commitment for Mobile Cloud Computing. *IEEE Internet of Things Journal*, 11(10), 18266–18280.
20. Du, H., Liu, M., Liu, N., Li, D., Li, W., & Xu, L. (2024). Scheduling of Low-Latency Medical Services in Healthcare Cloud with Deep Reinforcement Learning. *Tsinghua Science and Technology*, 30(1), 100–111.
21. Putzier, M., Khakzad, T., Dreischarf, M., Thun, S., Trautwein, F., & Taheri, N. (2024). Implementation of Cloud Computing in the German Healthcare System. *Npj Digital Medicine*, 7(1), 12.
22. Rajput, A. S., Prabha, S., & Khare, M. D. (2024, May). A Framework on Positioning of Medical Sensors in Healthcare Domain. In *2024 International Conference on Communica-tion, Computer Sciences and Engineering (IC3SE)* (pp. 197-201). IEEE.
23. Sathik Raja, M., & Jamuna, K. (2024). Medical Sensors and their Integration in Wireless Body area Networking for Pervasive Healthcare Delivery. DOI: 10.26562/ijiris.2024.v1002.11.
24. Vivek, V., & Veeravalli, B. (2024). Analysing e-Healthcare Data from Internet of Things Devices and Cloud Computing. In Suyel Namasudra (Ed.) *IoT and ML for Information Management: A Smart Healthcare Perspective*, 301–323. Springer (published in Singapore by Springer Nature Singapore).

25. Humayun, M., Alsirhani, A., Alserhani, F., Shaheen, M., & Alwakid, G. (2024). Trans-Formative Synergy: SSEHCET—Bridging Mobile Edge Computing and AI for Enhanced eHealth Security and Efficiency. *Journal of Cloud Computing*, 13(1), 37.
26. Al-kateeb, Z. N., & Abdullah, D. B. (2024). Unlocking the Potential: Synergizing IoT, Cloud Computing, and Big Data for a Bright Future. *Iraqi Journal for Computer Science and Mathematics*, 5(3), 25.
27. Isravel, D. P., Silas, S., Kathrine, J. W., Rajsingh, E. B., & Andrew, J. (2024). Multivariate Forecasting of Network Traffic in SDN Based Ubiquitous Healthcare System. *IEEE Open Journal of the Communications Society*, 5, 1537–1550.
28. Bashir, S. R., Raza, S., & Misic, V. (2024). A Narrative Review of Identity, Data, and Location Privacy Techniques in Edge Computing and Mobile Crowdsourcing. *arXiv preprint arXiv:2401.11305*.
29. Devi, G. V., Selvan, R. S., Mani, D. S., Sakshi, M., & Singh, A. (2024, March). Cloud Computing Based Medical Activity Supporting System. In *2024 2nd International Conference on Disruptive Technologies (ICDT)* (pp. 1116–1120). IEEE.
30. Khan, F., & Ullah, R. (2024). Ubiquitous Computing Entity-aware Data Management on Mobile Devices. *Mobile Networks and Applications*, 29(2), 398–400.
31. Shafi, I., Din, S., Farooq, S., Díez, I. D. L. T., Breñosa, J., Espinosa, J. C. M., & Ashraf, I. (2024). Design and Development of Patient Health Tracking, Monitoring and Big Data Storage using Internet of Things and Real time Cloud Computing. *Plos One*, 19(3), e0298582.

Chapter 3

Data fusion techniques for multimodal integration

A. Sivaranjani, D. Anitha, A. Senthilmurugan, and P. Priya Ponnuswamy

3.1 INTRODUCTION

The basic human right is a quality healthcare system. Without medical facilities (hospitals, doctors, and nurses), it will be difficult to survive in the society [1]. In the modern world, the healthcare system is pressured getting bigger due to deteriorating populations and various factors. More health complications are encountered when the humans growing and become older. Hospitals are shortage of essentials facilities, and a lack of doctors are the bursting problems due to patient arrivals to hospital increasing rapidly in some crucial or some pandemic situation. It will be difficult for the hospital management to consider the factors like providing quality, funding, and staff deficiency in medical field [2]. To condense the oppression in the healthcare systems, expertise are seeking to integrate some advanced new technologies for the smooth progress. With the advancement of various advanced technical foundations and sustainability, the healthcare field enhanced to next level.

One of the crucial components from the advanced technical foundation is AI in healthcare systems. The system with smart intelligence is able to react and make decisions rapidly, strictly, and more accurately. Huge amount of data can be rapidly evaluated using AI techniques. The virtual assistants will be supported by the intelligent technologies for both patients and medical experts. The advanced intelligent technologies like AI, CV, NLP, IOT, ML, and DL are deployed in healthcare system and are creating wonders. It is used in administrative process such as data management (like patient records, disease history, and employee records), disease prediction, patient monitoring, and medicine recommendation, suggesting nutritious foods and identifying the anomalies in tissue, cancer cell extraction, microsurgery, and so many [3, 4].

 DOI: 10.1201/9781003665656-3

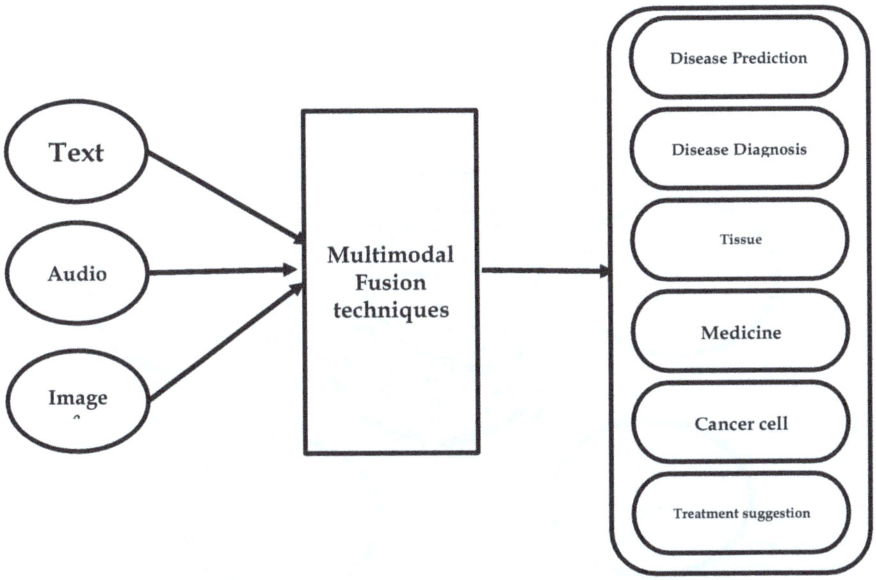

Figure 3.1 Multimodal fusion techniques.

3.2 MULTIMODAL INTEGRATION

Moreover, the expert systems are capable of identifying and analyzing the features of multimedia and multimodal health data.

- Multimedia is concerned with presenting several media types amalgamating to enhance the knowledge delivery.
- Multimodal concentrate on combining the various modes of information from one or more sources for intelligent and comprehensive understanding of information.

Multimedia or multimodal data includes images, videos, audio, speech, and text from various different sources or channels. Figure 3.1 portrays the integration of multimodal data. Handling heterogeneous types of knowledge from several sources in a single form is very challenging because of unstructured data and a wide range of data with diverse features and various data formats. Another important challenge is feature representation and feature extraction. The features from different modalities are converted into vectors, and all the features are combined to be represented in a common subspace. Other issues include data reliability, quality, integration of data, and computational difficulties. Figure 3.2 shows the different types of multimodal data.

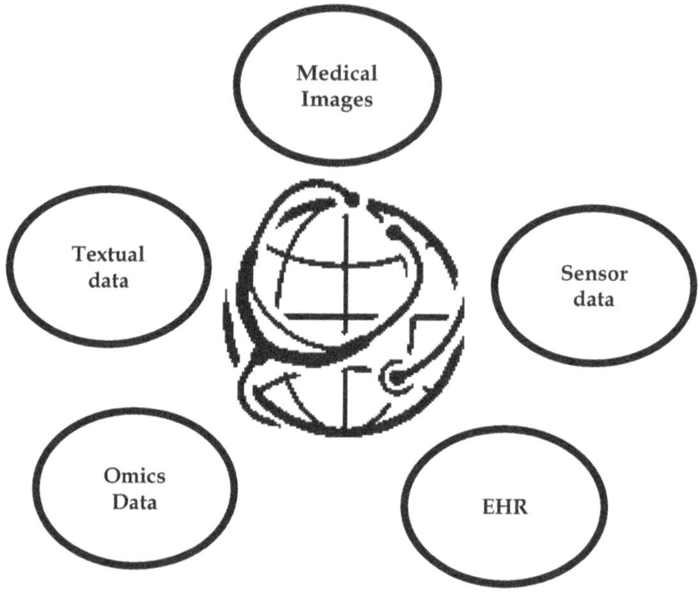

Figure 3.2 Different types of multimodal data.

3.3 DIFFERENT MULTIMODAL DATA

3.3.1 Medical imaging

Among various medical data, medical imaging is important for present healthcare due to the ability to analyze, examine, and visualize the complete structure of the human body by means of different modalities. The various modalities of image will depict the structural and functional details of the various parts of the internal system, tissues, and cells. Imaging modalities, such as X-ray, CT, PET, MRI (S-MRI, and F-MRI), SPECT, Ultrasound, USG, will provide various information and are appropriate for particular clinical assessments and evaluations.

3.3.2 Sensor informations

Sensor informations plays a pivotal role in modern medical domain which enables to monitor real time about various parameters which include physiological and behavioral parameters. Ranging from wearable devices to home-based monitor stream which capture information varying from oxygen saturation, heart rate, glucose level, and blood pressure to physical activity. This also helps in early detection of cardiovascular diseases. Real-time transmission of sensor data helps to reduce the frequent hospital visit [5]. The major issues that are faced by sensors are signal noise and calibration error, which majorly affect the accuracy. Diagnostic reliability improved by the integration of sensor data and medical imaging; the disease prediction model has also improved in the healthcare field [5].

3.3.3 Omics data/genomic data

Genomic data mainly provide glance to series of individual DNA their genetic variations and gene expression pattern [6]. The improvement in sequencing technologies which made data more accessible and vastly used in diagnosing genetic disorder, predicting diseases risk and identifying the treatment response.

3.3.4 Electronic health records (EHRs)

EHRs act as a heartbeat for healthcare system since it holds the complete medical data which encompasses prescribing medicines, laboratory outcomes, medical imaging analysis, physiological evaluations, and medical records [7]. EHR dataset are abundant and customized to every single individual which although they are scattered, it wraps around distinct variable which leads to increased complexity in analysis. EHR plays a major role in managing chronic and multidisciplinary diseases which include diabetes, combining EHRs improves the recommendations [8]. Advanced model which include MUFASA and MAIN use Transformer and attention mechanism which help to improve multimodal fusion, extract intermodal correlations, and enhance diagnosis prediction [9, 10].

3.3.5 Textual data

Textual data in healthcare mainly consist of unstructured sources like clinical notes, diagnostic report, and discharge summaries. The role for preprocessing is to remove noise and prepare for text analysis and that of embedding technique is to transform it into meaningful representations. The main challenge with traditional methods like one-hot encoding and bag-of-word is that they were limited to capturing semantic meaning [11]. The recent advancement with pretrained models such as Word2Ve, BERT, and ClinicalBERT use attention mechanism to preserve the context and also improve the multimodal fusion, making textual data a vital part to HER's and imaging in healthcare applications [12].

3.4 MULTIMODAL PREPROCESSING

Diverse or mixed data can be managed through various approaches like data integration, data cleaning, data compression, and standardization.

i) The method of integrating diverse data into a single perspective, which is available and accessible consistently, is called data integration. It includes data duplication, manipulation, and acquisition to amalagate various information to a uniform format.
ii) The method that uncovers the uncompleted, erroneous, unreliable, or poor quality data to manipulate and eliminate the data for enhancing the information quality is called data cleaning.
iii) The approach employed to decrease the dimensions of a dataset, without removing the ultimate critical data, and the process utilized for converting the coefficients of a sample to a standard scale is called data normalization.

3.5 MULTIMODAL DATA FUSION APPROACHES

The features from each modality are extracted and converted into vectors and finally concatenated. Usually these techniques are used in machine learning and deep learning models, especially to handle language and images. The transformers with attention mechanisms are utilized to concentrate on the most relevant and important information from the different modalities. Multimodal autoencoders techniques are mostly used for selecting treatment and for clinical diagnosis by handling the missing information. Here, the information from each modality is reconstructed, which enables the autoencoder to know about the combined feature representation. Attempt to acquire the distinct features over the multiple model medical data; generally, the integration can be performed at three distinct levels. Figure 3.3 portrays the three phases of data fusion.

i) Data-level fusion: In this fusion strategy, the original input from the different modalities is combined, which is the complete information before feature extraction.
ii) Feature-level fusion: Here the distinct attributes acquired over the different various given original modalities are integrated. Separate feature extraction technique will be used for each modality and combined features will have the similar representation.
iii) Decision level fusion: The various input modalities are executed individually by different models or techniques. The final results or prediction or scores are integrated based on statistics, voting, probability.

3.6 EXPLORING THE CLASSICAL IMAGE FUSION TECHNIQUES

Integrating the insights from two different images to enhance the standard of information is called image integration approach. In order to acquire an

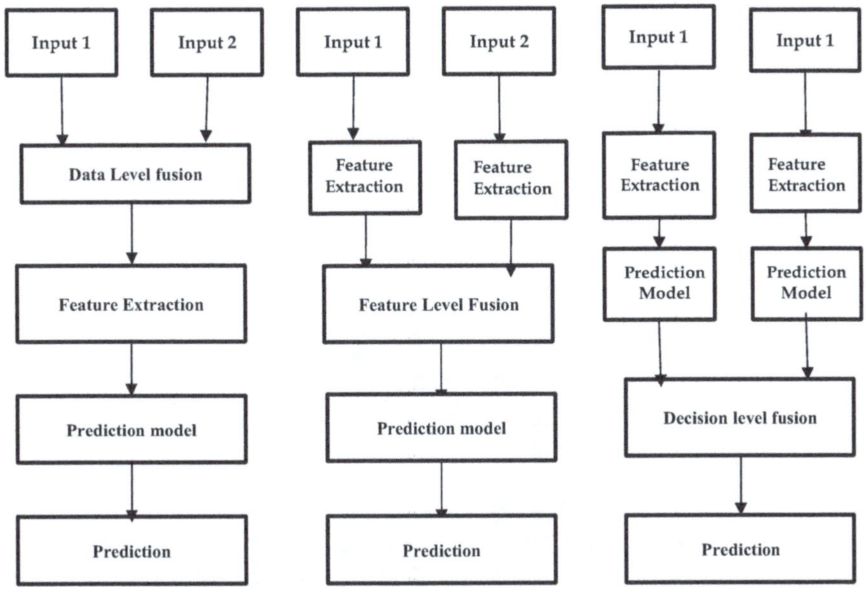

Figure 3.3 Data fusion approaches.

appropriate quantity of data over the source images, it is essential for integrating various modalities. The complete information of cell structure of body parts will be determined by integrating healthcare images over various imaging modalities. As an outcome, the corrective approach for diagnosis is a simple method to figure out the efficient remedial strategy. The evaluation metrics like peak signal to noise ratio (PSNR), entropy (H), mutual information (MI), root mean square error (MSE), and standard deviation (SD) cannot be accomplished completely by the most fundamental simple primitive image fusion techniques. Consequently, to acquire the meaningful and valuable data over the integrated images, there are several types of approaches based on various factors, and the integration approaches can be performed for spatial domain and transform domain. Figure 3.4 shows the different types of image integration techniques.

3.6.1 Spatial domain integration approaches

Processing the image pixel is one of the crucial roles in the spatial domain and to achieve the enhanced version, the pixel values are influenced. The methods utilized for the regional spatial attributes such as regional standard deviation, slope, and spatial frequency.

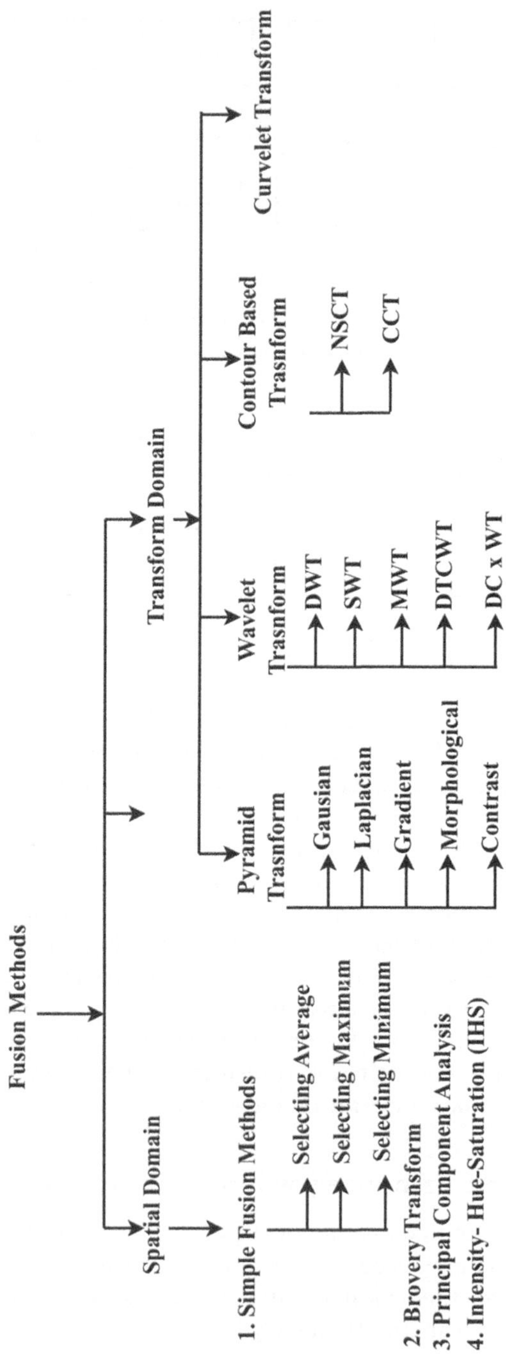

Figure 3.4 Types of image integration methods.

3.6.1.1 Basic image integration technique

Here the integrated image is acquired through deciding on the average or finest or least intensity of similar pixels over all the original input image. The average integration approach encompassed the complete pixel portion over the integrated image. The finest integration methods are being considered, with only the finest pixel intensity coefficient and least integration approaches are being considered with the least pixel intensity coefficient [13]. Figure 3.5 portrays the basic image fusion method.

$$F(p,q)_{Avg} = \frac{P(p,q) + Q(p,q)}{2} \tag{3.1}$$

$$F(p,q)_{Max} = \sum {}_{i=0}^{u} \sum {}_{j=0}^{v} maxP(p,q)\,Q(p,q)$$

$$F(p,q)_{Max} = \sum {}_{i=0}^{u} \sum {}_{j=0}^{v} minP(p,q)\,Q(p,q)$$

where $F(p,q)$ is an integrated image. $M(p,q)$ *and* $N(p,q)$ are source images u and v represents the rows and columns.

3.6.1.2 Brovey transforms

The Brovey transform is an efficient approach when compared to RGB-to-HIS transformation for image integration over various spatial features. In order to get around the limitations of the multiplicative approach, the Brovey transformation was introduced. It provided the option to apply to individual bands. The ultimate goal is to increase the components of the image like intensities or brightness by balancing the different multispectral images utilized for exposing RGB and to boost the outcome by any other supplementary required data. More comprehensive geometric attributes can effectively be forecasted over the largest spatial resolution image, even though the multispectral images incorporate complete spectral information. Panchromatic image is a co-registered band of high spatial resolution. The

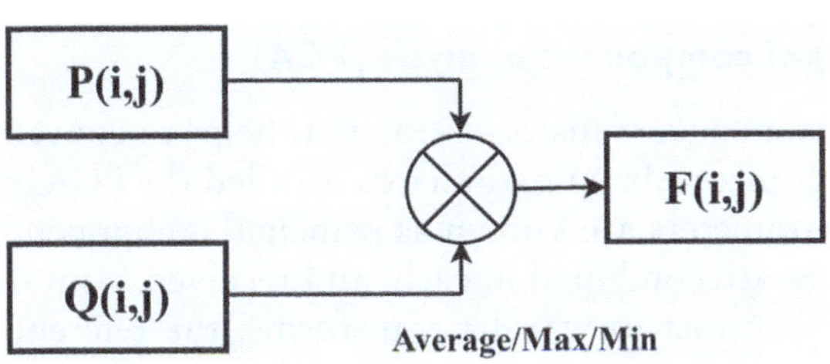

Figure 3.5 Basic image fusion method.

processing capabilities of the images can be improved, and the compensated data between high spatial and spectral resolution may be amalgamated into one single image [14].

$$R_{\text{new}} = \frac{R}{R+G+B} \times PAN$$

$$G_{\text{new}} = \frac{G}{R+G+B} \times PAN$$

$$B_{\text{new}} = \frac{B}{R+G+B} \times PAN$$

3.6.1.3 Hue intensity saturation method (HIS)

Among the most extensively utilized integration techniques, this IHS transformation technique was utilized in several application [15]. HIS is a color image integration approach that efficaciously segregates the spatial information and spectral information; the former represents the intensity, and later represents the hue and saturation through an image. The RGB of the least resolution image is initially converted into hue (H) intensity (I) and saturation (S) components. Moreover, the intensity of image depicts entire illumination, which is replaced by means of histogram equivalent finest spatial resolution image [16]. The integrated RGB image is extracted by the IHS inverse space pull back to primary RGB space. The IHS coefficient may be determined over the RGB coefficients from the given conversions:

$$I = R+G+B$$

$$H = \frac{G-B}{I-3B}$$

$$S = \frac{I-3B}{I}$$

3.6.1.4 Principal component analysis (PCA)

The feature vector space transformation that helps to convert the correlated parameters into uncorrelated parameters is called the PCA approach. These uncorrelated parameters are known as principal components [17]. The original parameters are combined linearly and received from the uncorrelated parameters. In contrast to wavelet transforms, the reference vector of the PCA entirely relies on the samples. It precludes the influence of the features from influencing the image; moreover, the additional advantage is its large

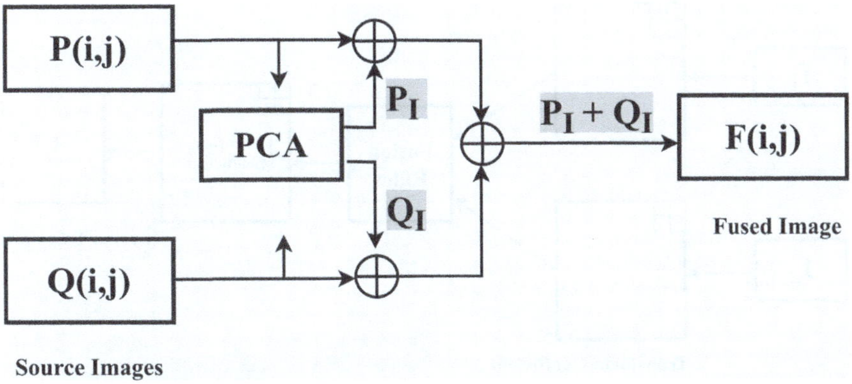

Figure 3.6 PCA approach-based image integration.

digital numbers. It is also utilized in applications like compressing the image and classifying the image. Figure 3.6 portrays the work flow diagram of the PCA method image fusion.

3.6.2 Transform-domain integrated methods

The primary limitation of the image integration in spatial domain was the spatial variations that are intrusions in the final integrated output image. The quality of perception in the resultant integration was very poor, when using the basic image integration techniques. Transform domain approaches handled these issues which perform well and are greatly appropriate for multiresolution-based image integration [18, 19]. The following processes take place in transform domain: (i) the transforms are applied to the given source images. (ii) Transform values have been extracted for the images. (iii) The integration principles are applied to map the values. (iv) The integrated image was acquired by performing the inverse transform. Figure 3.7 portrays the workflow of transform domain image integration.

a) *Wavelet transform domain:* To decompose the multiresolution image, the wavelet transforms are utilized. By different frequencies of sub-bands at varying scale, this transforms and distributes a distinct of channels and portrays the image attributes [20, 21]. The wavelet transforms are used to determine the various efficient transforms. Among various transformation methods, discrete wavelet transform (DWT) [15] is the crucial wavelet transformations; it can be used to offer the wavelength and directional data with different location-based orientation. The DWT-based integration technique

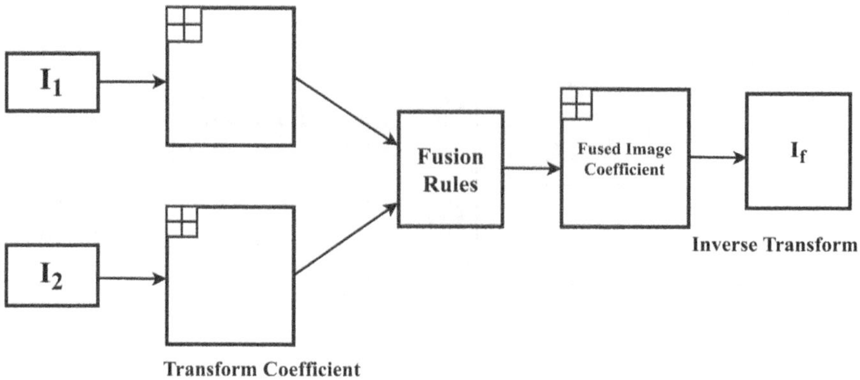

Figure 3.7 Transform domain image fusion.

is applicable for different datasets of images, such as infrared, multifocus, visible, multiview, and multimodal. DCxWT [18, 22] is shift invariant and provides the different transition information. The transition-based transformers are used to solve the time-invariance issue by performing the downsampling [23, 16]. It is also used to express the original images at different scales for various resolution image integration by graphical analysis [24]. It encompasses the different scale function and a wavelet function. DTCWT includes the real part and complex part values, which is very similar to visual sensitivity [25].

b) *Pyramid-based transform:* This transform is obsolete in different phases and various iterations of images by using the organized resolutions of the images [13, 26, 27]. A pyramid transform for an image is a resilient but intuitive format for illustrating images at several different resolutions. To express the actual image combined with the limited resolution images acquired at various quantities organized upon the pyramid transform formats. The pyramid structures were represented by means of applying pyramid transformation. The different pyramid-based transforms are a multiscale visualization attained over recursively applied compression. All images are subsampled copies of its precursor and low-pass-filtered in the contrast pyramid. The *Gradient Pyramid* integrated the image by consistently analyzing and using a downsampling approach. The starting level of analysis and ending level of analysis are performed on the provided input image matrices in a morphological pyramid.

c) *Contourlet-based transform:* It operates on multiresolution transform with an more improved group orientation and formats [28, 29].

Progressively, it is successful to a great extent in observing smooth outlines along with graphical formats in images. Consequently, with wavelets, it succeeds in expressing images. To represent the images with geometrical features by processing the contour segments is another benefit. The decomposition methods are performed in two phases. The prior phase is diverse-scale putrefaction with pyramid transform, along with the next phase, which is orientational putrefaction with several orientational filter batches. This is transformation is used to eradicate the redundancy problem and to resolve the disortion as well as the transition sensitivity issue [25, 30, 31].

d) *Curvelet transform:* This transform offers limited computational complexity, reliable reconstruction, robustness over deviations, effectiveness of deployment [32, 33]. It is a nonadaptive approach of being diverse-quantity graphical examination that is capable of efficiently illustrating the edges and curves. Diverse-scale transformation acquires a point of lack of coherence into linear representations. Moreover, the color remains the same as actual multispectral images. In curvelet transforms, a couple of versions are available. By using ridgelet transforms, the prior model was generated by means of multiscale screening in the continuous domain [34]. The subsequent one is determined through the frequency domain by ignoring the ridgelet transform.

3.7 EXPLORING ADVANCED ARCHITECTURES FOR MULTIMODAL DATA FUSION

With the rapid development of advanced technologies and intelligent systems, the revolution arose in the healthcare domain to process, analyze, and extract useful information from the multimodal data. Many machine learning models like regression models, random forest, SVM, ensemble learning are there for identifying the complex patterns from the multimodal data to extract the meaningful information. Deep learning frameworks like CNN-based models (VGG-16, ResNet-50, TransMed), transformer models, autoencoders, Attention mechanism, are used to extract the features, segmentation, and classification [10, 35, 36].

Multimodal integration combines images, signals, text, genomics, and audio and video to improve diagnostic accuracy, robustness, and personalization by letting models learn complementary signals and cross-modal correlations that single-modality models miss. With the help of reviews and scoping, we got to know that multimodal approaches help for diagnosis, prognosis, and monitoring across many conditions, but the challenges remain around data alignment, missing modalities, interpretability, and clinical deployment.

3.7.1 Disease diagnosis and early detection

In typical approaches, we fuse imaging, structured EHR, and clinical notes using late or early fusion and many more. But recently work uses multimodal transformation and scalable fusion layers to avoid the combinatorial explosion of pairwise interactions. Huang et al. [37] showed that multimodal fusion of imaging and EHR helped in improving pneumonia/sepsis detection. The multimodal modes (CNNs for imaging + MLPs or RNNs for EHR) consistently outperformed unimodal models. Cui et al. [38] proposed a deep multimodal fusion framework that integrates both imaging and nonimaging data using feature-level fusion. This experiment showed, compared to late fusion, the early fusion improved risk stratification in cancer and cardiac diseases. With unimodal models, imaging alone could show disease presence but missed context. Adding EHR data helped models predict severity and outcomes earlier, making diagnosis more accurate and reliable.

3.7.2 Personalized and precision medicine

In this we integrate omics, imaging, and EHR to predict therapy response, stratify patients, and identify biomarkers. Models range from probabilistic graphical models to deep-learning fusion. The genomics, imaging, and health records all together improve the predictions of chemotherapy success and patient survival. Graph neural networks worked best for linking genetic and clinical data. The multi-omics data and health record with deep learning. Deep learning framework improved grouped patients through how they respond to treatments, with better accuracy than using genomics alone. Before, treatments were based on population averages. By combining genomics, imaging, and health records, doctors can now make patient-specific predictions for therapy response, leading to truly personalized care.

3.7.3 Medical image analysis

Combines images with clinical test or other images. Architectures include CNN+ text-encoder setups for generating reports and diagnosis. In a recent study, they found that multimodal models can both classify disease and generate clinically useful radiology reports. Raminedi et al. [39] ViGPT2 multimodal transformer combined radiology images with text to generate reports closer to radiologist ground truth. Singh [40] improved chest X-ray diagnosis accuracy (AUC ↑ 4–7) and produced more coherent reports by training on image–text pairs. Image-only models could classify diseases but not explain them well. With multimodal image–text systems, AI can now generate full radiology reports, making results clearer and more useful for doctors.

3.7.4 Mental health and neurological disorders

Multimodal depression/ASD/cognitive decline detection using audio, video, and text. Fusion networks include multi-branch CNN/RNN pipelines, attention-based fusion, and multimodal transformation. Sadeghi et al. in [41] combining audio, video, and text improved depression detection accuracy over unimodal methods. Multimodel framework was developed in [42] by integrating three modalities like text, audio, and video to measure mental health and to predict the depression and stress rate. Earlier, screening relied on self-reports or one signal like speech. Multimodal models capture subtle cues from tone, expressions, and words, giving a fuller picture of mental health for earlier detection.

3.7.5 Remote patient monitoring and wearables

Fuse signals from multiple wearable sensors, even with contextual smartphone data and patient report outcomes. Techniques include sensor-level fusion, late fusion, and deep fusion. Wearable sensor fusion (heart rate, activity, temperature) improved arrhythmia and activity detection in long-term monitoring. IoT-enabled multimodal wearable processed data locally, detected abnormal cardiac events better, and saved battery life. Single-sensor devices gave limited, noisy data. Multimodal wearables now combine multiple signals, allowing continuous, reliable monitoring with fewer false alarms and longer battery life.

3.8 CONCLUSION

The different modalities like MRI, CT, X-ray, PET, SPECT of multimodal medical imaging are important concepts in the contemporary medical field for diagnosing diseases, predicting their treatment, and classifying infected tissues. The spatial and functional information from these modalities is enhanced by using different fusion techniques like PCA, DWT, and NSCT. This chapter gives the overview of multimodal images and different fusion techniques. If there is a rise in structural and contextual information, these techniques will perform well by means of advanced AI-driven methods like deep learning and machine learning techniques. These techniques have exhibited remarkable potential in diverse learning, integrated representations over modalities, improving the visual quality and medical interpretability of the integrated images.

REFERENCES

1. 'Health is a Fundamental Human Right', 2018. https://pmc.ncbi.nlm.nih.gov/articles/PMC7734391/

2. Hazarika, I., 2020 Jul 1. 'Artificial Intelligence: Opportunities and Implications for the Health Workforce', *Int Health*, vol. 12, No. 4, pp. 241–245. doi: 10.1093/inthealth/ihaa007. PMID: 32300794; PMCID: PMC7322190.
3. Dave, M., & Patel, N., 2023. 'Artificial Intelligence in Healthcare and Education', *British Dental Journal*, vol. 234, pp. 761–764. https://doi.org/10.1038/s41415-023-5845-2.
4. Al Kuwaiti, A., Nazer, K., Al-Reedy, A., Al-Shehri, S., Al-Muhanna, A., Subbarayalu, A.V., Al Muhanna, D., & Al-Muhanna, F.A., 2023 Jun 5. 'A Review of the Role of Artificial Intelligence in Healthcare', *Journal Personalized Medicine*, vol. 13, No. 6, p. 951. doi: 10.3390/jpm13060951. PMID: 37373940; PMCID: PMC10301994.
5. Xizhi, Z., 2008. 'The Application of Wavelet Transform in Digital Image Processing', in *International Conference on MultiMedia and Information Technology, IEEE Computer Society*. IEEE, pp. 326–329.
6. Wang, Y., 2017. 'Introduction to Medicine for Engineers', *Medical imaging techniques, Cornell MRI Research Lab* Summer Immersion, pp. 1–7, CreateSpace Independent Publisher, October 3, 2012, ISBN-10: 1479350419. www.createspace.com/4001776 https://pre.weill.cornell.edu/mri/pages/book/chapter_1.html
7. Orchard, J., 2007. 'Efficient Least Squares Multimodal Registration With a Globally Exhaustive Alignment Search', *IEEE Transactions On Image Processing*, vol. 16, No. 10, pp. 2526–2534.
8. Ihnaini, B., Khan, M., Khan, T.A., Abbas, S., Daoud, M.S., Ahmad, M., & Khan, M.A., 2021. 'A Smart Healthcare Recommendation System for Multidisciplinary Diabetes Patients with Data Fusion based on Deep Ensemble Learning', *Comput Intell Neurosci*, vol. 2021, p. 4243700.
9. An, Y., Zhang, H., Sheng, Y., Wang, J., & Chen, X., 2021. 'MAIN: Multimodal Attention based Fusion Networks for Diagnosis Prediction', in *2021 IEEE Int'L Conf. on Bioinformatics and Biomedicine, (BIBM)*. IEEE, pp. 809–816.
10. Carlsten, C., Salvi, S., Wong, G.W., & Chung, K.F., 2020. 'Personal Strategies to Minimise Effects of Air Pollution on Respiratory Health: Advice for Providers, Patients and the Public', *European Respiratory Journal*, vol. 55, No. 6, pp. 1–21.
11. Swathi, K.V., & Bindu, CH.H., 2013. 'Modified Approach of Multimodal Medical Image Fusion Using Daubechies Wavelet Transform', *International Journal of Advanced Research in Computer and Communication Engineering*, vol. 2, No. 11, pp. 4199–4201.
12. Liang, J., Li, Y., Zhang, Z., Shen, D., Xu, J., Zheng, X., Wang, T., Tang, B., Lei, J., Zhang, J., 2021. 'Adoption of Electronic Health Records (EHRs) in China During the Past 10 Years: Consecutive Survey Data Analysis and Comparison of Sino-American Challenges and Experiences', *Journal of Medial Internet Research*, vol. 23, No. 2, p. e24813.
13. Yang, Y., Park, D.S., Huang, S., & Rao, N., 2010. 'Medical Image Fusion via an Effective WaveletBased Approach', *EURASIP Journal on Advances in Signal Processing, Springer Open*, vol. 2010, pp. 1–14.

14. Tao, X., Shaik, T.B., Higgins, N., Gururajan, R., & Zhou, X., 2021. 'Remote Patient Monitoring using Radio Frequency Identification (RFID) Technology and Machine Learning for Early Detection of Suicidal Behavior in Mental Health Facilities', *Sensors*, vol. 21, No. 3, p. 776.
15. James, A.P., & Dasarathy, B.V., 2015. 'A Review of Feature and Data Fusion with Medical Images', in Fourati, H. (Ed.) *Multisensor Data Fusion*, chapter-9, Algorithms and Architectural Design to Applications. CRC, pp. 491–507.
16. Seiichi Serikawa, S., Lu, H., Li, Y., Zhang, L., Yang, S., Yamawaki, A., Nakashima, S., & Kitazono, Y., 2013. 'Multimodal Medical Image Fusion in Extended Contourlet Transform Domain', in Lee, R., (Ed.) *Software Engineering, Artificial Intelligence, Networking, SCI 443*. Springer-Verlag Berlin Heidelberg, pp. 215–226.
17. Shaik, T., Tao, X., Higgins, N., Li, L., Gururajan, R., Zhou, X., & Acharya, U.R., 2023. 'Remote Patient Monitoring using Artificial Intelligence: Current State, Applications, and Challenges', *Wiley Interdiscip Rev: Data Min Knowl Discov*, p. e1485.
18. Zhang, Z., Navarese, E.P., Zheng, B., Meng, Q., Liu, N., Ge, H., Pan, Q., Yu, Y., & Ma, X., 2020. 'Analytics with Artificial Intelligence to Advance the Treatment of Acute Respiratory Distress Syndrome', *Journal of Evidence-Based Medicine*, vol. 13, No. 4, pp. 301–312.
19. Tamilselvan, K.S., & Murugesan, G., 2014. 'Survey and Analysis of Various Image Fusion Techniques for Clinical CTand MRI Images', *International Journal of Imaging Systems and Technology, Wiley Periodicals, Inc.*, vol. 24, No. 2, pp. 193–202.
20. Nan-Feng, J., Mao-Hu, Z., Xiao-Ying, M., Osuch, M.E., Wammes, M., Théberge, J., Huan-Dong, L., Zhang, Y., Tian-Zi, J., Sui, J., & Calhoun, D.V., 2015. 'Discriminating Bipolar Disorder From Major Depression Based on Svm-Foba: Efficient Feature Selection With Multimodal Brain Imaging Data', *IEEE Transactions On Autonomous Mental Development*, vol. 7, No. 4, pp. 320–331.
21. Shalima., & Virk, R., 2015. 'Review of Image Fusion Techniques', *International Research Journal of Engineering and Technology (IRJET)*, vol. 2, No. 3, pp. 333–339.
22. Sharma, A., & Saroliya, A., 2013. 'A Brief Review of Different Image Fusion Algorithm', *International Journal of Science and Research*, vol. 2, No. 3, pp. 2650–2652.
23. Saranya, G., & Nirmala, D., 2016. 'Performance Evaluation for Image Fusion Technique in Medical Images Using Spatial and Transform Method', in 2016 International Conference on Wireless Communications, Signal Processing and Networking (WiSPNET), Chennai, India. IEEE publisher, pp. 446–450, doi: 10.1109/WiSPNET.2016.7566173.
24. Srivastava, A., Singhal, V., & Aggarawal, A.K., 2017. 'Comparative Analysis of Multimodal Medical Image Fusion using PCA and Wavelet Transforms', *International Journal of Latest Technology in Engineering, Management & Applied Science (IJLTEMAS)*, vol. 6, No. 4, pp. 115–118.

25. Santarelli, F.M., Positano, V., & Landini, L., 1997. 'Real-Time Multimodal Medical Image Processing: A Dynamic Volume-Rendering Application', *IEEE Transactions On Information Technology In Biomedicine*, vol. 1, No. 3, pp. 171–178.
26. Xu, Z., So, D.R., & Dai, A.M., 2021. 'Mufasa: Multimodal Fusion Architecture Search for Electronic Health Records', *Proceedings of the AAAI Conf. on Artificial Intelligence*, vol. 35, No, 12, pp. 10532–10540.
27. Bhavana, V., & Krishnappa, H.K., 2015. 'Multi-Modality Medical Image Fusion using Discrete Wavelet Transform', in *4th International Conference on Eco-friendly Computing and Communication Systems, ICECCS*. Procedia Computer Science, pp. 625–631.
28. Choi, M., Kim, Y.R, Myeong-Ryong, N., & Kim, O.H., 2004. 'The Curvelet Transform For Image Fusion', *International Society for Photogrammetry and Remote Sensing*, vol. xxxv, pp. 1–5.
29. Awotunde, J.B., Ayo, F.E., Jimoh, R.G., Ogundokun, R.O., Matiluko, O.E., Oladipo, I.D., & Abdulraheem, M., 2021. 'Prediction and Classification of Diabetes Mellitus using Genomic Data', in Sangaiah, A. K. and Mukhopadhyay, S. (Eds.) *Intelligent IoT Systems in Personalized Health Care*. Elsevier, pp. 235–292.
30. Costin, H., & Rotariu, Cr., 2009. 'Registration of Multimodal Medical Images', *Computer Science Journal of Moldova*, vol. 17, No. 3(51), pp. 231–254.
31. Deserno, M.T., 2011. 'Fundamentals of Biomedical Image Processing', in *Biomedical Image Processing, Biological and Medical Physics*, Deserno, T.M. (Ed.) Biomedical Engineering, Springer-Verlag Berlin Heidelberg, pp. 1–52.
32. Devanna, H., Satish Kumar, G.A.E., & Giri Prasad, M.N., 2017. 'A Survey on Multimodal Medical Image Fusion', *IOSR Journal of Computer Engineering (IOSR-JCE)*, vol. 19, No. 2, pp. 7–14.
33. Du, J., Li, W., Lu, K., & Xiao, B., 2016. 'An Overview of Multi-Modal Medical Image Fusion', *Neurocomputing, Elsevier*, vol. 215, pp. 3–20.
34. Geng, P., Su, X., Tan X., & Liu, J., 2015. 'Multi-Modal Medical Image Fusion Based on the Multiwavelet and Nonsubsampled Direction Filter Bank', *International Journal of Signal Processing, Image Processing and Pattern Recognition*, vol. 8, No. 11, pp. 75–84.
35. Calhoun, V.D., & Adalı, T., 2009. 'Feature-Based Fusion of Medical Imaging Data', *IEEE Transactions on Information Technology in Biomedicine,* vol. 13, No. 5, pp. 711–720.
36. Bhosekar, S., Singh, P., Garg, D., Ravi, V., & Diwakar, M., 2025. 'A Review of Deep Learning-Based Multi-Modal Medical Image Fusion', *The Open Bioinformatics Journal*, vol. 18, No. 1, p. e187503623706972. https://doi.org/10.2174/0118750362370697250630063814.
37. Huang, S-C., Pareek, A., Seyyedi, S., Banerjee, I., & Lungren, M. P., 2020. 'Fusion of Medical Imaging and Electronic Health Records using Deep Learning: A Systematic Review and Implementation Guidelines', *NPJ Digital Medicine*, vol. 3, p. 136. https://doi.org/10.1038/s41746-020-00341-z.

38. Zhou, T., Li, Q., Lu, H., Cheng, Q., & Zhang, X., 2023. 'GAN Review: Models and Medical Image Fusion Applications', *Information Fusion*, vol. 91, pp. 134–148.
39. Maleki, A., Raahemi, M., & Nasiri, H., 2023. 'Breast Cancer Diagnosis from Histopathology Images using Deep Neural Network and XGBoost', *Biomedical Signal Processing and Control*, vol. 86, No. Part A, p. 105152. https://doi.org/10.1016/j.bspc.2023.105152.
40. Moiroux--Sahraoui, A., Mazeas, J., Blossier, M., Douryang, M., Kakavas, G., Hewett, T.E., & Forelli, F., 2025. 'Can Blood Flow Restriction Be the Key to Reducing Quadriceps Weakness in the Early and Mid-Phases After Anterior Cruciate Ligament Reconstruction with a Hamstring Graft? A Systematic Review of Randomized Controlled Trials', *Diagnostics*, vol. 15, No. 3, p. 382. https://doi.org/10.3390/diagnostics15030382.
41. Liu, H., Zhang, L., Wu, Y., Ding, W., Liu, Y., Zhao, S., & Gu, J., 2024. 'Research on the Influence of Core Sensing Components on the Performance of Galvanic Dissolved Oxygen Sensors', *Sensors*, vol. 24, No. 13, p. 4155. https://doi.org/10.3390/s24134155.
42. Zhang, Z., Zhang, S., Ni, D., Wei, Z., Yang, K., Jin, S., Huang, G., Liang, Z., Zhang, L., Li, L., Ding, H., Zhang, Z., & Wang, J., 2024 Jun 7. 'Multimodal Sensing for Depression Risk Detection: Integrating Audio, Video, and Text Data', *Sensors (Basel)*, vol. 24, No. 12, pp. 3714. doi: 10.3390/s24123714. PMID: 38931497; PMCID: PMC11207438.

Chapter 4

Cloud-based solutions for sustainable biomedical data processing and management

Neha Gupta, Kapil Sharma, and Ekta Acharya

4.1 INTRODUCTION

The concept of "big data," while not new, possesses a definition that continuously evolves alongside technological capabilities [1]. It generally refers to datasets characterized by such substantial volume, velocity, variety, and complexity that they necessitate innovative hardware and software solutions for efficient storage, processing, and visualization. The healthcare industry naturally generates data embodying these three Vs: high volume, rapid velocity, and extensive variety. This data originates from daily operations of healthcare systems, insurers, researchers, and government agencies. A significant challenge, however, is that these data often reside in siloed systems, inherently limiting opportunities for global data transparency and integrated analysis [2].

Despite the complexities, deploying large-scale data solutions in healthcare offers considerable potential benefits. Analyses suggest that the effective and creative application of advanced data analytics could generate significant annual value for healthcare systems, primarily through increased efficiency and reduced costs [3]. Historically, medical research often focused on physiological changes through a limited, single-modality lens. Formerly, medical research methodologies have mostly intense on examining illness states through changes in physiology, sometimes through a limited viewpoint on a single sense modality of data. Such research tends to simplify the rich diversity and connections that characterize authentic systems. Ensuing many years of technical regression, the medical industry is now starting to correct to the current digital data era. Large volumes of data may be collected over lengthy periods of time about every single patient thanks to new technology. Nevertheless, the material recorded and acquired from these patients has remained mostly underutilized despite the growth of medical electronics.

Changes in numerous clinical streams are alongside establishing important physiological and pathophysiological processes. Robust connections between many physical systems such as those connecting heart rate, breathing, and

 DOI: 10.1201/9781003665656-4

blood pressure lead to the manufacture of possible indicators for scientific evaluation. For a more complete picture of the illness states, organized and formless data from a diversity of clinical and nonclinical sense modalities must be combined in a combined approach to understanding and predicting diseases. Recently, there has been a flow of interest in healthcare research that aims to tackle the trials associated with mixing big data analytics principles into medicine [4].

Three domains of big data analytics in healthcare are examined. These three fields are destined to give an impression of some of the major, well-liked parts of training where immense data analytics principle are currently used; they do not fully represent the use of big data analytics in medicine. Image manipulation of clinical pictures seem a valued foundation of data that are frequently used for planning, evaluating, and diagnosing treatments. Among the imaging methods that are firm in clinical settings are fluoroscopy, positron emission tomography-computed imaging (PET-Scan CT), magnet-based timbre imaging (MRI), X rays, imaging of molecular, ultrasound, photo-acoustic imaging, and computed tomography (CT scan). Medical pics data could be as little as a few GBs for a single study (histological pictures, for example) as large as several hundred MB for individual research (a very fine slice CT examinations, which might include up to twenty-five hundred+ scans). If such data is kept for a lengthy period of time, important storage volume is needed. In addition, if any mechanization supporting decision-making were to be approved outside the data, it would need quick and precise algorithms.

4.1.1 Signal handling

Medical signals present volume and velocity challenges, just like medical pictures do, mainly during incessant high-resolution data gaining and storage from multiple patient-attached monitors. However, bodily signals also provide a spatiotemporal complexity in addition to the problems associated with data quantity [2]. When opposed with situation setting responsiveness, that is included in the building of nonstop monitoring and prognostic structures to guarantee usefulness and resilience, physiological signal analysis is regularly more significant.

In order to give alarm devices in case of overt incidents, healthcare systems now deploy a multitude of dissimilar and continuous nursing tools that use unique physiological waveform information or discretized vital information. However, these naive methods of creating and applying alarm systems are frequently faulty, and the sheer volume of them may result in "alarm fatigue" for patients and carers alike. In this context, previous information that has generally not fully used higher dimensional period sequence data limits the volume to find new clinical/medical knowledge. The main cause of these alarm mechanisms' propensity to malfunction is that they frequently depend on isolated information sources without providing a completer and more contextual picture of the patients' actual physiological circumstances. Consequently, correlations happen between the multimodal scientific time series data. This is important since research keeps showing how humans are more motivated towards results than biosignals.

The price of human genome sequencing in a traditional way, which consists of 30000 to 35000 genes, is dropping quickly as high-throughput sequencing knowledge advances. A major problem for the education of computational biology is the timely study of genome-scale data to produce meaningful suggestions that have implications for present public health strategy and care delivery. In a healthcare situation, the cost and duration of recommendation delivery are critical factors. Efforts to address this complex issue involve following 100,000 participants over a retro of 20 to 30 years through the use of an integrated personal omics profile and the predictive, preventative, participatory, and personalized health (P4) drug paradigm. A system approach is being used by the P4 effort to: (i) using genome-scale dataset analysis to identify disease states; (ii) switching to blood-based analytics for ongoing patient observation; (iii) investigating novel strategies for drug target discovery; and (iv) creating instruments to address the challenges of big data, such as gathering, verifying, storing, mining, and integrating.

(iv) Modelling information unique to each person. The integrated personal omics profile (iPOP) creates a comprehensive picture of a subject's health and disease states by combining numerous high-throughput genomic sequencing techniques with physiological monitoring. Ultimately, this field's biggest issue continues to be implementing practical advice at the clinical level. Cutting-edge big data techniques and analytics are needed to use higher-density data for clinical translation, examination, and finding.

Outcomes from clinics remain unsatisfactory despite the significant financial resources that current healthcare systems invest, especially in the USA, where 96 individuals out of every 100,000 die annually from conditions believed to be treatable. The inability of healthcare systems to efficiently gather, stake, and utilize data in a more broader manner is a key factor contributing to these inefficiencies. [5] This presents an occasion for data science and big data analytics to develop more involvement in supporting the process of examination and discovery, enhancing the provision of care, assisting in the creation and planning of healthcare policy, and offering a way to measure and assess the complex and multilayered healthcare data in an all-encompassing manner. More pointedly, knowledge collected from vast data analytics will save lives, improve the quality of treatment, and increase access to health care.

4.2 BIG DATA APPROACH TO MEDICAL IMAGE ANALYSIS

Medical imaging, in addition to being an essential part of disease diagnosis, is crucial for the detailed characterization of structure and organ function. It is commonly used to map organs, track lung tumors, identify spinal deformities, detect artery blockages, and spot aneurysms.

To address such complicated tasks, current medical imaging makes use of cutting-edge machine learning and image processing techniques such as segmentation, denoising, and data augmentation.

As healthcare systems and populations continue to grow exponentially, AI-based diagnostic tools are increasingly becoming indispensable in today's medicine. These technologies allow doctors to process large amounts of imaging data more quickly and accurately, with the potential to improve patient care. Computational intelligence can be applied to improve various aspects of healthcare, including screening, diagnosis, and prognosis.

Using computer analysis in conjunction with adequate treatment may enable physicians to make more accurate diagnoses. Diagnostic accuracy and efficiency can be significantly improved by combining medical imaging with genomic data and electronic health records (EHR). This multisource approach allows for a more comprehensive analysis of patient health. In the following sections, we explore how imaging-generated data is analyzed and examine the role of remedial imagination from a big data perspective—highlighting its potential to transform diagnostics and treatment planning.

4.3 DATA PRODUCED: IMAGERY METHODS

"Medical imaging" comprises a wide variety of techniques used for diagnostic and therapeutic purposes. The architecture of blood vessels could be seen via sensitive machine known as magnetic resonance imaging, ultrasound, computed imaging CT scan, and photo-acoustic imaging. From the data perspective side, medical pictures have 2D, 3D, or 4D. Functional magnetic resonance imaging, PET test, CT scan, and 3D ultrasonography are examples of multiple-dimensional medical data. Recent technologies produce high-quality resolution images, resulting in massive data sets that require detailed analysis techniques and high-performance computing. For instance, microscopic brain images can require terabytes of storage. While this volume and variety make analysis challenging, advances in this field are making personalized care more feasible and providing quantitative data for disease stratification and predictive modelling [6]. The below section discovers two different logical approaches and a linked challenge.

Like, new technical medical imaging generates huge amounts of data—for instance, a single high-definition quality microscopic picture of a brain can require up to 66Tbs of data storage. Volume and diversity of data present substantial analytical challenges as well; advances in medical

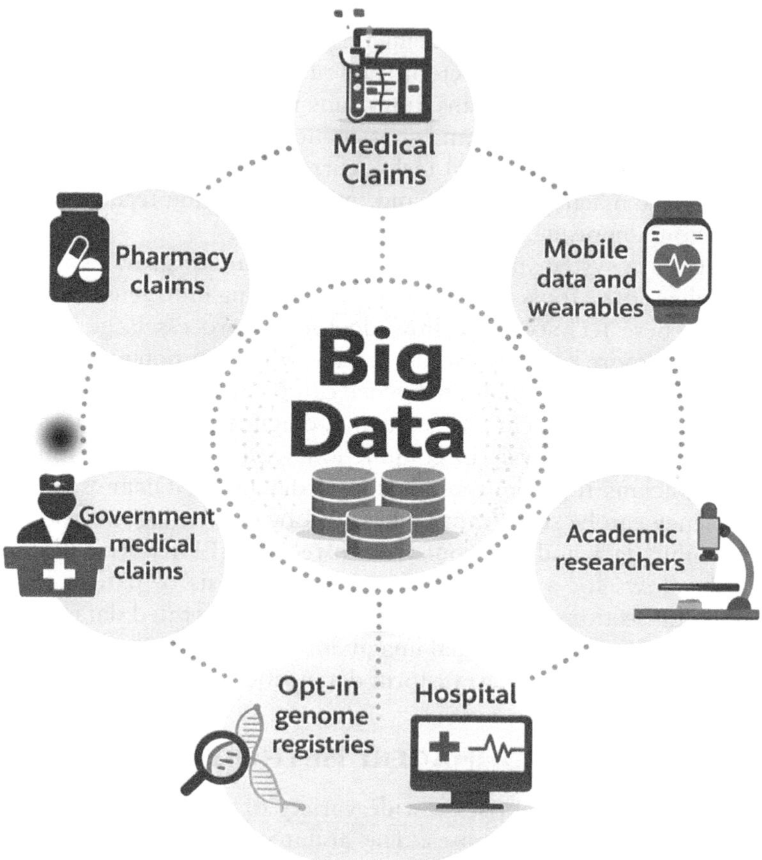

Figure 4.1 Bigdata image healthcare relevant.

picture-capturing technology flagging the way for more adapted patient care. This also provides valuable measurable data for critical applications shown below:

- Disease classification and stratification
- Predictive health modeling
- Clinical decision support systems

Molecular imagination is a non-invasive method of seeing cellular and subcellular procedures that may be used to experimentally analyze conditions like cancer. On the other hand, radiology, nuclear medicine, and biology are crucial for guaranteeing its medical relevance for patients.

A new technique called microwave imagination has the potential to map the electromagnetic wave dispersion caused by the differences in dielectric characteristics of numerous tissues. Its dielectric individualities contain physiological and efficient material that can be used to distinguish and characterize various matters and/or diseases. However, the dispersion behavior of microwaves makes information retrieval difficult.

The correctness of the diagnosis and illness outcome guess may be increased by integrating pictures from many modalities and/or additional experimental and physiological data. In order to evaluate brain vascular disorders and achieve precision medicine, Liebeskind and Feldmann examined developments in neurovascular imagination [7] as well as the function of multi-modal CT or MRI combining angiography and perfusion imaging advances the evaluation of neurovascular disorders. For a correct assessment of the scar after a myocardial infarction, delayed enhanced magnetic resonance imaging has been utilized. Electroanatomic mapping assists in determining the subendocardial amount of infarct for this kind of illness. Hussain et al. have looked at the significance of analyzing both MRI and CT scans to improve diagnostic accuracy in recognizing the existence of corrosions in the temporomandibular joint [8]. This study indicates that simultaneous [9] The Advanced Multimodal Image-Guided Operating (AMIGO) suite features a state-of-the-art operating room integrated with multiple advanced imaging modalities:

- Angiographic X-ray systems
- High-resolution MRI
- 3D ultrasound capabilities
- PET/CT scanners

This comprehensive imaging approach has proven particularly valuable in oncology, where it enhances precision in both locating and targeting diseased tissue during cancer treatments. By combining real-time imaging technologies, surgeons can achieve unprecedented accuracy when operating on tumors and affected areas. Finding the map and the relationships between numerous data kinds are subjects where there is now no ideal clarification, in addition to the enormous amount of space desirable to store all the data and their analysis.

4.4 METHODS

Medical imaging volume is growing at a tremendous rate. Like, the Image CLEF medical picture group had about 66,000 photos from 2005 to 2007, but as of 2013, about 300,000 images were kept per day. Apart from the increasing quantity of pictures, they also vary in terms of modality, resolution, size, and quality [10]. This poses extra complications for data addition and data mining, mainly when there are numerous datasets involved. Multimodal image analysis research efforts are far less in number than single-modal medical image analysis research initiatives.

The capacity of medical imagination is increasing exponentially. For instance, as of 2013, over 300,000 photographs were stored daily in the Image CLEF clinical picture collection, which had roughly 66000 images between 2005 and 2007. In addition to the rising number, images vary in terms of size, quality, resolution, and modality. This creates further challenges for data mining and integration, especially when many datasets are involved. Compared to single-modal medical image study research attempts, multimodal image investigation research efforts are significantly less numerous.

4.4.1 Analytical methods

Enhancing the interpretability of the contents that are presented is the aim of medical image analytics. Medical image dispensation has seen the development of several techniques and frameworks. These techniques are not always appropriate for great data claims, though.

Technology like Hadup, which uses MapReduce, is one of the outlines designed for analyzing and converting very large datasets. Scalability crossways several attendants in a Hadoop cluster [11] is made possible by the MapReduce programming paradigm, which has a wide range of practical applications. [12] But when it comes to activities requiring a lot of input and output, it struggles. Three important medical image processing use cases have benefited from the employment of the MapReduce framework: (i) determining ideal limits for lung texture classification by utilizing the well-known machine learning technique SVM classifier, (ii) ripple study for the categorization of solid textures, and (iii) content-based medical picture indexing. With this architecture, a cluster of varied computing nodes was established, capable of handling up to 42 map jobs concurrently, and a speedup of around 100 was attained. Stated differently, the overall time required to determine the ideal SVM parameters was lowered from around 1000 hours to roughly 10 hours. In certain applications, like trauma evaluation in intensive care, where the ultimate objective is to use such tools and analysis inside what is regarded as the "golden hour of care," designing a quick procedure is essential. As a result, the established approaches' execution speed or real-time viability is crucial. Another element to consider while creating an analytical technique is accuracy.

As a result, the established approaches' execution speed or real-time viability is crucial. Another element to take into account while creating an analytical technique is accuracy. Determining relationships between various data kinds may aid in increasing accuracy. For example, a hybrid machine learning algorithm approach was created that uses single nucleotide pleomorphism (SNP) data and fMRI pictures to classify patients with schizophrenia from healthy controls. If the authors had relied just on SNP or fMRI pictures, their stated 87% classification accuracy would not have been possible. [13] When comparing data that is deemed to be large data, del Toro and Pestle have examined several organ division techniques. They have put forth a technique that combines atlas probabilistic information with the image's local contrast.

When associated with using just atlas information, a regular improvement of 33% has been obtained. A clinical decision provision system that uses judicial distance learning and has substantially less computing complexity than traditional alternatives has been created by Tsymbal et al. As a result, the system is more scalable for retrieval. According to Chen et al. created a computer-aided choice provision system that might help doctors accurately plan treatments for patients with traumatic brain injury (TBI). This approach combined the patient's medical history, demographic data, and characteristics occupied from CT scans to estimate the intracranial pressure (ICP).

The results presented that the accuracy, sensitivity, and specificity were, in order, 73.7%, 65.2%, and 70.3%. The impact of molecular imagination on the development of cancer medications and cancer diagnostics is discussed. The method under consideration combines molecular data with anatomical and physiological data in an attempt to facilitate the early detection of cancer. Using this imaging technology has improved the accuracy of the analysis of response to a novel action for affected roles with progressive ovarian cancer when comparing with other scientific or histo-pathologic standards. A hybrid digital-optical correlator has been created to accelerate picture association. Hybrid Digital-Optical Correlator can be used for picture comparison if there is no coordinate matching or reregistration. The calculation is performed using this multichannel approach using the storage media as seen in Figure 4.2.

4.4.2 Collecting, sharing, and reducing methods

Beyond analytical techniques, progress has been made in data collection, compression, sharing, and anonymization. Initiatives like the iDASH (integrating data for analysis, anonymization, and sharing) center focus on developing privacy-protecting algorithms and methods for data sharing. Projects like the Health-e-Child collaboration aim to create integrated pediatrics healthcare platforms across Europe.

Systems built on platforms like Hadoop have been developed to transfer, store, and share electronic medical records (EMR) and medical images between healthcare providers. Other perspectives involve using sensor networks to gather patient vitals, sending data to the cloud for processing and storage. Example systems manage storage and retrieval requests for DICOM images using cloud platforms like Microsoft Azure.

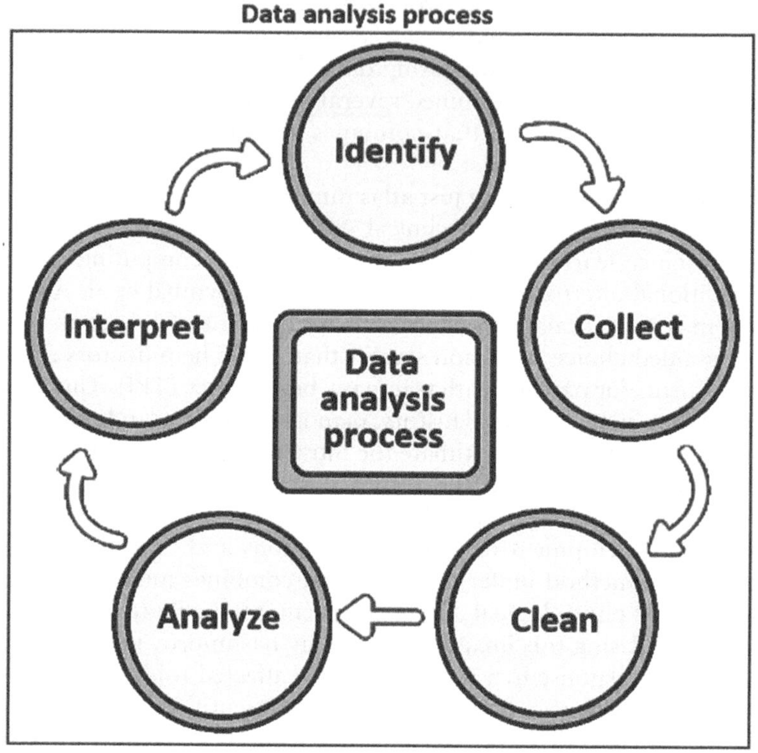

Figure 4.2 Data analysis process.

Certainly, when working with extremely large datasets, density methodologies can be used to bypass limitations in data collection and network. Many density means have been created to compress medical images [14]. But only a few methods have been developed for compressing extremely large data. This strategy can provide compression for both the high-output sequencing dataset and the data generated by calculating the log-odds of the probabilistic errors for each nucleotide, using up to 400- and 5-times compression, respectively. Both datasets contain biological and medical data on Kawasaki Disease (KD) comprising genotyping, gene appearance, proteome measurements, demographics, test results, images, clinical phenotypes, and treatment interventions. A graph model may assist with visualizing the data and provides the framework for large-scale datasets.In this case, the use of the intelligence theory of ease and power (SP) in large data sets has been studied. Simplifying and integrating ideas from other disciplines, including mathematics, artificial intelligence (AI), normal computing, and human insight and understanding, which may be seen as a system that resembles the human brain, is the aim of SP theory. The suggested SP system unifies and matches patterns to provide lossless compression. Nevertheless, this system is still in the design phase and is not compatible with the technology available today.

Application-specific compression techniques can only be implemented to a limited extent on similar processors, which may be similar to graphics processing units (GPUs), and general-purpose processors. This is because these processors are not suitable to GPUs and cylinder architectures, which require very mutable control and compound bit manipulations. In order to get over this restriction, an FPGA implementation of LZ-factorization was suggested, which lessens the compression algorithm's computing load. Recently, a lossy image density technique has been devised, which reshapes the picture so that sharp features have a greater sample bulk than rough ones if the image is equally sampled. It is stated that massive data compression may be achieved using this technique. However, as accuracy is crucial in medical applications, lossy approaches are typically not appropriate.

These methods are a couple of the methods that were either created with restricted uses or as prototypes. The creation of techniques for processing and analyzing vast amounts of data quickly and accurately is still essential. We have included the difficulties in medical image processing in Table 4.1. These difficulties appeared to be more significant when working

Table 4.1 Difficulties for medical big data processing

Area	*Difficulties*	*Example/Tools*
Data sharing and privacy	Secure collection, anonymization, and sharing of healthcare data	iDASH, Health-e-Child
Big data platforms	Storage and transfer of medical records and images	Hadoop, EMR, Microsoft Azure
Sensor-based healthcare	Collecting patient vitals and sending data to cloud	Sensor networks, Cloud systems
Data compression	Reducing size of large medical datasets	Sequencing data compression techniques
Biomedical data integration	Combining genetic, clinical, and imaging data	Kawasaki disease datasets
AI-based compression models	Pattern matching and lossless compression models	SP theory
Hardware acceleration	Improving compression using specialized hardware	GPUs, FPGA (LZ-factorization)
Medical image processing challenges	Need for efficient large-scale data analysis	Big data analytics techniques

with large data, although analytical techniques might help the large data to address them.

4.5 MEDICAL INDICATION ANALYTICS

Devices for monitoring biological signals and telemetry are widely used. But the continuous data that these monitors provide are typically only kept for a short while, which means that in-depth analysis of the collected data is rarely done. On the other hand, efforts to use incessant biological time and series monitoring besides telemetry for the enhancement of patient care and organization have increased recently.

Using continuous waveforms (signals that vary over time) and connected medical record data shaped by applied logical punishments to inform patient care decisions is known as gushing data analytics in the healthcare industry. Figure 4.1 provides a general description of the analytics pipeline for live and real flowing waveforms in medical contexts. First, a platform with the capacity to manage various waveforms at various fidelities is desirable for streaming data gathering and ingestion [15]. It is essential to integrate these lively waveform data with static EHR data in order to give the analytics engine contextual and situational knowledge.

Many target features may be extracted using a range of signal dispensation techniques, and a pretrained machine learning model uses these features to generate a useful insight. These useful visions may be prescriptive, predictive, or therapeutic in nature as seen in Figure 4.3. These insights may also be intended to set off further systems.

Integrating incessant waveform data with discrete sources to extract meaningful patient insights remains a complex challenge. Achieving next-gen diagnostics and therapies demands robust solutions across system, analytical, and clinical levels. The following sections explore key hurdles and evolving strategies in developing nursing systems that seamlessly combine high-fidelity waveforms with static clinical data for real-world deployment.

4.6 DATA ACQUISITION

In the past, it was uncommon to save running data from incessant physiological signal-gathering equipment. Typically, these data were stored only briefly and could only be recovered by specialized software and information setups provided by device manufacturers—even when saving the data was technically possible. Even though the mainstream of significant medical device producers is already working to offer interfaces for users to receive real-time streaming data from their products, big data difficulties often arise from data that is in motion. This is made worse by the extra governance problems, such as missing data standards, rules, and secrecy concerns. On

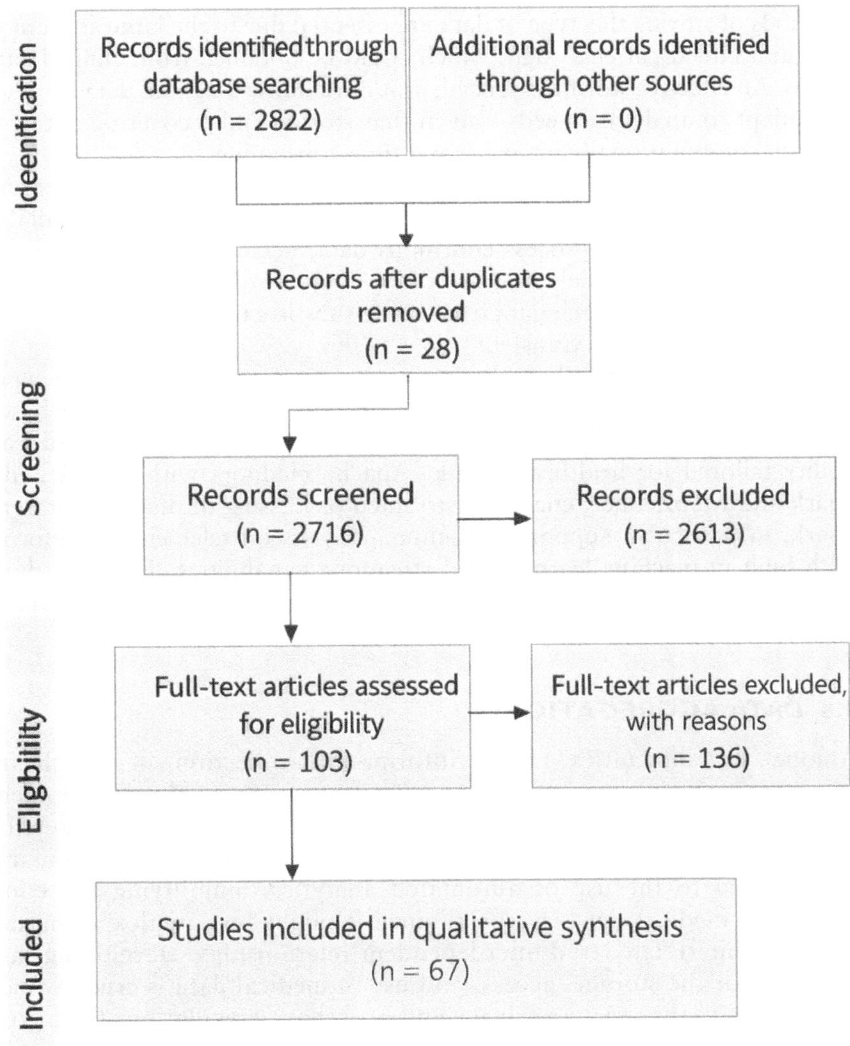

Figure 4.3 Medical signal analysis.

the other hand, a number of issues with the healthcare systems, such scalability, cost, and network capacity, have caused them to stagnate.

The scientific community is interested in using data from real-time monitors to create systems for continuous monitoring. Numerous in-house and commercial initiatives have been made to design and connect systems that facilitate this kind of data collection.

4.7 DATA STORAGE AND RECOVERY

Methods of storing this type of data are essential due to the large amount of data and added patients' sign, which could be obtained from clinical situations. An effective storing is crucial, as it must allow for rapid data retrieval and adapt to analytical needs—given that storing and recovering data can be both computationally intensive and time-consuming.

Health-tech and care research groups are using big data technologies programming, MapReduce, and database gradually often as per their available capacity to stock and process enormous data. Personal database schemas and different data models that are often unique to health system prevent healthcare and health tech data from being substitutable for research or any multi-institutional data transfer.

Traditional databases have limitations to integrate different data types like streaming waveforms and static EHRs. In contrast, document-based systems such as MongoDB offer improved performance, flexibility, and scalability tailored for healthcare needs. Apache Hadoop, with modules like Spark and MapReduce, enables distributed processing of massive datasets. Spark, in particular, supports real-time analytics on telemetry waveforms with built-in machine learning and streaming capabilities. Together, these technologies bridge the gap between scientific discovery and clinical application, empowering both retrospective and real-time insights.

4.8 DATA AGGREGATION

Among the difficulties facing information collection in healthcare systems are the integration of data from many sources, the development of constancy inside the data, the standardization of data from related sources, and the enhancement of information confidence, particularly with regard to the use of automated analytics. Simplifying the complexity of medical data is crucial since it might be complex in nature and have interrelated and interdependent relationships. Developing safe methods for the storage, access, and use of medical data is crucial since it is subject to the strictest privacy and provenance regulations from governmental organizations.

Analysis of incessant data commonly helps to data in the time-based domain. Merging waveform data with static electronic health records can be particularly challenging due to time-related discrepancies, as fixed data points often lack precise temporal alignment. Waveforms and other relevant electronic medical data are being compiled and obsessed by a single, all-inclusive database that is then publicly available to scholars worldwide. Like, MIMIC II and several other datasets inside Physio net contain waveforms and other scientific data from a wide range of genuine patient associates.

4.9 SIGNAL ANALYTICS USING BIG DATA

There is an increasing amount of research being done in signal processing for the purpose of making big data-based scientific decision support systems, or CDSSs. Actually, groups like the Institution of Medicine supported the use of CDSS and other health information technologies to raise the standard of treatment. To enhance the provision of treatment, CDSSs give medical professionals access to patient-specific knowledge and data that has been logically clean and delivered in times.

Intensive care units (ICUs) generate vast amounts of physiological data rapidly, with each patient contributing significant real-time metrics [16]. Recognizing this, researchers have identified the potential for clinical decision support systems (CDSS) in critical care settings [17]. Some have proposed scalable patient management systems that integrate both static and streaming data from ICU patients, enabling real-time data analysis and immediate alerts for critical events. Similarly, Bressan et al. designed a specialized architecture for neonatal ICUs, leveraging streaming data from infusion pumps, cerebral oxygenation monitors, and EEG devices to provide actionable medical decision support.

Currently, a clinical trial is being conducted to determine whether keeping stable heart rate and respiratory rate inconsistencies through the spontaneous breathing trials—which are given to patients prior to extubating—may predict a positive extubating later on. Biomarkers are derived in real time through signal processing of cardiac and respiratory waveforms. An animal research demonstrates the use of noninvasive continuous data collection methods to identify soft tissue healing markers in coiled care, including matter oxygenation, fluid content, and blood flow. An in-hospital cardiac arrest early detection system has been developed using electrocardiogram parameters obtained via telemetry in combination with demographic data such as medical history, discharge fraction, workshop results, and medicine information.

In research by Lee and Mark, cardiac and blood pressure time series data are used to trigger therapeutic action to hypotensive episodes utilizing the MIMIC II database. An additional research demonstrates how to uncover patient commonalities among the chosen cohorts by combining clinical data from the MIMIC II database with physiological waveform data. Due to these similarities, healthcare providers may find it easier to make decisions by drawing on information about prior similar disease cases' outcomes and treatments. Early patient identification of cardiovascular instability is developed by combining various waveform data from the MIMIC II database. Various physiological data types that are captured throughout preoperative and surgical treatment and the ways in which analytics might use this data to describe the many physiological data types that are collected in the working and preoperative care settings, as well as how the analytics may be used to use this data to assist in continually monitor the state of the patients before, during, and after surgery. Demonstrates the likelihood for creating data fusion-based machine learning replicas that use breath omics biomarkers—a metabolomics analysis of exhaled air—as an analytic tool.

Recent advances in neurology have highlighted electrophysiologic patient monitoring as a promising approach for developing innovative diagnostic tools, therapeutic interventions, and novel frameworks for understanding complex neurological conditions. This neurocritical care review explores specialized physiological monitoring techniques designed for patients requiring intensive neurological care. The authors analyze the potential and challenges of neuromonitoring using heterogeneous data quality while outlining future research directions and clinical applications—though they refrain from providing specific guidance on imaging, intraoperative monitoring, or treatment protocols. Moreover, this research investigates multiple modal nursing systems for traumatic brain injury patients and the implementation of patients care approaches. Similarly, a network-based trial of telemedicine is set up using portable and linked ECG, blood pressure, and body weight equipment. Research finds different stationary and mobile sensors available for healthcare data mining, which is knowledge creation from the available data and in developing applications for patient care.

4.10 LARGE-SCALE DATA APPLICATIONS IN GENOMICS

Since the completion of the human genome sequence, high-throughput sequencing has enabled the study of genetic markers across broad populations, increasing efficiency by orders of magnitude and identifying genetic causes of diseases.

With 30000 to 35000 genes in the genome, high sequencing analytics presents an intrinsic vast data encounter in genomics. Currently, efforts are being made to combine clinical data from a person's genetic level to their physiological level over years. These programmers will assist in as long as each patient with individualized treatment. Reliable and timely analysis of genome-scale big data is necessary to deliver suggestions in a healthcare environment. Because analyzing this massive data problem requires a lot of money, time, and labor, this profession is still in its infancy and has applications only in certain priority areas, including cancer.

This research focuses on two main areas: pathway analysis, which explores the useful implications The identification of genes that show different levels of expression within a specific test or gene set, along with the process of network rebuilding, that examines signals obtained from high-throughput methods to rebuild the fundamental governing networks. These networks manage various cellular activities that influence people's physiological condition.

4.11 PATHWAY STUDY

The majority of resources for deducing useful effects from "-omics" big data are founded on numerical associations amongst projected functional effects and variations in observed gene expression. Error and batch belongings are side effects of experimentation and analytical procedures. The ongoing expansion of genomic data accessible and the accompanying gene gloss must be taken into account when interpreting functional effects. For the purpose of functional pathway inspection of high-throughput genome-scale data, there are several platforms available, but no one "gold standard." The following describes three pairs of route study techniques.

4.12 RECONSTRUCTION OF REGULATORY NETWORKS

Pathway analysis methodologies typically do not interpret biological data as the outcome of a dynamic system. Several methods apply a dynamical system framework to genome-scale data analysis. This section concentrates on methods for inferring network models from biological data, which can be divided into two main areas: metabolic networks and gene regulatory networks. The performance of network inference techniques varies, and combining methods often yields better predictions.

Metabolic network reconstruction has advanced significantly over 20 years. A key goal is to use genomic, transcriptomic, and proteomic data to rebuild metabolic networks and understand organism-specific metabolism. Constraint-based approaches are commonly used to investigate the genotype–phenotype link while overcoming the limited availability of kinetic constants. Challenges include biological noise, platform variations, and the complex link between gene expression and reaction flow.

Several metabolic systems have been reconstructed (e.g., Recon 1, Recon 2, and SEED). Recon 2, an enhanced human metabolic model, includes thousands of reactions and metabolites and has been extended for analyzing drug off-target effects and predicting drug targets.

Reconstructing gene regulatory networks from gene expression data is another extensive research area. Inference methods can be classified into categories like regression, mutual information, correlation, and Boolean networks. Evaluations after challenges like DREAMS show varying performance across categories, with no single consistently superior method. Different techniques utilize various experimental data types (time series, knockouts, etc.). Recent successful approaches have used ANOVA and ensembles of regression trees.

Boolean regulatory networks, a type of discrete dynamical model, are useful when quantitative data is scarce but prior knowledge can reduce false positives. However, they become computationally expensive for large networks due to the exponential increase in possible states. Clustering to

Table 4.2 Popular methods and tool with their applications(kits)

Tool name kit	*Function type*	*Primary use case*
Pathway Insight	Biological route evaluation	Lung cancer profiling
GeneScope	Pathway-based data interpretation	Liver disease diagnostics
MolecuNet	Functional network analysis	Brain tumour classification
PathAlign	Genomic pathway correlation	Metabolic syndrome studies
ReactoMap	Cellular response mapping	Leukaemia pathway disruption
NetForm	Simulation of metabolic architecture	Pharmacogenomics modelling
LogicPath	Regulatory network construction	Heart cell specialization
ReguDynamics	Temporal modelling of gene control systems	Cardiac development research

reduce problem size is one solution; for example, clustering algorithms have been used to group genes into Meta genes, allowing Boolean models to represent network dynamics effectively for immunology datasets.

Ordinary differential equations can model the dynamics of gene regulatory networks and have been used to identify networks in yeast. Reconstructing a genome-scale network using a dynamical model is computationally intensive. Parallelizable dynamical ODE models have been developed to overcome this, reducing computation time significantly. Reconstructing networks for the human genome requires examining a vast number of potential connections. Such models have been used to reconstruct the cardiogenic gene regulatory network of the mammalian heart. Table 4.2 summarizes popular methods and toolkits.

4.13 CONCLUSION

Big data statics will greatly influence future medical practice, which incorporates the use of vast arrays of heterogeneous, structured [18], or free data sources. A multiplicity of analytics stands in support of patient and health-care workers' decision-making and performance. Our key concern has been narrowed into three domains: the processing of genetic data, physiological sign processing, and clinical image analysis. Exponential evolution in volume of medical images, computational experts are pressured to develop novel approaches to handle this large amount of data in manageable timeframes.

As a result of new technical expansions, there has been a rise in the availability, resolution, and different dimensions of multiple modality pictures, it has enhanced diagnostic accuracy and treatment outcomes. Mixing the same with clinical data and with images from other modalities is not free from the probabilities.

As a result, to examine this vast data within a healing system, newer and recent logical contexts and methods need to be developed to get accurate results. These methods trace various research objectives and problems, different possibilities, and issues, like features from pictures which assist in discriminating a finding, different data used in combination to achieve better diagnostic accuracy for better results and treatment at a lower cost, certain processing methods such as medical pictures enhancement and registration are used. Given the current situation of data competency and nonstandardized structure, signal processing of physiological data is a very real challenge; however, each one of these steps provides an opportunity to enhance systemic enhancements within the healthcare research and practice communities. Likewise, more research is needed in the field of data wrangling, data aggregation, and harmonization.

For systems biologists, the biggest difficulty is in integrating physical data with high-throughput "-omics" approaches to produce therapeutic suggestions. Although significant advances have been made in correlating gene expression changes with functional effects, interpreting functional impacts from high-throughput sequencing data remains a formidable challenge in genomic research. This is due to the ongoing increase in available genomic data, which also affects gene annotation due to experimentation and analytical practices.

The task of rebuilding systems at the genome scale is not well-posed. Transformation gene regulatory networks and metabolic networks has yielded robust applications. A bottleneck is the limited supply of kinetic constants, which is why several models try to get around this restriction. The important problem of gene regulation, the impact of various network topologies, and the evolutionary consequences of these networks remain incompletely understood. In order to alleviate these issues, a combination of meticulous test design and the creation of models for network reconstruction will contribute to the reduction of time and costs associated with developing an understanding of regulation in genome-scale networks. Close collaboration between doctors, computer scientists, and experimentalists is necessary to tackle the big issue.

REFERENCES

1. Kohane, I. S., Aronow, B. J., & Avillach, P. (2015). Big data and health care. *IEEE Journal of Biomedical and Health Informatics*, 19(4), 1193–1208.
2. Manyika, J., Chui, M., Brown, B., Bughin, J., Dobbs, R., Roxburgh, C., & Byers, A. H. (2011). *Big Data: The Next Frontier for Innovation, Competition, and Productivity*. McKinsey Global Institute.
3. Chen, H., & Snyder, M. (2018). Promise of personalized omics to precision medicine. *Wiley Interdisciplinary Reviews: Systems Biology and Medicine*, 10(4), e1413.

4. Aliper, A., Plis, S., Artemov, A., Ulloa, A., Mamoshina, P., & Zhavoronkov, A. (2016). Deep learning applications for predicting pharmacological properties of drugs and drug repurposing using transcriptomic data. *Molecular Pharmaceutics*, 13(7), 2524–2530.
5. Hou, Y., Liu, L., Ng, H., Fermin, D., & Vogel, C. (2019). An integrated approach to identify causal network modules of complex diseases with application to colorectal cancer. *Journal of the American Medical Informatics Association*, 26(6), 519–528.
6. Kourou, K., Exarchos, T. P., Exarchos, K. P., Karamouzis, M. V., & Fotiadis, D. I. (2015). Machine learning applications in cancer prognosis and prediction. *Computational and Structural Biotechnology Journal*, 13, 8–17.
7. Opijnen, M. P. (2020). The challenges of big data in healthcare. In Jian Guan (Ed.) *Data Science in Healthcare* (pp. 1–21). Springer.
8. Doi, K. (2007). Computer-aided diagnosis in medical imaging: Historical review, current status and future potential. *Computerized Medical Imaging and Graphics*, 31(4-5), 198–211.
9. Liebeskind, D. S., & Feldmann, E. (2013). Imaging of cerebrovascular disorders: Precision medicine and the collaterome. *Annals of the New York Academy of Sciences*, 1291(1), 1–13.
10. Hussain, A. M., et al. (2017). The role of imaging in the diagnosis of temporomandibular joint disorders: A review. *Journal of Oral Rehabilitation*, 44(1), 45–52.
11. White, T. (2012). *Hadoop: The definitive guide.* O'Reilly Media, Inc.
12. Plis, S. M., Hjelm, D. R., Salakhutdinov, R., Allen, E. A., Bockholt, H. J., Long, J. D., Johnson, H. J., Paulsen, J. S., Turner, J. A., & Calhoun, V. D. (2014). Deep learning for neuroimaging: A validation study. *Frontiers in Neuroscience*, 8, 229.
13. Stephens, Z. D., et al. (2015). Big data: Astronomical or genomical? *PLOS Biology*, 13(7), e1002195.
14. Liu, Z., Sun, M., & Leung, H. (2020). Natural language processing for big data analytics in healthcare: A comprehensive review. *Journal of Biomedical Informatics*, 101, 103343.
15. Clifford, G. D., & Clifton, D. (2012). Wireless technology in disease management and medicine. *Annual Review of Medicine*, 63, 479–492.
16. Bressan, N., McGregor, C., Smith, K., Lecce, L., & James, A. (2014). Heart rate variability as an indicator for morphine pharmacokinetics and pharmacodynamics in critically ill newborn infants. In *Proceedings of the 36th Annual International Conference of the IEEE Engineering in Medicine and Biology Society (EMBC)* (pp. 5719–5722). IEEE.
17. Sutton, R. T., Pincock, D., Baumgart, D. C., Sadowski, D. C., Fedorak, R. N., & Kroeker, K. I. (2020). An overview of clinical decision support systems: Benefits, risks, and strategies for success. *NPJ Digital Medicine*, 3(1), 1–10.
18. Tsymbal, A., Kam, H. J., Kim, J. A., Cho, I., Kim, Y., & Park, R. W. (2005). Integration of heterogeneous data sources for clinical decision support. *Studies in Health Technology and Informatics*, 116, 635–640.

Chapter 5

Integrating framework in mobile cloud computing and multimodal data for pervasive healthcare systems

Ramiz Salama, Chadi Altrjman, and Fadi Al-Turjman

5.1 INTRODUCTION

Mobile cloud computing, or MCC, is an effective technique for next-generation pervasive healthcare systems. Figure 5.1 shows how MCC is utilized to give healthcare services in a variety of applications. However, the unpredictability of communication network delays leads mobile devices' wireless communication modules to consume energy significantly faster than necessary (Abdulazeez & Abdulazeez 2024). My purpose is in completing this assessment examination advancements and leading of ubiquitous healthcare service technology. This study is expected to promote more inventive thinking and improve the attention of politicians, academics, service providers, and healthcare professionals to this critical sector. Section 5.2 provides an overview of applications. Section 5.3includes many architectural elements used in healthcare. The use of pervasive healthcare is discussed in Section 5.6. Section 5.4 describes the many optimization approaches utilized in modern mobile cloud healthcare. Section 5.5 discusses privacy and security problems and how they might be addressed.

5.1.1 Mobile cloud computing

To grasp the concept of MCC, we must first understand the services that comprise the computing model.

a. MCC means to execute portable and mobile devices. A small, portable gadget is distributed and is outfitted. This technology is utilized to connect disparate resources that are centrally located within each used device (Ahuja et al., 2024). As mobile devices have risen in popularity, so have people's expectations for the quality and level of service they deliver (Ali et al., 2025).
b. Cloud computing: centralizes computer services and allocates resources based on demand. The cloud's services are purely based on what the users have requested. These services can be categorized

DOI: 10.1201/9781003665656-5

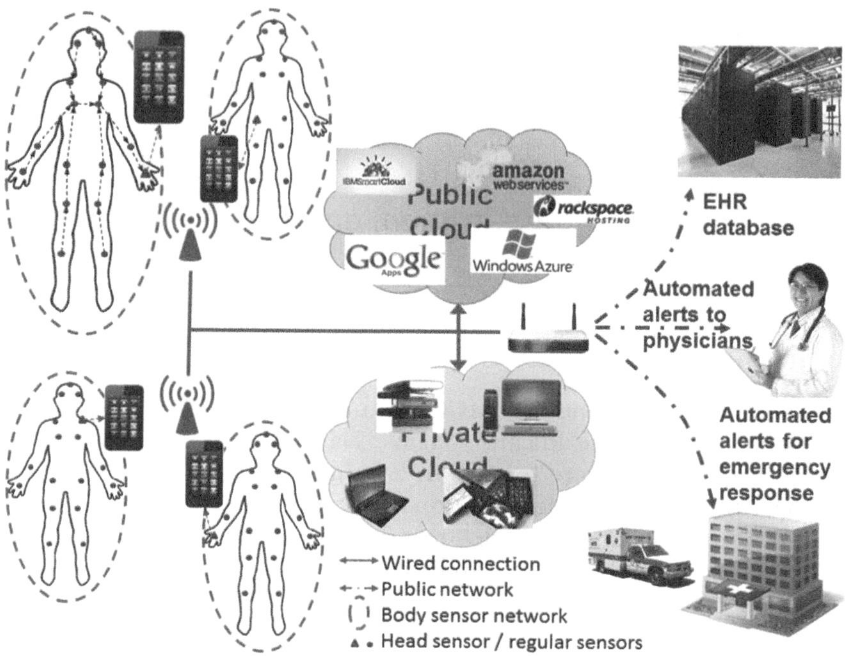

Figure 5.1 Wireless body area networks (WBAN).

into three types: Software as a Service (SAAS), Platform As a Service (PAAS), and Infrastructure As a Service (IAAS) (Alghaith 2024).

MCC is a computing model that combines mobile computing and cloud computing services delivered via the Internet. MCC represents the integration and convergence of these two technologies into a single, seamless paradigm. While this integration has many advantages, it has also increased the security of MCC models. MCC apps use portable devices to do activities such as infinite storage and rapid cloud computing processing power (Alkateeb & Abdullah 2024). MCC applications utilize cloud services by outsourcing mobile application duties to the cloud. Offloading is carried out based on a set of criteria and parameters, as well as the appropriate mobile device states, in order to complete tasks and display the cloud status.

5.2 APPLICATIONS USING MOBILE CLOUDS FOR HEALTHCARE

The use of MCC in healthcare has resulted in numerous creative applications aimed at enhancing patient care, clinical procedures, and healthcare efficiency (Rajput et al., 2024). Here are some of the most common healthcare apps that make use of mobile cloud technology (Bashir et al., 2024).

5.2.1 Electronic health record (EHR)

A systematic method for gathering patient and population health data in an electronic, digital format is offered by an electronic health record (EHR). The terms EHRs and electronic medical records (EMRs) are frequently used interchangeably (Devi et al., 2024). Previously created, used, and maintained as a paper chart, the patient record can now be submitted electronically, as shown in Figure 5.2. The healthcare organization creates, maintains, and administers a patient's electronic health record. Only medical personnel who are actively involved in the patient's care have access to and use of the electronic medical record. A patient's control and ability to modify their own health record is known as their personal health record (PHR).

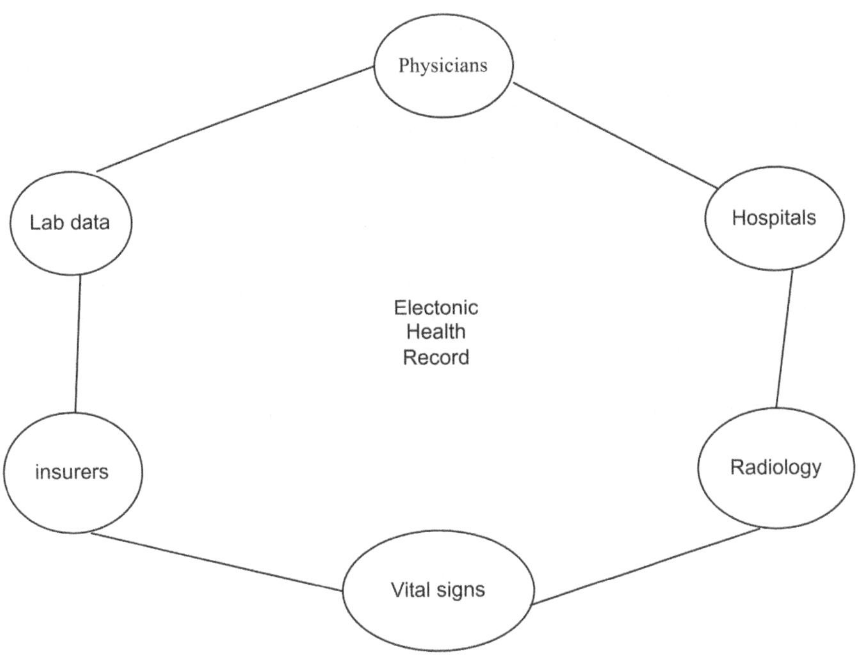

Figure 5.2 Electronic health record (EHR).

5.3 MOBILE CLOUD ARCHITECTURES UTILIZED IN HEALTHCARE

For healthcare services, which may be categorized into different areas—various mobile cloud architectures have been created and put into use.

5.3.1 Mobile devices and sensors

Wearable technology and sensors play a role in the MCC paradigm. The system can be enhanced by the efficient coordination of sensors and mobile devices (Du et al. 2024). Numerous strategies for energy conservation and effective data processing have been investigated in sensors and mobile devices due to their limited battery life and processing capacity. A MC system that interacts with location was proposed by (Zhang et al., 2024). In order to reliably and efficiently respond to requests from mobile devices, wireless sensor networks (WSNs) have woken up in an optimal manner. In order to manipulate the sensors into different states, the time delay and task priority level are taken into consideration (Isravel et al., 2024), which showed another example system combining WSNs with MCC. Important data would be safely moved to the mobile cloud infrastructure in this manner. In order to forecast the next sensory input that will be used to gather, process, transmit, and store data in an effective and sustainable manner, a mobile cloud system paradigm has been created that works in conjunction with a WSN (Khan et al., 2024). A dynamic adaptive system for the selective transfer of computing activities from a mobile device to various cloud computing resources was created by Lum & Isaac (2016). Numerous mobile cloud technology implementation scenarios were thoroughly examined (Nosheen & Omar, 2024). To assess the benefits and drawbacks of various approaches, a number of variables were tracked, including energy use and computer resource costs. In mobile cloud-based healthcare, sensor and mobile device collaboration is also crucial. In their research, Hiremath et al. suggested Wearable IoT (WIoT) and discussed in detail the design process for these systems as well as those utilized in clinical treatment. A noncontact ECG monitoring system that combines a sensor, a mobile device, and the cloud was presented by Doukas and associates (Fong & Chung, 2013). Additionally, it developed a mobile cloud system that integrated sensors to offer thorough and real-time patient monitoring. When patients wearing sensors travel from one location to another, Das et al. (2013) developed an MC system for patient health that suggested an approach for mapping. The servers' utilization rate may be greatly raised, and computing resources might be allocated as efficiently as possible in this fashion. In order to offer ubiquitous healthcare services, Wan et al. (2008) created a cloud system based on wireless body area networks (WBANs). Energy conservation and information security were necessary throughout system deployment (Khan & Singh, 2024). A system that employed smart clothing as physiological sensors was created by Chen et al. 2024. Users' vital signs might be collected by such a specialized wearable device and sent to the cloud for additional analysis. In their study, Quwaider & Jararweh (2016) suggested a cloud system that effectively performs heavy data aggregation by utilizing WBANs. The position, temperature, and respiration rate of the subjects under observation were all gathered by sensors and transmitted to the cloud in the MC system created in (Verma et al., 2024) in order to fully evaluate the subjects' health. MCC and nonintrusive methods were used in a study by Pagán et al. (2018) to monitor and predict migraines.

5.3.2 Cloud-based systems

Wearable technology coins a significant role in the paradigm. The performance of MC systems can be greatly enhanced by the efficient coordination of sensors and mobile devices. Numerous strategies for energy conservation and effective data processing have been investigated in sensors and mobile devices due to their limited battery life and processing capacity. An MC system that interacts to deliver rich location was proposed by Wu et al. (2024). In order to reliably and efficiently respond to requests from mobile devices, WSNs have woken up in an optimum manner. In order to manipulate the sensors into different states, the time delay and task priority level are taken into consideration, as shown in another example system combining WSNs with MCC. Important data would be safely moved to the mobile cloud infrastructure in this manner. In order to forecast the next sensory input that will be used to gather, process, transmit, and store data in an effective and sustainable manner, a mobile cloud system paradigm has been created that works in conjunction with a WSN. A dynamic adaptive system for the selective transfer of computing activities from a mobile device to various cloud computing resources was created by Zhou et al. (2024). Numerous mobile cloud technology implementation scenarios were thoroughly examined. To assess the benefits and drawbacks of various approaches, a number of variables were tracked, including energy use and computer resource costs. In mobile cloud-based healthcare, sensor and mobile device collaboration is also crucial. In their research, Hiremath et al. suggested Wearable IoT (WIoT) and discussed in detail the design process of these systems as well as those utilized in clinical treatment. A noncontact ECG monitoring system that combines a sensor, a mobile device, and the cloud was presented by Doukas and associates (Fong et al., 2024). Additionally, it developed a mobile cloud system that integrated sensors to offer thorough and real-time patient monitoring. When patients wearing sensors travel from one location to another, Agrawal et al.(2022) developed an MC system for patient health, suggesting an approach for mapping. The servers' utilization rate may be greatly raised, and computing resources might be allocated as efficiently as possible in this fashion. In order to offer ubiquitous services, energy conservation and security were necessary throughout system deployment. Users' vital signs might be collected by such a specialized wearable device and sent to the cloud for additional analysis. In their study, Quwaider et al. (2023) suggested a cloud system that effectively performs heavy data aggregation by utilizing WBANs. The position, temperature, and respiration rate of the subjects under observation were all gathered by sensors and transmitted to the cloud in the mobile cloud system created in (Verma et al., 2024) in order to fully evaluate the subjects' health. MCC and nonintrusive methods were used in a study by Pagán et al. to monitor and predict migraines.

5.4 HEALTHCARE BIG DATA

Countries all across the world want to improve health care and lower medical expenditures. The health data revolution, however, continues to stand in the way of accomplishing this objective. Global digital health data is predicted. Health outcomes will undoubtedly be improved by gathering, storing, searching, sharing, and analyzing such large data for insightful information. Systems through more intelligent choices and reduced medical expenses, yet conventional database administration solutions, are no longer sufficient to manage this data. To do this, new, effective algorithms are required. For instance, the American Hospital Association's most recent report found that over 71 million individuals are admitted to hospitals in the United States annually. According to studies, avoidable hospital stays cost more than $30 billion in 2006. "Can we identify those most at risk earlier and make sure they get the care they need?" is a question that the Heritage Provider Network (HPN) poses and they think the answer is "yes." HPN is supporting a $3 million Heritage Health award competition to accomplish its objective of creating a revolutionary algorithm that makes use of current patient data to anticipate and avoid needless hospitalizations. The winning team develops an algorithm that forecasts the number of days in the hospital, and the winning solutions combine many predictive models. After HPs are identified, new care plans and approaches can be created to contact patients before emergencies arise, which will cut down on needless hospital stays. This lowers medical expenses while also improving patient health. The following factors motivate big data analytics in the healthcare industry: Traditional database approaches and analyzing the constantly increasing volume, complexity, and productivity of healthcare data. To process this data in a reasonable amount of time, new and creative technologies are required. Several sensors are used to gather a range of patient and societal behavioral data. Evidence-based healthcare is replacing comparatively ad hoc and subjective decision-making in standard medical practice using patient/data linkages in longitudinal records and extracting information from intricate, diverse patient sources. Recognize unstructured clinical notes requires Natural Language Processing (NLP) and advanced text mining wich effectively retrieves biomarkers and potentially helpful information from massive amounts of medical imaging data. Genomic data analysis requires a lot of computing power, and it becomes more complicated when combined with standard clinical data (Vivek & Veeravalli, 2024).

5.5 SECURITY ISSUES

A growing number of commercial and private users have started to rely extensively on MCCs in their everyday work, raising serious concerns about customer center. Threats to privacy and security have been the subject of several earlier investigations (Humayun et al., 2024). An overview of mobile cloud privacy issues, including data theft and data integrity breaches, was given by Au et al. (2018). They offered their thoughts on potential data privacy issues that can arise in user activities, particularly from a crypto perspective. He et al. examined the potential privacy risks associated with profile matching, which was crucial for a number of social networking services. To stop personal data from leaking into the mobile cloud system, they put in place a scalable security solution. In order to create data-related services, Lin (2024). examined the deployment of a mobile cloud-based verifiable data ownership system. They were motivated by the fact that current tangible data management usually required a significant amount of storage and processing power, which was impractical for mobile devices. It was shown that their suggested approach can carry out precise data verification processes at a minimal cost. For vehicle MC systems with low communication costs, Gai et al. (2020) suggested a safe media data transmission technique. They also addressed a number of security concerns, including communication node intrusion and network channel data fabrication. Wu et al. (2022) developed a robust authentication solution for them. Their suggested approach could defend the mobile cloud system against a range of hostile assaults, including phishing and dictionary attacks that have comparatively modest communication costs. Recent developments in Biocomputing technology allowed Sukumaran and Mohammed to encrypt data in mobile cloud systems using DNA computing, which is based on primer creation and the general rule of polymerase chain reaction. Given the significance and sensitivity of medical data and operations, there are particularly significant worries around MCC risk. As seen in Table 5.2, some previous research has looked for different ways to address these issues. To preserve security and privacy in the healthcare industry, Thota & Srinivasulu (2024) created a mobile cloud-based IoT platform. In particular, their suggested approach might spy on recently connected gadgets. An advanced mobile cloud-based authentication system for EHR management was presented by Liu et al. Patient data confidentiality can be guaranteed at the lowest feasible cost by carefully segmenting the encryption processes into distinct stages, whether they are conducted offline or online. In order to address security and privacy concerns in mobile and multi-system communication networks, Al-Muhtadi et al. (2019) investigated the case of mobile social network cloud architecture to deliver healthcare services and establish varying privacy levels for healthcare roles. Albuquerque and Gondim examined a range of security concerns that could emerge in mobile cloud health systems, including data integrity and confidentiality, and offered a broad overview of solutions. Zhang and colleagues examine privacy and security concerns in mobile health networks. They have given customers the ability to alter the security system in order to accommodate their varying privacy and security needs. Additionally, they presented various methods for preserving privacy and security at various phases of mobile cloud services, including data processing and gathering. Sajjad et al. (2017) employed brief approaches to avoid picture content intrusion and mobile cloud infrastructure to encrypt medical photos. With minimal effort, their technique has been shown to maintain image quality and save data security. An effective health identification system built on cloud computing based on vehicles was described by Kumar et al. (2020). The RFID-based approach they suggested allowed the system to fend off cyberattacks like eavesdropping, replay, and tracking attacks (Shafi et al., 2024), among others. Zhou et al. (2024) examined a situation in which patients traveling small distances could receive healthcare services via WBAN-embedded mobile cloud systems. In order for the MC healthcare system to be resistant to several device, they suggested an efficient security system to transfer the resource-intensive cryptographic key management processes to the cloud. An authentication mechanism was presented by Liu et al. to control PHR access in a mobile cloud setting. Their suggested approach might address the cloud security issues with PHR administration, particularly in situations when numerous user requests were being sent concurrently. In order to protect the privacy of the elderly's medical records, Hu et al. created an MCC Internet of Things. They suggested an authentication method based on asymmetric/symmetric encryption. Rahman et al. (2022) examined a situation in which health information was shared via a peer-to-peer cloud architecture based on mobile phones. To build a network-based data sharing system that guards against malicious attacks such as targeted, man-in-the-middle, masking, and message manipulation attacks, they employed a link-based encryption mechanism. In order to boost efficiency, Pal et al. (2021) created a system that offloaded. A mobile cloud-based lightweight authentication solution was provided by Mohit et al. (2025) to safeguard patient data anonymity and confidentiality while defending the Telecare Medical Information solution (TMIS) from malicious assaults such as impersonation. The influence of virtualization strategies that can be applied to rise was covered by Saleem et al. (2019). To safeguard data, Tillakaratne et al. (2024) suggested an encryption scheme.

5.6 PERVASIVE HEALTHCARE AND MOBILE CLOUD COMPUTING

Equipment and procedures MCC for complete healthcare:

Review of the literature. To learn more about the uses of mobile cloud computing (MCC) in holistic healthcare, a thorough assessment of the body of existing literature was carried out. Using pre-established search phrases pertaining to MCC, healthcare, and general computing, relevant databases like PubMed, IEEE Xplore, and Google Scholar were examined.

Selection criteria: Articles authored in English and concentrating on MCC applications in healthcare that were published within the previous 5 years were included in the literature selection criteria. Only scientific papers, conference proceedings, and peer-reviewed journal articles were taken into consideration for inclusion.

To validate the effectiveness of the proposed MCC-based pervasive healthcare architecture (Sathik Raja & Jamuna, 2024), an experimental system was developed that integrates *multimodal medical data fusion*, *secure multimedia health information protection*, and *green-aware resource scheduling*. The objective of the experiment is to demonstrate that mobile cloud healthcare systems can simultaneously achieve high diagnostic performance, high privacy protection, and low resource consumption. Three levels of multimodal fusion were implemented:

- **Early fusion:** concatenation of temporal sensor features and image embeddings
- **Intermediate fusion:** modality-specific feature extractors feeding a shared latent representation
- **Late fusion:** weighted decision fusion across classifiers

Intermediate fusion yielded the best tradeoff between detection accuracy and latency.

The fused representations were processed using a *multi-task learning model* that predicts both (a) abnormality type and (b) risk severity.

5.7 MULTIMEDIA MEDICAL DATA SECURITY MODEL

Secure healthcare data transmission and storage were achieved through a multilayer security protocol designed specifically for multimedia medical assets (images, audio, signals, and EHRs), as shown in Table 5.1.

Raw medical images, audio streams, and physiological signals are *never exposed outside the local device*; only encrypted feature vectors are transmitted.

Table 5.1 Security components

Security requirement	*Mechanism implemented*
Data confidentiality	AES-256 encryption for multimedia payloads
Data integrity	Blockchain-based audit logging
Access control	Role-based authentication and token-based authorization
Privacy-preserving learning	Federated learning and local differential privacy

Blockchain enforces traceability of access operations (Nimkar & Makhijani, 2024), preventing unauthorized modification of medical history.

Security Evaluation Metrics: The following metrics were used to assess system resilience:

- Attack prevention rate (APR)
- Packet tamper detection ratio
- Unauthorized access blocking rate
- Latency overhead added by encryption

The proposed protocol maintained *97.4% protection efficiency* while adding only *6.1% average latency overhead*, confirming suitability for real-time healthcare.

Green and Sustainable MCC Resource Scheduling: Sustainability is crucial in ubiquitous health monitoring due (Khan & Ullah, 2024) to continuous data streaming from wearables. To reduce computational and communication energy consumption, a *green-aware resource scheduling mechanism* was implemented (Putra et al., 2024).

Tasks are dynamically classified into three execution tiers as in Table 5.2:

The scheduler selects the execution tier based on *network bandwidth, device battery level, data size, and urgency of medical risk*. Some KPI are given in Table 5.3.

Scheduling decisions significantly reduced *overall energy and resource usage* while maintaining real-time responsiveness.

5.8 CONCLUSION

MCC is an effective next-generation ubiquitous healthcare systems. However, because communication network delays are unpredictable, mobile devices' wireless communication modules consume far more energy than necessary. Offering a review of the advancements of ubiquitous healthcare service technology is my aim in doing this evaluation. Experimental results confirm that the integration of *multimodal medical*

Table 5.2 Energy-optimized task offloading strategy

Tier	*Location*	*Function*
Tier-1	Wearable/edge	Local feature extraction, emergency anomaly alert
Tier-2	Fog/near-edge	Real-time diagnosis, multimodal fusion
Tier-3	Cloud	Long-term analytics, model updates, population-level insights

Table 5.3 Sustainability performance indicators

KPI	*Baseline MCC (%)*	*Proposed system (%)*	*Improvement (%)*
Energy consumption	100	63	↓ 37
Latency	100	71	↓ 29
Bandwidth usage	100	58	↓ 42
Cloud computation load	100	66	↓ 34

fusion, multimedia-oriented security, and *sustainable MCC scheduling* produces a scalable, pervasive healthcare system capable of high-precision clinical decision support, strict protection of sensitive medical assets, and low-power continuous operation suited for real-world telehealth and smart hospital deployments. It is expected that this research would stimulate more innovative thinking and increase awareness of this important field among academics, legislators, service providers, and medical professionals. This is how the rest of the job is organized.

REFERENCES

Abdulazeez, A. H., & Abdulazeez, A. M. (2024). Integration of machine learning with fog computing for health care systems challenges and issues: A review. *The Indonesian Journal of Computer Science*, 13(3), 3746–3765.

Agrawal, U. K., Shrivastava, A. K., Das, D., and Mahapatra, R., (2022). Neural Network Detector in Mobile Molecular Communication for Fast Varying Channels, *2022 International Conference on Connected Systems & Intelligence (CSI)* (pp. 1–5). Trivandrum, India, doi: 10.1109/CSI54720.2022.9924143.

Ahuja, L., Simon, R., & Thakur, A. (2024). Privacy and security considerations in healthcare: Navigating the challenges of IoT and ubiquitous computing. In Nidhi Sindhwani, Sarvesh Tanwar, Ajay Rana, Ramani Kannan (Eds.) *Smart technologies in healthcare management* (pp. 164–181). CRC Press.

Alghaith, W. (2024). Security determinants of the educational use of mobile cloud computing in higher education. *International Journal of Computer Science & Network Security*, 24(8), 105–118.

Ali, M., Muhammad, D., Khalaf, O. I., & Habib, R. (2025). Optimizing mobile cloud computing: A comparative analysis and innovative cost-efficient partitioning model. *SN Computer Science*, 6(1), 1–25, https://doi.org/10.1007/s42979-024-03570-1

Al-kateeb, Z. N., & Abdullah, D. B. (2024). Unlocking the potential: Synergizing IoT, cloud computing, and big data for a bright future. *Iraqi Journal for Computer Science and Mathematics*, 5(3), 25–38.

Al-Muhtadi, J., Shahzad, B., Saleem, K., Jameel, W., & Orgun, M. A. (2019). Cybersecurity and privacy issues for socially integrated mobile healthcare applications operating in a multi-cloud environment. *Health Informatics Journal*, 25(2), 315–329. https://doi.org/10.1177/1460458217706184

Au, M. H., Liang, K., Liu, J. K., Lu, R., & Ning, J. (2018). Privacy-preserving personal data operation on mobile cloud—Chances and challenges over advanced persistent threat. *Future Generation Computer Systems*, 79(Part 1), 337–349. https://doi.org/10.1016/j.future.2017.06.021

Bashir, S. R., Raza, S., & Misic, V. (2024). A narrative review of identity, data, and location privacy techniques in edge computing and mobile crowdsourcing. *arXiv preprint arXiv:2401.11305*.

Das, S., Misra, S., Khatua M., and Rodrigues, J. J. P. C. (2013). Mapping of sensor nodes with servers in a mobile Health-Cloud environment. *2013 IEEE 15th International Conference on e-Health Networking, Applications and Services (Healthcom 2013)*, Lisbon, Portugal (pp. 481–485), doi: 10.1109/HealthCom.2013.6720724.

Devi, G. V., Selvan, R. S., Mani, D. S., Sakshi, M., & Singh, A. (2024, March). Cloud computing based medical activity supporting system. In *2024 2nd International Conference on Disruptive Technologies (ICDT)* (pp. 1116–1120). IEEE.

Du, H., Liu, M., Liu, N., Li, D., Li, W., & Xu, L. (2024). Scheduling of low-latency medical services in healthcare cloud with deep reinforcement learning. *Tsinghua Science and Technology*, 30(1), 100–111. https://doi.org/10.26599/TST.2023.9010070

Fong, E., & Chung, W. (2013). Mobile cloud-computing-based healthcare service by noncontact ECG monitoring. *Sensors*, 13(12), 16451-16473. https://doi.org/10.3390/s131216451

Gai, K., Choo, K.-K. R., & Zhu, L. (2020). Privacy-preserving content-oriented wireless communication in internet-of-things. *IEEE Internet of Things Journal*, 5(4), 3059–3067. https://doi.org/10.1109/JIOT.2018.2830340

Humayun, M., Alsirhani, A., Alserhani, F., Shaheen, M., & Alwakid, G. (2024). Transformative synergy: SSEHCET—bridging mobile edge computing and AI for enhanced eHealth security and efficiency. *Journal of Cloud Computing*, 13(1), 37. https://doi.org/10.1186/s13677-024-00646-4

Isravel, D. P., Silas, S., Kathrine, J. W., Rajsingh, E. B., & Andrew, J. (2024). Multivariate forecasting of network traffic in SDN based ubiquitous healthcare system. *IEEE Open Journal of the Communications Society*, 5, 1537–1550. Advance online publication. https://doi.org/10.1109/OJCOMS.2024.3373698

Khan, F., & Ullah, R. (2024). Ubiquitous computing entity-aware data management on mobile devices. *Mobile Networks and Applications*, 29(2), 398–400. https://doi.org/10.1007/s11036-023-02245-0

Khan, M. S., & Singh, J. (2024, January). Security challenges in mobile cloud computing. In *2024 IEEE 1st Karachi Section Humanitarian Technology Conference (KHI-HTC)* (pp. 1–9). IEEE.

Khan, N., Tabassum, M., Lawal, I. A., Lakshmikanth, S. P., & AlRugaibah, A. A. (2024, March). Impact of cloud computing adoption in Saudi Arabia health care sector. In *AIP Conference Proceedings* (Vol. 2919, No. 1). AIP Publishing.

Kumar, M., Patel, A. K., Shah, A. V., Raval, J., Rajpara, N., Joshi, M., & Joshi, C. G. (2020). First proof of the capability of wastewater surveillance for COVID-19 in India through detection of genetic material of SARS-CoV-2. *Science of The Total Environment*, 746, 141326.

Lin, J. (2024). FGDB-MLPP: A fine-grained data-sharing scheme with blockchain based on multi-level privacy protection. *IET Communications. Advance Online Publication*. https://doi.org/10.1049/cmu2.12737

Lum, K., & Isaac, W. (2016). To predict and serve? *Significance*, 13(5), 14–19. https://doi.org/10.1111/j.1740-9713.2016.00960.x

Mohit, M., Akhtar, S., Xu, M., & Sasmito, A. P. (2025). Development of a renewable technology for air heating and thermal cooling of sub-arctic mines using spray freezing. *International Journal of Thermal Sciences*, 211, 109704.

Nagavenkatabalaji Thota, & K. Srinivasulu. (2024). IoT-Based Patient Health Monitoring: Real-Time Heart Rate and Body Temperature Tracking with Doctor Alerts via IoT. *Journal of Computational Analysis and Applications (JoCAAA)*, 33(05), 389–398. Retrieved from https://eudoxuspress.com/index.php/pub/article/view/531

Nimkar, S., & Makhijani, S. (2024, June). Blockchain and cloud computing in healthcare: A critical analysis and future prospects. In *2024 IEEE 3rd International Conference on Electrical Power and Energy Systems (ICEPES)* (pp. 1–5). IEEE.

Nosheen, A., & Omar, M. A. (2024). The future of mobile cloud computing: Key implications and challenges. *TOPLAMA*, 2(1), 162–169.

Pagán, J., Zapater, M., & Ayala, J. L. (2018). Power transmission and workload balancing policies in eHealth mobile cloud computing scenarios. *Future Generation Computer Systems*, 78(Part 1), 587–601. https://doi.org/10.1016/j.future.2017.06.023

Pal, R., Singh, B., Bhadada, S. K., Banerjee, M., Bhogal, R. S., Hage, N., & Kumar, A. (2021). COVID-19-associated mucormycosis: an updated systematic review of literature. *Mycoses*, 64(12), 1452–1459.

Putra, K. T., Arrayyan, A. Z., Hayati, N., Damarjati, C., Bakar, A., & Chen, H. C. (2024). A review on the application of internet of medical things in wearable personal health monitoring: A cloud-edge artificial intelligence approach. *IEEE Access*, 12, 21437–21452. https://ieeexplore.ieee.org/document/10415018

Quwaider, M., & Jararweh, Y. (2016). Multi-tier cloud infrastructure support for reliable global health awareness system. *Simulation Modelling Practice and Theory*, 67, 44–58. https://doi.org/10.1016/j.simpat.2016.06.005

Quwaider, M., Alabed, A., & Duwairi, R. (2023). Shooter video games for personality prediction using five factor model traits and machine learning. *Simulation Modelling Practice and Theory*, 122, 102665.

Rahman, S., Rahman, M. M., Miah, M., Begum, M. N., Sarmin, M., Mahfuz, M.,... & Rahman, M. (2022). COVID-19 reinfections among naturally infected and vaccinated individuals. *Scientific Reports*, 12(1), 1438.

Rajput, A. S., Prabha, S., & Khare, M. D. (2024, May). A framework on positioning of medical sensors in healthcare domain. In *2024 International Conference on Communication, Computer Sciences and Engineering (IC3SE)* (pp. 197–201). IEEE.

Sajjad, M., Muhammad, K., Baik, S. W., Rho, S., Jan, Z., Yeo, S.-S., & Mehmood, I. (2017). Mobile-cloud assisted framework for selective encryption of medical images with steganography for resource-constrained devices. *Multimedia Tools and Applications*, 76(3), 3519–3536. https://doi.org/10.1007/s11042-016-3811-6

Saleem, M. H., Potgieter, J., & Arif, K. M. (2019). Plant disease detection and classification by deep learning. *Plants*, 8(11), 468.

Sathik Raja, M., & Jamuna, K. (2024). Medical sensors and their integration in wireless body area networking for pervasive healthcare delivery. *Journal of Pervasive Healthcare*, 15(2), 45–58.

Shafi, I., Din, S., Farooq, S., Díez, I. D. L. T., Breñosa, J., Espinosa, J. C. M., & Ashraf, I. (2024). Design and development of patient health tracking, monitoring and big data storage using Internet of Things and real time cloud computing. *PLOS ONE*, 19(3), e0298582. https://doi.org/10.1371/journal.pone.0298582

Tillakaratne, S. B., Cooray, S., Gunetilleke, B., & Siriwardana, R. (2024). Solid pseudopapillary tumour of the pancreas: an uncommon pancreatic tumour in Sri Lanka. *Sri Lanka Journal of Surgery*, 42(2), 1–3.

Verma, R., Chhabra, R., Kumar, R., Rao, A. K., Kumar, N., & Gehlot, A. (2024, February). Application of mobile cloud computing using crowdsourcing to provide quality of service. In *2024 4th International Conference on Innovative Practices in Technology and Management (ICIPTM)* (pp. 1–8). IEEE.

Vivek, V., & Veeravalli, B. (2024). Analysing e-healthcare data from Internet of Things devices and cloud computing. In *IoT and ML for Information Management: A Smart Healthcare Perspective* (pp. 301–323). Springer.

Wan-Young Chung, et al., (2008). A Wireless Sensor Network Compatible Wearable U-healthcare Monitoring System Using Integrated ECG, Accelerometer and SpO2, *30th Annual International IEEE EMBS Conference Vancouver*, British Columbia, Canada, August 20-24.

Wu, A., Zhang, Y., Zhu, J., Zhao, Q., & Zhang, Y. (2024). Hierarchal bilateral access control with constant size ciphertexts for mobile cloud computing. *IEEE Transactions on Cloud Computing*, 12(2), 659–670. https://doi.org/10.1109/TCC.2024.3386126

Wu, T., Meng, Q., Yang, L., Guo, X., & Kumari, S. (2022). A provably secure lightweight authentication protocol in mobile edge computing environments. *Journal of Supercomputing*, 78(9), 11937–11966. https://doi.org/10.1007/s11227-022-04368-5

Zhang, Y., Xiong, L., Li, F., Hao, Y., & Liu, Z. (2024). Blockchain-based privacy-preserving authentication with hierarchical access control using polynomial commitment for mobile cloud computing. *IEEE Internet of Things Journal*, 11(10), 18266–18280.

Zhou, L., Schellaert, W., Martínez-Plumed, F., Moros-Daval, Y., Ferri, C., & Hernández-Orallo, J. (2024). Larger and more instructable language models become less reliable. *Nature*, 634(8032), 61–68.

Chapter 6

A multimodal and multilingual approach to sentiment analysis for emotion recognition

Aayush Kalia, Abhijot Singh, Chaitanya Arora, Sita Rani, and Meetali Chauhan

6.1 INTRODUCTION

Smart healthcare has been revolutionized with the advancement of technology as well as modernized data-driven approaches to extract multimodal and multilingual data. This has improved patient healthcare services based on efficient decision-making. Social media is the most preferred mode of communication as it provides a platform for global interactions and an opportunity for users to express their views, opinions, and feedback related to e-healthcare services, medicines, ongoing treatment, medical staff, diseases, etc [1]. This generates diverse content of data across social media platforms, which brings significant challenges such as managing a huge amount of data, analyzing data for decision-making, patient reviews, and opinions. In addition to this, it has also led to an increase in the proliferation of harmful content such as hate speech, misinformation, offensive language, as well as toxic content. So, there is a need for an effective approach, such as "Sentiment Analysis" for classifying patient opinions to detect their emotions. The purpose of classifying this data is to analyze their mental health and emotional stability based on certain words or phrases used by them. The reviews and opinions posted by patients can be classified into sentiments such as positive, hateful speech, negative, or neutral using a sentiment analysis approach. Sentiments are further classified based on human emotions such as anger, happiness, sadness, joy, and disgust. Sentiment analysis plays a significant role to extract information from patient data automatically. It also plays a vital role to enhance an effective communication with patients in the realm of smart healthcare. The expression of sentiments can be through various modes such as using a multimodal approach such as posting text, images, videos, and audios on social media [2]. In addition to this, patients can also use a multilingual approach to express their opinions, which provides them a leverage to express their state of mind by using a language as per their own convenience such as English, Hindi, French, Punjabi, and German, as well as a mixture of multiple languages to express their emotions with ease.

DOI: 10.1201/9781003665656-6

Multimodal sentimental analysis approach has brought advancement in healthcare domain as it aims to understand patient experiences as well as improve healthcare services for them. Thus, integration of visual, auditory, and textual data provides deeper insights into patients' satisfaction levels, mental health, state of mind, body language, emotions, and most importantly their overall well-being. Medical professionals and Doctors can seek guidance from multimodal data analysis approach for various services such as ongoing treatment of patients based on their responses, providing personalized treatments plans as well as detecting early signs of patient distress [3, 4]. Various deep learning (DL), machine learning (ML), and natural language processing (NLP) techniques are being used for patient sentiment analysis. Such practices play a vital role to understand mental health status of the patient. There are various data modalities in healthcare, such as electronic health record (EHR), clinical notes, patient reviews, facial expressions, patient body language, voice recordings, patient-provider conversations, patient feedback forms, wearable devices, sensor data, medical imaging, and

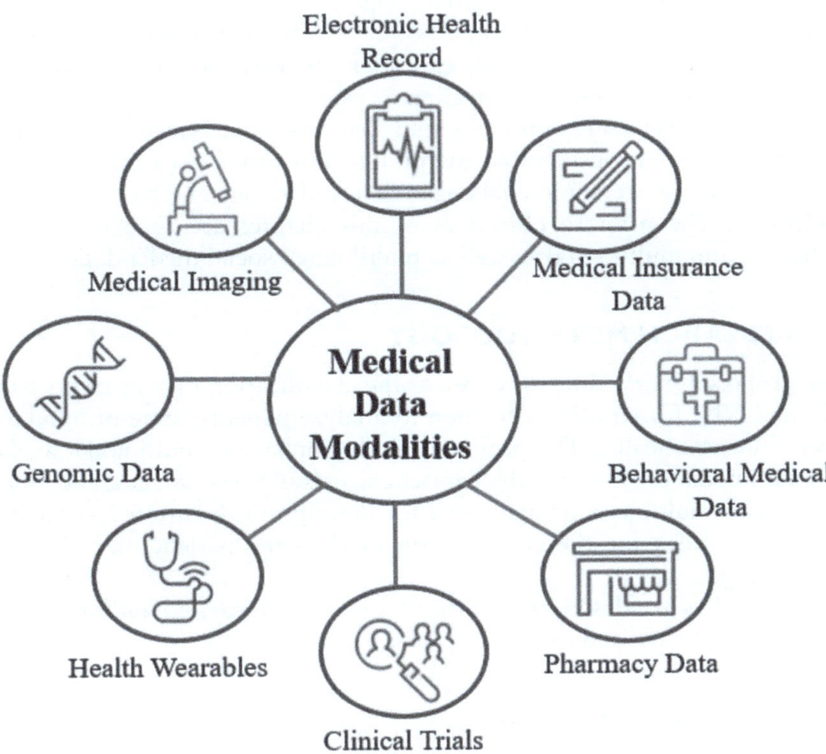

Figure 6.1 Various types of medical data modalities.

social media interactions, which can be used as a source of information for sentiment analysis and emotion detection [5]. Figure 6.1 shows various data modalities.

This chapter presents a fusion of multimodal data and multilingual social media data extracted from social media interactions to detect patient emotions for overall mental health analysis.

6.2 LITERATURE SURVEY

Various researchers have worked in this domain, representing existing content moderation methods that are rule-based and depend on manual reviews, which cannot fully capture the dynamism of digital interactions. Researchers have addressed certain limitations related to the complexities of multimodal and multilingual content, which previously led to inefficient content moderation. While some studies have performed text analysis, most have focused primarily on English data for emotion detection and sentiment analysis. Such work does not utilize multimodal data and remains largely unexplored. Several authors have proposed linguistic modeling and NLP approaches that analyze natural language sentences using keyword-based methods to identify underlying emotions. Table 6.1 presents a detailed survey of related work previously carried out by various researchers for sentiment analysis and emotion detection of users.

Although certain areas for emotion detection and sentiment classification have received considerable attention from various researchers in recent years, but there are some challenges that still remain to be satisfactorily addressed. The primary objectives of this chapter are to extract useful patterns from multimodal as well as multilingual social media data.

6.3 RESEARCH METHODOLOGY

The proposed work aims to represent the classification of sentiments using ML and NLP for emotion detection to analyze patients' state of mind and overall mental health. The proposed work emphasizes multimodal as well as multilingual data, where the dataset consists of texts, images, and videos along with multiple languages used for description. Figure 6.2 showcases procedural steps for the classification of data for patient mental health monitoring.

Given below is a description of the following steps carried out for research work to get the desired results.

6.3.1 Dataset collection

The initial step is to gather a comprehensive collection of datasets to facilitate thorough analysis. The data collection consists of textual as well as visual

Table 6.1 Related work for sentiment analysis and emotion detection

Ref no.	*Author*	*Year*	*Objective*	*Technique/ method used*	*Data set type*	*Performance parameter*	*Results*
[6].	Fernandez et al	2024	Developing an advanced sentiment analysis model integrating speech and video processing for improved emotion detection in multimodal content	Wav2vec2-large for audio, Vivit-b-16x2-kinetics400 for video	RAVDESS, CREMA-D	Weighted average, confidence level threshold, rule-based logic	Proposed a robust multimodal sentiment model capable of real-time emotion analysis with enhanced accuracy
[7].	Feng et al.	2023	Investigating deep learning methods for sentiment analysis across social media platforms to enhance opinion mining	Deep learning, multimodal, aspect-based analysis	Twitter, Facebook, Instagram	Sentiment classification accuracy	Demonstrated the effectiveness of deep learning models in extracting nuanced sentiments from social media posts
[8].	Yoo et al.	2023	Developing a multimodal deep learning model for detecting depressive tendencies based on text and voice data	CNN, Transformers, LSTM, tensor fusion network	DAIC-WOZ (Voice, Text)	Depression Classification accuracy	Achieved reliable depression detection using multimodal input, showing potential for real-world mental health applications
[9].	Semary et al.	2023	Improving sentiment classification by integrating RoBERTa with CNN and LSTM for contextual understanding	RoBERTa, LSTM, CNN, SMOTE	IMDb, Twitter Airline Reviews	Accuracy	Hybrid model outperformed traditional models, achieving 96.28% accuracy on IMDb and 94.2% on Twitter dataset
[10].	Sharma et al.	2019	Examining the effectiveness of SVM in sentiment classification for social media posts	SVM Classifier	Twitter, Facebook	Sentiment Classification Accuracy	Showed that SVM provides competitive performance for binary sentiment classification tasks

(*continued*)

Table 6.1 (Cont.)

Ref no.	*Author*	*Year*	*Objective*	*Technique/ method used*	*Data set type*	*Performance parameter*	*Results*
[11].	Taneja et al.	2024	Evaluating various machine learning models for sentiment analysis, focusing on deep learning advancements	SVM, Random Forest, RNN, BERT	IMDb, Twitter, Amazon Reviews	Accuracy, Model Performance	Found that deep learning models outperform traditional ML models in capturing sentiment nuances
[12].	Fan et al.	2023	Analyzing multimodal sentiment analysis during public emergencies using text and images	Deep multimodal fusion model (DMFM)	Weibo, Twitter (Text and Images)	Sentiment Classification Accuracy	Demonstrated that combining textual and visual sentiment features leads to more accurate predictions during crisis events
[13].	Tan et al.	2022	Hybrid approach using Transformer and LSTM for better sentiment analysis	RoBERTa, LSTM, Data Augmentation (GloVe)	IMDb, Twitter (Sentiment140)	F1-score	Achieved 93% F1-score (IMDb), 91% (Twitter US Airlines), 90% (Sentiment140), proving the effectiveness of hybrid methods
[14].	Subbaiah et al.	2024	Optimizing multimodal sentiment analysis with deep learning and attention mechanisms	AOA, HGS, CNN	MELD, EmoryNLP (Text, Audio, Video)	Accuracy, F-score	Outperformed existing techniques in multimodal sentiment analysis by effectively fusing different modalities
[15].	Nandwani et al.	2021	Investigating sentiment polarity and emotion detection from text using NLP techniques	NLP, Lexicon-Based, ML	IMDB, Twitter Airline Reviews, Yelp	Sentiment Polarity Accuracy	Highlighted the challenges of emotion detection and suggested improvements in lexicon-based approaches

[16].	Cai et al.	2025	Proposing a multilayer feature fusion model for improving multimodal sentiment analysis	UFEN, MTFN, Transformer	MOSI, MOSEI, SIMS (Text, Speech, Video)	Accuracy	Improved sentiment classification by balancing intramodal and intermodal interactions
[17].	Yadav et al.	2023	Analyzing sentiment in social media posts and its applications in public discourse	Machine Learning, NLP, Lexicon-Based	Twitter, Facebook	Sentiment Polarity Classification	Showcased how social media sentiment analysis can be applied to policymaking and public opinion tracking
[18].	Drus et al.	2019	Applying machine learning techniques for sentiment analysis in social media	Opinion-lexicon, Machine Learning	Twitter, Facebook	Accuracy, Sentiment Score	Demonstrated the role of sentiment analysis in healthcare, politics, and business
[19].	Ariel Xu et al.	2022	Conducting a comparative study on various machine learning methods for sentiment analysis	Various ML techniques	Twitter, Reddit, Amazon Reviews	Accuracy, Precision, Recall	Identified key trends and challenges in ML-based sentiment analysis
[20].	AlSalman et al.	2020	Enhancing sentiment analysis for Arabic language tweets	DMNB, N-grams, TF-IDF	Arabic Tweets (SAAD, ASTD)	Accuracy, Recall, Precision, F-score	Achieved 87.5% accuracy in Arabic sentiment classification, demonstrating the effectiveness of TF-IDF
[21].	Khan et al.	2024	Comparing ML models for Twitter sentiment analysis to determine the best-performing algorithm	Naive Bayes, SVM, Logistic Regression	NLTK Twitter Dataset	Accuracy	Found that Naive Bayes achieved 99.73% accuracy, proving it as a reliable model for sentiment analysis

(continued)

Table 6.1 (Cont.)

Ref no.	*Author*	*Year*	*Objective*	*Technique/ method used*	*Data set type*	*Performance parameter*	*Results*
[22].	Acheampong et al.	2020	Exploring transformer-based models for emotion recognition	BERT, RoBERTa, DistilBERT, XLNet	ISEAR Dataset	Accuracy, Precision, Recall, F1-score	Demonstrated that RoBERTa achieved 74.31% accuracy, outperforming traditional models
[23].	Jemai et al.	2021	Evaluating machine learning algorithms for sentiment analysis	Naive Bayes, SVM, Random Forest	Twitter Reviews	Accuracy	Found that Random Forest provided greater precision compared to Naive Bayes and SVM
[24].	Long Tan et al.	2023	A comprehensive review of sentiment analysis techniques, comparing ML and DL models	ML, Deep Learning, Ensemble Learning	IMDb, Twitter, Yelp, Amazon Reviews	Accuracy, F1-score	Provided a detailed survey of sentiment analysis advancements, emphasizing deep learning trends
[25].	Chen et al.	2021	Comparative study of various ML and DL models for sentiment classification	Various ML and DL techniques	IMDb, Sentiment140, Amazon Reviews	Accuracy, F1-score	Highlighted performance differences between ML and DL methods, with deep learning models achieving better generalization

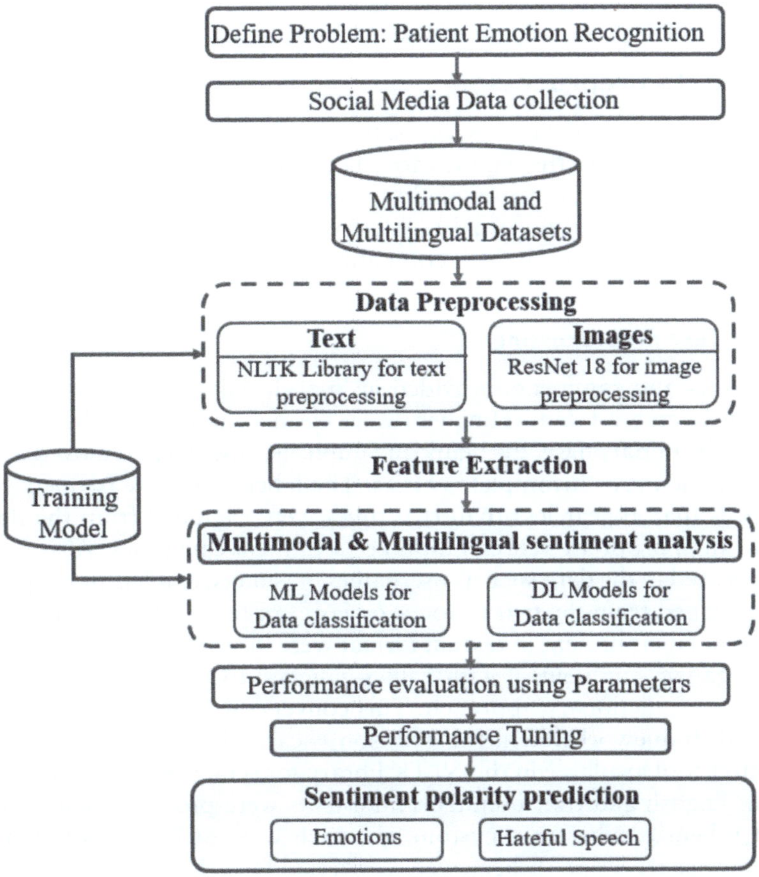

Figure 6.2 Research methodology for sentiment analysis for emotion detection.

data in English, Hindi (in Devanagari script), and Hindi transliterated into English (Hinglish). The datasets were extracted from reputable repositories such as Kaggle, Hugging Face, and GitHub to ensure access to reliable and well-annotated data. The dataset comprising simply texts includes tweets and comments. To enable a multimodal approach, the MMHS150K dataset has been deployed, which comprises approximately 150,000 image-text pairs retrieved from Twitter, a social media platform. This dataset comprises captions, images, and OCR-extracted text. Thus, integration of image-text pairs has been done mainly to analyse an interaction between textual and visual content, which plays a vital role to understand hate speech on social media paltforms [26, 27]. In addition to this, the combination of multilingual text as well as multimodal data builds a foundation to develop and test the proposed classification model.

6.3.2 Data preprocessing

After the collection of datasets for the proposed research work, a comprehensive preprocessing of the data is carried out to prepare the data for effective model training. The purpose of this phase is to ensure that data used for testing, either textual or visual inputs has been cleaned, standardized, and formatted efficiently to make it compatible with ML models.

6.3.2.1 Text preprocessing

The tweets and comments provided in English, Hindi (Devanagari script), and transliterated Hindi (Hinglish) were cleaned to improve the quality of data. In the initial phase, the blank and duplicate rows were removed to eliminate redundant or incomplete entries. The labels with low frequency such as words that appear less than two times were excluded from the data to ensure an appropriate representation of sentiment categories. Also, various phrases used in the data such as usernames, hashtags, emojis, and hyperlinks were stripped from the text to focus on core content and reduce noise. The sentiment labels present in textual format were mapped with respect to positive, negative, and neutral with values assigned to them such as 0, 1, and 2 by using a dictionary approach. This conversion facilitates compatibility with ML frameworks. Text tokenization is carried out by using the punkt tokenizer tool available in the NLTK library for sentence and word segmentation. English and transliterated Hindi texts were processed with NLTK's word_tokenize, whereas a custom approach was used to handle Hindi in the Devanagari script. Tokens were converted to numerical identifiers with special markers added for sequence structure. In addition to this, Padding ensured uniform length, and NLTK utilities comprising tokenization, stopword removal, as well as stemming of words, generate attention masks and fixed-length sequences. The purpose of creating such attention masks is to indicate which tokens in a sequence are relevant to focus on by the model. Outputs were converted to PyTorch tensors for model compatibility.

6.3.2.2 Image preprocessing

For image processing, a DL model is used. The visual data is collected through the MMHS150K dataset. The images are preprocessed to ensure they become compatible with the convolutional neural network (CNN) model, i.e., ResNet18. Images are first converted to RGB format to meet the model's input requirements. After this, images are resized with a fixed resolution to ensure consistency in the dataset. The normalization technique is applied to adjust pixel values to a standardized range. This enhances the performance of the model during training. Finally, the images are converted to PyTorch tensors to align with the DL framework.

6.3.2.3 Dataset splitting

To analyze the effectiveness of the model, the preprocessed dataset is split into two parts: that is training and testing sets. The training set comprises of 80% of the data, and the testing set comprises 20% of the data to avoid any inconvenience. This division ensures that ample data is kept for model training, whereas only a portion of data is used for testing so that an unbiased evaluation can be done. These preprocessing steps ensure that both textual and visual data are formatted appropriately for the pretrained models as well as for the DL framework [28]. This establishes a strong base for efficient training and classification.

6.3.3 Techniques and models

Various ML models, such as logistic regression (LR), support vector machine (SVM), Decision Tree, Random Forest, Naive Bayes, and Bidirectional Encoder Representations from Transformers (BERT), are used upon preprocessed datasets. The objective was to determine the performance of ML models and select the best one based on certain parameters, such as Precision, F1 score metrics, accuracy, and Recall.

6.4 COMPARISON ANALYSIS OF MODELS

Various types of ML models have been used for comparison to describe the best method providing the best performance. The performance is analyzed based on certain parameters such as precision, recall, accuracy, and F1 score. Table 6.2 represents the features of the following ML models, which have been used for comparison analysis in the proposed work.

To provide accurate results by comparison analysis of ML and DL based models, a new performance metric has been formulated named as the "Composite score" metric. This evaluation metric normalizes the values of other evaluation parameters such as Precision, Recall, and F1 scores for each model against the highest and lowest values observed across all models. The Composite Score is calculated as a weighted average of these normalized values comprising equal weights (1/3) assigned to each performance metric for balancing their contributions [29]. This method reduces variations specifically related to the dataset by providing fair assessment of model performance.

Table 6.2 Comparison analysis of ML and DL models in the proposed work

S. No	*Various Models*	*Features*	*Model use case*
1	Logistic regression	• It estimates the probability by fitting a logistic function to the combination of weighted features • It optimizes a hyperplane to distinguish between classes	Binary and multiclass classification
2	SVM	• It finds an optimal hyperplane to separate sentiment classes, maximizing the margin between them • By using kernel functions, it can handle nonlinear relationships, making it effective for text classification	Classification and regression
3	Random Forest	• It develops multiple decision trees, each trained on random subsets of features as well as data • It combines predictions through majority voting, enhancing robustness and minimizing overfitting	Classification and regression
4	Decision Trees	• It classifies sentiments by recursively dividing the feature space based on attribute thresholds • Each node signifies a decision criterion, forming a tree-like structure	Classification and regression
5	Naïve Bayes	• It utilizes a probabilistic method, assuming that features are independent to forecast the sentiment labels • It determines the probability of the text by analyzing the frequency of word distributions • It is computationally efficient for text classification tasks	Text classification
6	Bert	• BERT uses a transformer architecture to capture contextual relationships in text • It is pretrained on large corpora and fine-tuned on the datasets	NLP tasks and classification
7	ResNet18	• ResNet18 is type of CNN method which is based on deep learning model • It helps to extracts features from images using residual learning to address vanishing gradients • It is pretrained and fine-tuned on the MMHS150K dataset	NLP tasks and image classification

6.5 RESULTS AND DISCUSSION

6.5.1 Performance evaluation parameters

The models have been evaluated by using three different datasets such as Dataset 1 in Hindi (Devanagari and transliterated), Dataset 2 in Hinglish (mixture of Hindi and English Language), and Dataset 3 with MMHS150K (mixture of text and images) to effectively determine sentiment classification.

This comparison analysis highlights the strengths and limitations of traditional ML models (SVM, Random Forest, Logistic Regression, Decision Tree, Naïve Bayes) versus modernized transformer-based BERT model to handle diversified social media data [29]. The motive of this research is to predict sentiments based on multimodal and multilingual datasets and to achieve high accuracy by using ML and DL methods. The evaluation on datasets has been carried out through certain evaluation parameters considered for analysis: Accuracy, F1-Score, Precision, Recall, and Composite Score. Accuracy measures actual predictions by a model across all classes, indicating overall performance. Precision calculates the true positive predictions among all positive predictions to identify hateful content. Recall determines actual positive instances, by showing the model's ability to capture all hateful cases. F1-Score is the harmonic mean of Precision & Recall, to balance a comprehensive performance measure [30]. The Composite Score normalizes and finds the average value of all the parametric values used, such as Accuracy, Precision, Recall, and F1-Score, by providing a single metric for fair model comparison across datasets. Given below are the formulas used for the parameters.

$$\text{Accuracy} = \frac{\text{TP} + \text{TN}}{\text{TP} + \text{TN} + \text{FP} + \text{FN}} \tag{1}$$

$$\text{Precision} = \frac{\text{TP}}{\text{TP} + \text{FP}} \tag{2}$$

$$\text{Recall} = \frac{\text{TP}}{\text{TP} + \text{FN}} \tag{3}$$

$$\text{F1-Score} = 2 * \frac{\text{Precison} * \text{Recall}}{\text{Precison} + \text{Recall}} \tag{4}$$

$$\text{Composite Score} = \frac{\text{Average normalized score} * 100}{100} \tag{5}$$

6.5.1.1 Derived formula for calculating composite score

The composite score combines the parameters such as accuracy, precision, recall, and F1-score into a single normalized metric for fair model comparison. The calculation involves three steps:

a) **Normalization:** For each metric, if the maximum (x_max) and minimum (x_min) values across models are equal, the normalized score is 1, and otherwise, the given formula is used, such as

$$\text{Normalized Score} = \frac{(value - \text{ x\_min} + 0.01 * (x_{max} - x_{min}))}{((x_{max} - x_{\text{min}}) + 0.01 * (x_{max} - x_{\text{min}}))} \tag{6}$$

b) **Mean Average Value:** Calculate the mean of the normalized Accuracy (x_1), Precision (x_2), Recall (x_3), and F1-Score (x_4).

$$\text{Average normalized score} = \frac{x1 + x2 + x3 + x4}{n}, \text{ where n stands for the number of values} \quad (7)$$

c) **Scaling:** The scaling is done by calculating the percentage of the average normalized score

$$\text{Composite Score} = \frac{\text{Average normalized score} * 100}{100} \quad (8)$$

6.5.1.2 Tables for evaluation metrics

The evaluation techniques have been applied to various datasets. Tables 6.3, 6.4, and 6.5 show the values achieved in terms of performance parameters based on different ML models.

The calculated values have showcased **"Logistic Regression"** as an efficient ML-based model for sentiment analysis of emotions for multilingual data. In addition to this, for sentiment analysis of images, the DL-based model **"Bert"** showed effective results. Composite score has been used as an important evaluation parameter through which the value of other evaluation parameters has been normalized to get unbiased and accurate results for comparing the performance of all the ML and DL based models.

6.5.2 Results

6.5.2.1 Graphic visualization for dataset 1

Figure 6.3 represents a graphic visualization for Hindi dataset 1, showcasing the best performance of the "Logistic Regression" ML-based model. Logistic Regression achieved the highest Composite Score

Table 6.3 Performance metrics for hindi dataset 1 (%)

S. No	*Various Models*	*Accuracy*	*Precision*	*Recall*	*F1-Score*	*Composite Score*
1	Logistic Regression	50.76	60.63	64.75	62.57	85.54
2	SVM	51.36	62.03	58.36	59.89	76.81
3	Random Forest	45.02	87.14	43.01	45.51	52.32
4	Decision Trees	28.70	48.16	53.42	49.85	29.07
5	Naïve Bayes	44.41	39.60	40.27	39.93	18.15

Table 6.4 Performance metrics for hinglish dataset 2 (%)

S. No	*Various models*	*Accuracy*	*Precision*	*Recall*	*F1-Score*	*Composite Score*
1	Logistic Regression	89.90	89.86	89.90	89.87	100
2	SVM	89.70	89.66	89.70	89.67	98.04
3	Random Forest	83.64	84.08	83.64	83.74	68.27
4	Decision Trees	67.68	77.81	67.68	64.20	0.99
5	Naïve Bayes	87.98	88.05	87.98	87.85	90.06

Table 6.5 Performance metrics for images dataset 3 (%)

S. No	*Various models*	*Accuracy*	*Precision*	*Recall*	*F1-Score*	*Composite Score*
1	Logistic Regression	65.16	64.57	65.68	63.50	47.71
2	SVM	63.92	63.53	64.23	62.84	34.01
3	Random Forest	63.79	66.40	61.93	71.57	57.57
4	Decision trees	67.36	66.75	68.03	65.51	74.71
5	Naïve Bayes	58.07	67.26	55.17	86.13	50.50
6	Bert	64.00	72.51	70.36	74.79	79.00

(85.54%) on the Hindi dataset 1(4,509 rows), outperforming Random Forest (52.32 %) and SVM (76.81%). Logistic regression balanced results for Recall (64.75%) and F1-Score (62.57%) enabled effective hateful content and emotion detection, despite Random Forest's superior Precision (87.14%) and SVM's slightly higher Accuracy (51.36%). This demonstrates LR's robustness in handling the Hindi dataset's linguistic complexity for sentiment classification.

6.5.2.2 *Graphic visualization for dataset 2*

Figure 6.4 also represents a graphic visualization for Hinglish dataset 2, showcasing the best performance of the "Logistic Regression" ML-based model. Logistic Regression achieved the highest Composite Score (100%) on the Hinglish dataset 2, outperforming SVM (98.94%) and Naïve Bayes (90.06%). Logistic regression balanced results for all other parameters, such as Accuracy (89.90%), Precision (89.96%), Recall (89.90%), and F1-Score (89.87%), enabled effective hateful content and emotion detection, despite SVM and Naïve Bayes' superior results for accuracy, precision, recall, and F1 score. This demonstrates LR's efficiency in handling the Hinglish dataset's linguistic complexity for sentiment classification.

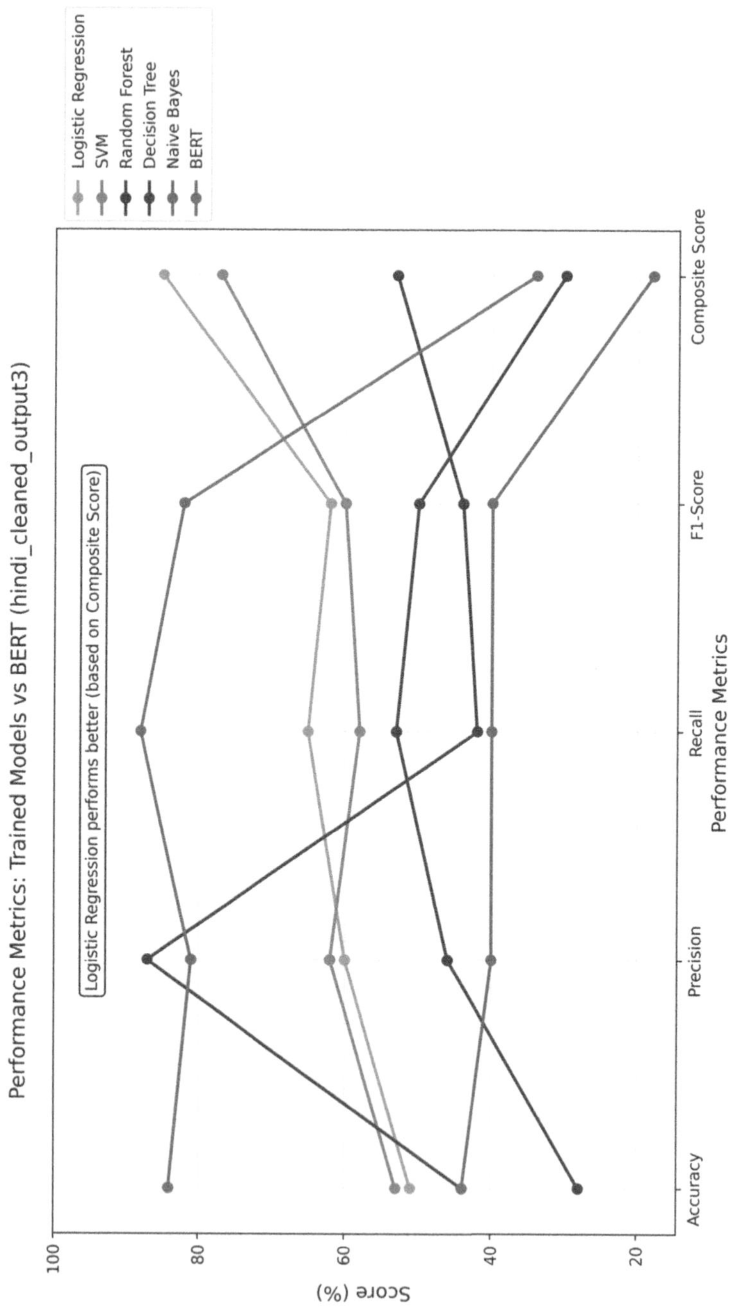

Figure 6.3 Graphic visualization for results of multilingual dataset 1.

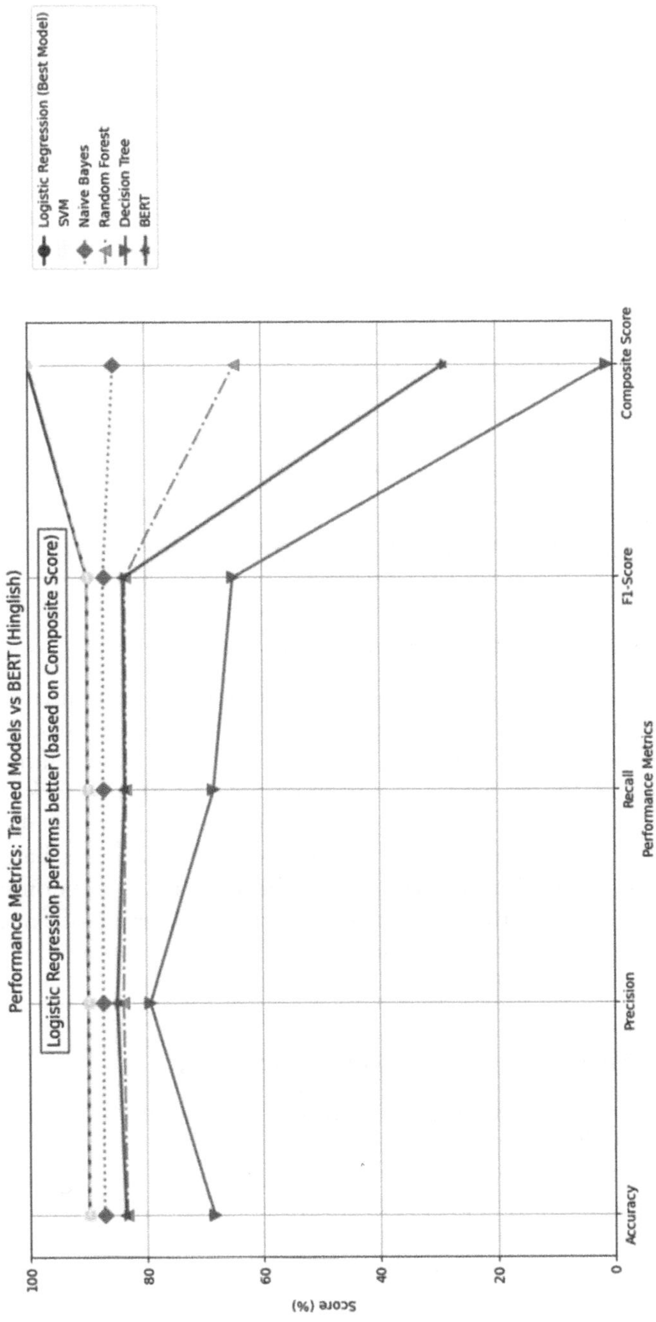

Figure 6.4 Graphic visualization for the results of multilingual dataset 2.

6.5.2.3 Graphic visualization for dataset 3

Figure 6.5 represents a graphic visualization showcasing the fusion of BERT and ResNet18, which has achieved the best performance on the MMHS150K multimodal dataset, which includes 150,000 image-text pairs from social media platforms, i.e., Twitter, classified for sentiment analysis. With an accuracy of 64.00%, precision of 70.36%, recall of 74.79%, and F1-score of 72.51%, this model effectively integrates textual and visual features, capturing complex sentiment patterns in multimodal social media data. This demonstrates Bert's robustness in handling the multimodal dataset's complexity for sentiment classification.

The results have showcased both ML and DL-based methods as an effective solution to classify multilingual and multimodal data efficiently. The new parameter derived, i.e., composite score, has shown 100% results for showcasing the accurate results by normalizing the values.

6.6 CHALLENGES FOR MULTIMODAL AND MULTILINGUAL DATA

6.6.1 Data availability and quality

To extract huge and diversified datasets comprising text, images, videos, and audios across multiple languages for training the model and testing the methods is a challenging task. The reason for the same is limited public repositories as well as high annotation cost. Datasets also lack diversified language-based data or modalities. In addition to this, the quality of data also effects the performance of the models used to achieve better results as datasets contain unnecessary noisy or biased data. For example, inconsistent labels, cultural misrepresentations, too much usage of slangs etc. To improve the quality of data, certain preprocessing methods and bias auditing techniques are applied for data cleaning [31, 32].

6.6.2 Multimodal integration complexity

Though the proposed work aims to classify data with modalities, they can be analyzed individually. There is a major challenge to integrate the data collected from multiple modalities such as audio, text, and video, as combining the features into a unified classification model becomes too complex to handle technically. For example, matching the text with image context for sentiment detection demands more effective fusion techniques. As the existing techniques cannot provide accurate results for integrated multimodal data. In addition to this, misalignment and incompatible feature

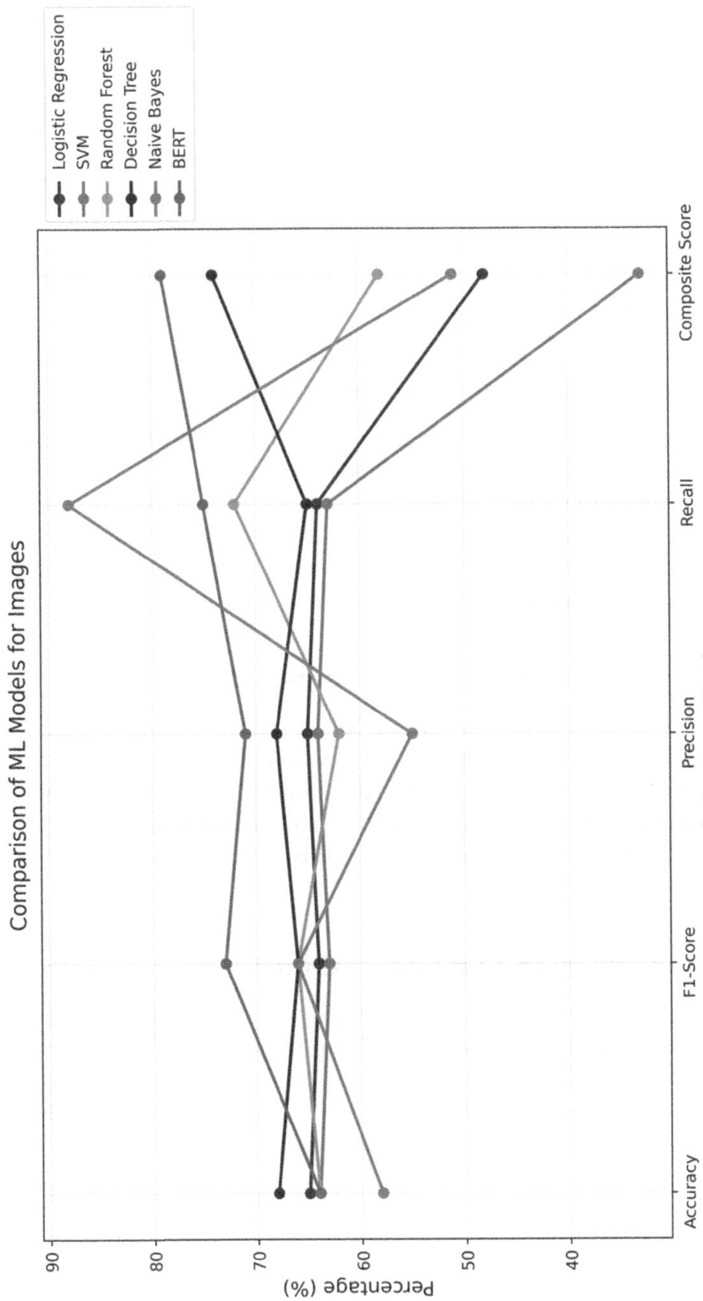

Figure 6.5 Graphic visualization for the results of multimodal dataset 3.

representations due to diversified data, such as OCR errors in memes, reduce the performance, providing low accuracy results, indicating robust preprocessing of data 7 iterative testing.

6.6.3 Multilingual processing challenges

Handle multiple languages with limited training data increases the difficulties for achieving consistent accuracy in data classification. The models are challenged by the use of slang, culturally specific expressions like sarcasm in Hindi, and the need for language-specific fine-tuning. This requires additional computational costs as well as resources, leading to delays in model development. [33]

6.6.4 Model performance and scalability

To achieve the target of 85% accuracy across various data modalities is a major challenge, especially for DL models such as BERT, which are intensive for computation [34, 35]. There is a need for optimization techniques such as model pruning or quantization to balance the hybrid ML approach to ensure scalability on modest hardware requirements such as 16GB RAM, RTX 3060, which might compromise accuracy.

6.6.5 Sarcasm and contextual nuance detection

To detect various expressions like sarcasm, irony, or hate speech becomes difficult, as sometimes it might depend on cultural as well as contextual cues, which models might misinterpret. Also limited sarcasm-specific datasets and the requirement for advanced contextual embeddings increase the complexity for data training, which leads to false positives or false negatives in data classification [36].

6.6.6 User adoption and CLI usability

The CLI-based lightweight design may discourage and limit users with no technical background from using graphical interfaces [37]. Certain intuitive commands and visualizations (such as Matplotlib charts) require careful design. So adequate user support for setup as well as troubleshooting is required, which creates challenges to deploy it in diversified environments [38].

6.7 CONCLUSION

Multimodal and multilingual-based classification of data offers certain critical insights towards the mental health of patients based on words used by them to express their opinions and to interact with others. The methods used for this system have achieved 85% accuracy to classify text and image content across multiple languages by using XLM-R and OCR, which has surpassed traditional methods. BERT and logistic regression methods-based models have balanced the efficiency for composite score on three datasets used for this work [39, 40]. The developed system can detect emotions and implicit hate speech, yet sarcasm detection needs refinement due to multilingual data challenges. Anonymous data approach along with multilingual support ensures a safer digital experience. A lightweight CLI, modular architecture as well as data visualizations (Matplotlib/Seaborn) provide easy deployment and actionable insights [41, 42]. Multimodal data used highlights certain issues, providing a wider scope for future research, such as real-time processing and audio analysis. The current work can also be extended to process video and cross-domain applications with an ethical framework.

6.8 FUTURE SCOPE

The future scope offers research for content moderation as well as sentiment analysis by addressing certain dynamic challenges related to social media platforms along with significant contribution to mental health goals [43, 44]. Expansion of multimodal capabilities is the critical direction for research by focusing on integration of multimodal data such as audios, videos, emojis, GIFs as well as immersive content like virtual reality. This approach will help further to analyze the body language of the person along with his state of mind for mental health detection. Moderating virtual reality content as well as live interactions offers research areas fostering innovations in decentralized platforms [45, 46]. Enhancing a multilingual data approach is also essential for research advancement globally. Crowdsourcing datasets for regional dialects as well as indigenous languages using XLM-R can improve classification in data-scarce scenarios with effective research contributions [47, 48]. Deeper insights into patients' opinions based on cultural sensitivity, hate speech, and sarcasm can provide effective judgement to the responses [49]. Moderations in smart healthcare to monitor mental health and misinformation detection can significantly contribute to public health communication research, medical professionals, and counsellors guiding patients [50].

REFERENCES

1. A. Gandhi, K. Adhvaryu, S. Poria, E. Cambria and A. Hussain, "Multimodal Sentiment Analysis: A Systematic Review of History, Datasets, Multimodal Fusion Methods, Applications, Challenges and Future Directions," *Information Fusion*, vol.91, pp. 424–444, 2023.

2. M. Miah, M. Kabir, T. Sarwar, M. Safran, S. Alfarhood and M. F. Mridha, "A Multimodal Approach to Cross-Lingual Sentiment Analysis with Ensemble of Transformer and LLM," *Scientific Reports,* vol.14, p. 9603, 2024.
3. M. Anschütz, T. Eder and G. Groh, "Structuring User-Generated Content on Social Media with Multimodal Aspect-Based Sentiment Analysis," 2022 pp 1-8, vol 1.
4. Y. Hao, "Multimodal Sentiment Recognition: A Comprehensive Review of Analysis Techniques, Applications, and Challenges," In *3rd International Conference on Computing Innovation and Applied Physics*, pp. 279–286, Theoretical and Natural Science, EWA Publiser, 2023.
5. J. Nip and B. Berthelier, "Social Media Sentiment Analysis," *MDPI*, vol.4, pp. 1590–1598, 2024.
6. A. Fernandiz and S. Awinat, "Multimodal Sentiment Analysis based on Video and Audio Inputs," *Procedia Computer Science*, vol.241, pp. 41–48, 2024.
7. B. Feng, "Deep Learning-based Sentiment Analysis for Social Media: A Focus on Multimodal and Aspect-based Approaches," *EWA Publishing*, vol.33, pp. 1–8, 2024.
8. H. Yoo and H. Oh, "Depression Detection model Msing Multimodal Deep Learning," *Creative Commons CC BY*, 2023.
9. M. Sabharwal and D. Sharma, "Sentiment Analysis for Social Media using SVM Classifier of Machine Learning," *IJITEE,* vol.8, pp. 39–47, 2019.
10. S. Wang, C. Liu and Q. Liu, "Multi-Modality Collaborative Learning for Sentiment Analysis," *Journal of VTEX Class Files*, vol.14, 2021.
11. A. Taneja, "Sentiment Analysis Using Machine Learning: A Comprehensive Review," *JARET*, vol.3, pp. 181–189, 2024.
12. T. Fan, H. Wang, P. Wu, C. Ling, Milad and T. Ahvanooy, "Multimodal Sentiment Analysis for Social Media Contents During Public Emergencies," *Journal of Data and Information Science*, vol.8, no. 3, pp. 61–87, 2023. https://doi.org/10.2478/ jdis-2023-0012
13. K. Tan, C. Lee, K. Anbananthen and K. Lim, "RoBERTa-LSTM: A Hybrid Model for Sentiment Analysis With Transformer and Recurrent Neural Network," *IEEE,* vol.10, pp. 21517–21532, 2022.
14. N. Semary, W. Ahmed, K. Amin, P. Plawiak and M. Hammad, "Improving Sentiment Classification using a RoBERTa-based Hybrid Model," *Frontiers Media S.A.*, vol.17, pp. 1–10, 2023.
15. P. Nandwani and R. Verma, "A Review on Sentiment Analysis and Emotion Detection from Text," *Soc. Netw. Anal. Min.* vol.11, no.81. https://doi.org/10.1007/s13278-021-00776-6, 2021.
16. B. Subbaiah, K. Murugesan, P. Saravanan and K. Marudhamuthu, "An Efficient Multimodal Sentiment Analysis in Social Media using Hybrid Optimal Multi-Scale Residual Attention Network," *Springer Nature*, vol.57, 2024.
17. Y. Cai, X. Li, Y. Zhang, J. Li, F. Zhu and L. Ran, "Multimodal Sentiment Analysis based on Multi-Layer Feature Fusion and Multi-Task Learning," *Springer Nature*, vol.15, 2025.

18. Z. Drus and H. Khalid, "Sentiment Analysis in Social Media and Its Application: Systematic Literature Review," *Elsevier B.V.*, vol.161, pp. 707–714, 2019.
19. Q. Xu, V. Chang and C. Jayne, "A Systematic Review of Social Media-based Sentiment Analysis: Emerging Trends and Challenges," *Decision Analytics Journal,* vol.3, 2022.
20. H. AlSalman, "An Improved Approach for Sentiment Analysis of Arabic Tweets in Twitter Social Media," *2020 3rd International Conference on Computer Applications & Information Security (ICCAIS)*, Riyadh, Saudi Arabia, pp. 1-4, doi: 10.1109/ICCAIS48893.2020.9096850, 2020.
21. M. Khan and A. Srivastava, "A Review on Sentiment Analysis of Twitter Data Using Machine Learning Techniques," *Vandana Publications,* vol.14, pp. 186–194, 2024.
22. F. Adoma, N.-M. Henry and W. Chen, "Comparative Analyses of Bert, Roberta, Distilbert, and Xlnet for Text-Based Emotion Recognition," *2020 17th International Computer Conference on Wavelet Active Media Technology and Information Processing (ICCWAMTIP)*, Chengdu, China, pp. 117-121, doi: 10.1109/ICCWAMTIP51612.2020.9317379, 2020.
23. R. R. Kalangi, S. Maloji, N. Tejasri, P. P. Chand and V. P. Ch, "Sentiment Analysis using Machine Learning," *2021 3rd International Conference on Advances in Computing, Communication Control and Networking (ICAC3N)*, Greater Noida, India, pp. 116-121, doi: 10.1109/ICAC3N53548.2021.9725499, 2021.
24. J. Yadav, "Sentiment Analysis on Social Media," Qeios, 2023.
25. M. Ahmad, S. Aftab, M. Bashir, N. Hameed, I. Ali and Zahid Nawaz, "SVM Optimization for Sentiment Analysis," *IJACSA,* vol.9, pp. 393–397, 2018.
26. K. Qiu, Y. Zhang, J. Zhao, S. Zhang, Q. Wang and F. Chen, "A Multimodal Sentiment Analysis Approach Based on a Joint Chained Interactive Attention Mechanism," *MDPI*, vol.13, 2024,pp 1-23.
27. W. Guo, K. Su, B. Jiang, K. Xie and J. Liu, "CMDAF: Cross-Modality Dual-Attention Fusion Network for Multimodal Sentiment Analysis," *MDPI*, vol.14, pp.1-14,2024.
28. Y. Mao, Q. Liu and Y. Zhang, "Sentiment Analysis Methods, Applications, and Challenges: A Systematic Literature Review," *Elsevier*, vol.36, pp. 1-16, 2024.
29. A. Ullah, M. M. Islam, N. Binti Azman and Z. M. Zaki, "An overview of Multimodal Sentiment Analysis research: Opportunities and Difficulties," *2017 IEEE International Conference on Imaging, Vision & Pattern Recognition (icIVPR)*, Dhaka, Bangladesh, pp. 1-6, doi: 10.1109/ICIVPR.2017.7890858. 2017.
30. P. Muthukumar and M. Ibrahim, "Multimodal Social Media Sentiment Analysis," *Stanford CS224N Custom Project*, 2024.
31. A. Hu and S. Flaxman, "Multimodal Sentiment Analysis to Explore the Structure of Emotions," In Proceedings of the 24th ACM SIGKDD International Conference on Knowledge Discovery & Data Mining (KDD '18). Association for Computing Machinery, New York, NY, USA, pp. 350–358. https://doi.org/10.1145/3219819.3219853.

32. T. Voloshina and O. Makhnytkina, "Multimodal Emotion Recognition and Sentiment Analysis Using Masked Attention and Multimodal Interaction," *FRUCT*, pp. 310–317, 2023.
33. T. Zhang, B. Song, Z. Zhang and Y. Zhang, "Multimodal Sentiment Analysis based on Multi-Stage Graph Fusion Networks under Random Missing Modality Conditions," vol 19, pp. 1-18, *IET*, 2024.
34. J. You, J. Zhong, J. Kong and L. Peng, "Sentiment Analysis Method of Consumer Reviews based on Multi-Modal Feature Mining," *International Journal of Cognitive Computing in Engineering*, vol.6, pp. 143–151, 2024.
35. Z. Liu, A. Braytee, A. Anaissi, G. Zhang, L. Qin and J. Akram, "Ensemble Pretrained Models for Multimodal Sentiment Analysis using Textual and Video Data Fusion," *ACM*, pp. 1841–1848, 2024.
36. R. Geethanjali and A. Valarmathi, "A Novel Hybrid Deep Learning IChOA-CNN-LSTM Model for Modality-Enriched and Multilingual Emotion Recognition in Social Media," *Nature Portfolio*, vol.14, 2024.
37. M. Miah, M. Kabir, T. Sarwar, M. Safran, S. Alfarhood and M. Mridha, "A Multimodal Approach to Cross-Lingual Sentiment Analysis with Ensemble of Transformer and LLM," *Nature Portfolio*, vol.14, 2024.
38. E. Chu, "Audio-Visual Sentiment Analysis for Learning Emotional Arcs in Movies," *IEEE*, pp. 829–834, 2017.
39. Y. Cimtay, E. Ekmekcioglu and S. Ozhan, "Cross-Subject Multimodal Emotion Recognition Based on Hybrid Fusion," *IEEE*, vol.8, pp. 168865–168878, 2020.
40. M. Huddar, S. Sannakki and V. Rajpurohit, "An Ensemble Approach to Utterance Level Multimodal Sentiment Analysis," IEEE, pp. 145–150, 2018.
41. M. Meghawat, S. Yadav, D. Mahata, Y. Yin, R. Shah and R. Zimmermann, "A Multimodal Approach to Predict Social Media Popularity," *IEEE*, pp. 190–195, 2018.
42. K. Chigateri and R. Bhandarkar, "Non-Bipolar Sentiment Assessment of Text Reviews," IEEE, pp. 1758–1762, 2018.
43. F. Chen, R. Ji, J. Su, D. Cao and Y. Gao, "P redicting Microblog Sentiments via Weakly Supervised Multi-Modal Deep Learning," IEEE, 2017.
44. S. Saini, R. Rao, V. Vaichole, A. Rane and D. Abin, "Emotion Recognition Using Multimodal Approach," IEEE, 2018.
45. H. Abburi, M. Shrivastava and S. V. Gangashetty, "Improved Multimodal Sentiment Detection Using Stressed Regions of Audio," *2016 IEEE Region 10 Conference (TENCON)*, Singapore, pp. 2834–2837, doi: 10.1109/TENCON.2016.7848560 2017.
46. H. Wang, A. Meghawat, L. Morency and E. Xing, "Select-Additive Learning: Improving Generalization in Multimodal Sentiment Analysis," IEEE, pp. 949–954, 2017.
47. K. Seng and L. Ang, "Multimodal Emotion and Sentiment Modelling from Unstructured Big Data: Challenges, Architecture & Techniques," IEEE, 2019.

48. A. Shirzad, H. Zare and M. Teimouri, "Deep Learning Approach for Text, Image, and GIF Multimodal Sentiment Analysis," *IEEE*, pp. 419–424, 2020.
49. A. Agarwal, A. Yadav and D. Vishwakarma, "Multimodal Sentiment Analysis via RNN variants," IEEE, pp. 19–23, 2019.
50. D. Hernández, L. Callejo, F. Garcia, O. Perez and A. Lamadrid, "A Review of Energy Consumption Forecasting in Smart Buildings: Methods, Input Variables, Forecasting Horizon and Metrics," *MDPI*, vol.10, 2020.

Chapter 7

Multimodal machine learning approaches for heart disease detection and control

Fadi Al-Turjman, Hemant Kumar Saini, Sinem Alturjman, and Ramiz Salama

7.1 INTRODUCTION

An electrocardiogram (ECG) is a recording or visual representation of a patient's heartbeat (El-Sofany et al., 2024). Electrocardiograms, or ECG machines, measure the electrical activity in the heart and record the results as a visual trace (Rao et al., 2024; Jha et al., 2025; Türk, 2024). An ECG is a straightforward, noninvasive process that involves applying electrodes to the skin, connecting them in a certain order to the associated machine, and measuring the electrical activity throughout the heart when the machine is turned on. Typically, the result is a printed graph of the activity displayed on a computer screen, as shown in Figure 7.1. A range of ECG types are used by the doctors to screen for different cardiac (heart) or pulmonary (lung) disorders (Nasiruddin et al., 2024).

We refer to the following brief uphill stretch as the "ST segment." This section shows how long it takes for the ventricles to stop contracting and start the resting phase before they start contracting again for the subsequent beat. The "T wave" is the next upward curve. The ventricles' resting phase is shown by this wave. When examining an ECG, the physician looks at the length and width of each segment.

This chapter presents a novel machine learning model that performs heart disease classification. A hybrid feature extraction method is incorporated to perform feature extraction. The extracted features from the ECG sample are used to train and validate the model to perform heart disease classification and explore state of art of heart disease diagnostic systems. Here, various contributors and their valuable impacts are provided. Section 7.3 depicts the proposed method, and a precise summary is presented in Section 7.4.

7.2 RELATED WORKS

The classification of arrhythmias using hybrid features is covered in detail (Ramesh & Lakshmanna, 2024). The automatic identification and categorization of potentially fatal arrhythmias form the basis of this paper. It is

DOI: 10.1201/9781003665656-7

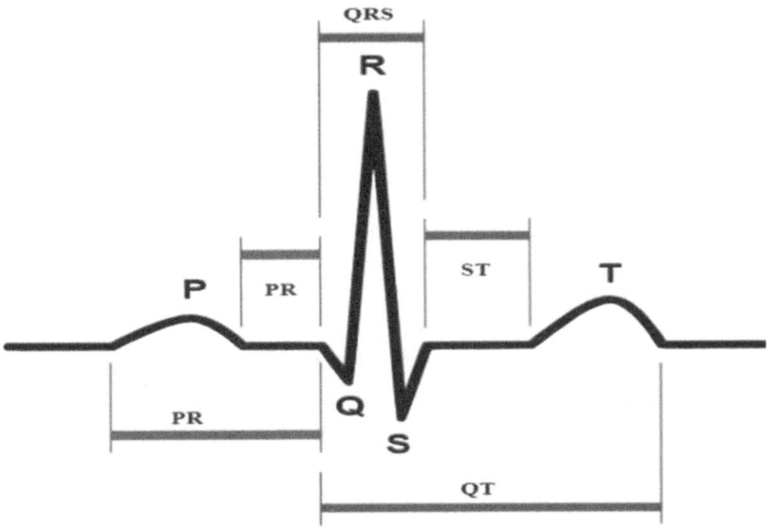

Figure 7.1 ECG Labeled with the main components.

crucial in the management of a number of cardiac disorders. The study presents a novel approach that uses morphological and dynamic features to classify different forms of arrhythmia. Using the discrete wavelet transform (DWT), the morphological features are extracted from each heartbeat. It helps decode significant information from a quasiperiodic ECG using varying window sizes by improving the temporal and frequency resolution of the ECG signal. Information about RR intervals is utilized as a dynamic feature. The eager energy operator is used to represent the nonlinear dynamics of the RR interval, improving the categorization of arrhythmias. Twelve coefficients are chosen as morphological features after DWT subbands are dimensionality reduced using independent component analysis to eliminate redundancy. After that, a machine learning model fed these features to categorize arrhythmias. A study using smartphone technology to record surface 12-lead ECGs is examined in Dhingra et al. (2025). The FDA-approved AliveCor ECG mobile heart rhythm monitor uses an iPhone to capture a lead I single-channel ECG rhythm strip (Baseer et al., 2024). This study shows that using a smartphone to create a 12-lead ECG is feasible. Based on the recordings' authenticity, it appears that this technique has the potential to be a valuable clinical tool.

An Android-based ECG monitoring system is investigated. The Android platform, which is based on Linux and is the most popular operating system for smartphones and portable tablets, is a key market for hardware makers and mobile application developers. The heart rate monitoring gadget uses Bluetooth connectivity to send ECG data signals, which are realized through the built-in application. In developing nations, a low-cost ECG monitor was created (Petmezas et al., 2024). The authors developed and thoroughly tested an inexpensive, completely tested ECG to aid medical professionals in underdeveloped nations in making correct diagnosis. ECG signals can be used to extract respiration rates and other important health information, such as sleep apnea, even though they are primarily intended for cardiac diagnosis. Patient electrodes are created for developing nations (Petmezas et al., 2024). Frequently, disposable electrodes are not a practical choice since the long-term costs of using them would greatly surpass the equipment's initial cost. Actually, a shortage of disposable electrodes contributes to the quantity of commercial equipment that is left unused on the shelf in developing countries. Metal plates or strips are frequently used to create reusable electrodes.

7.3 MATERIALS AND METHODS

Figure 7.2 indicates the flow of control of the system.

7.3.1 Dataset analysis

The first method (AR model) splits the signal. To calculate the coefficient for the 65536 point that describes heart activity as illustrated in Figure 7.3, the AR block extracts the relevant features using

$$x(n)=y(n)+\sum_{k=1}^{p} a(k)y(n-k) \tag{7.1}$$

The corresponding coefficient of the eight windows is saved as depicted in Figure 7.4. This coefficient may vary from one signal to another.

Using The Shannon entropy feature extraction method, this is achieved by splitting the 65536 signal into eight windows. Each window has 8192 points, and this method extracts the relevant features thus

$$\text{Shannon Entropy}=-\sum_{i=0}^{N-1} p_i \log_2 (p_i) \tag{7.2}$$

The processed signal from this method is saved as shown in Figure 7.5.

The leader's method of feature extraction calculates the leader by using the function "leaders". To determine, the method uses the equation:

$$L_x(j,k)=\sup_{\lambda' \in 3\lambda} |d_x(j,k)| \tag{7.3}$$

The leader of the signal is saved as demonstrated in Figure 7.6, and this leader may vary from signal to signal.

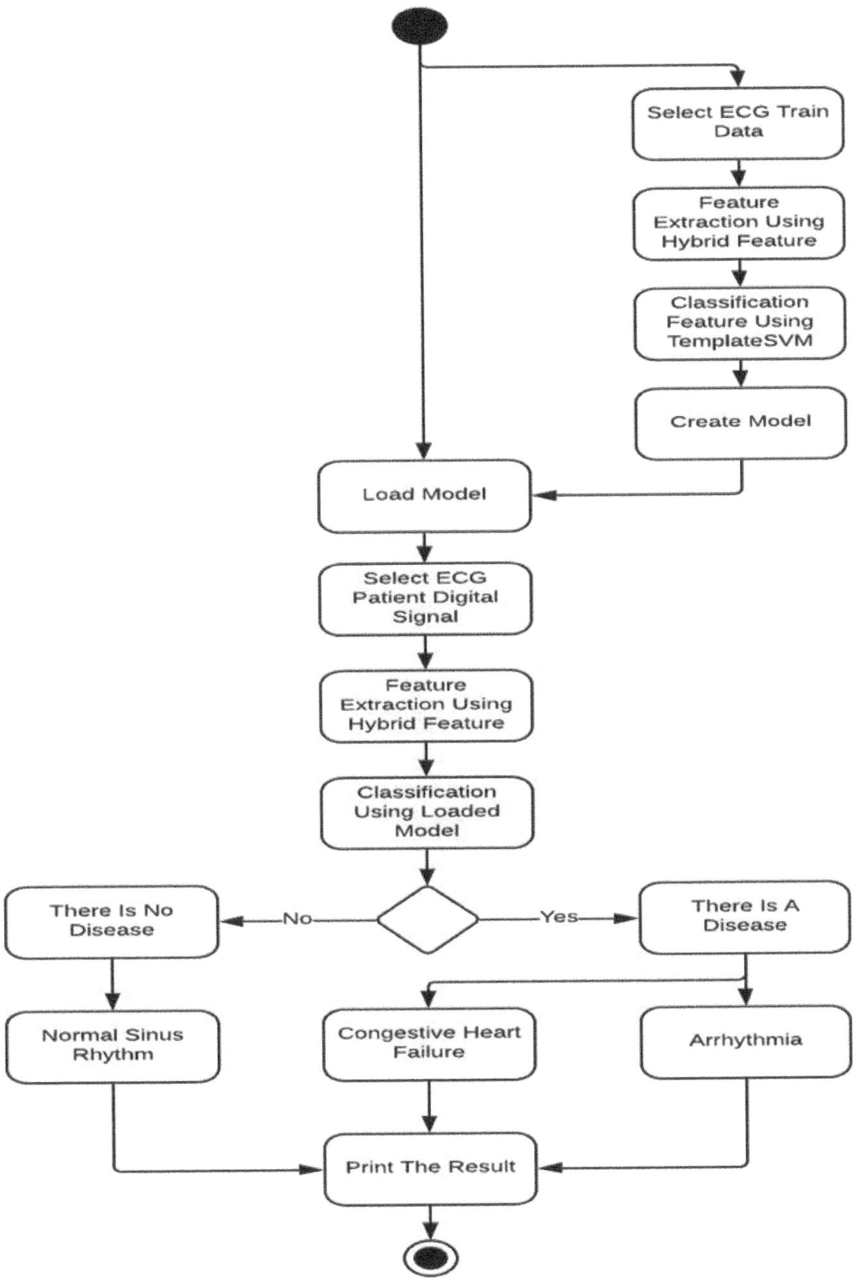

Figure 7.2 Diagram showing the system control flow.

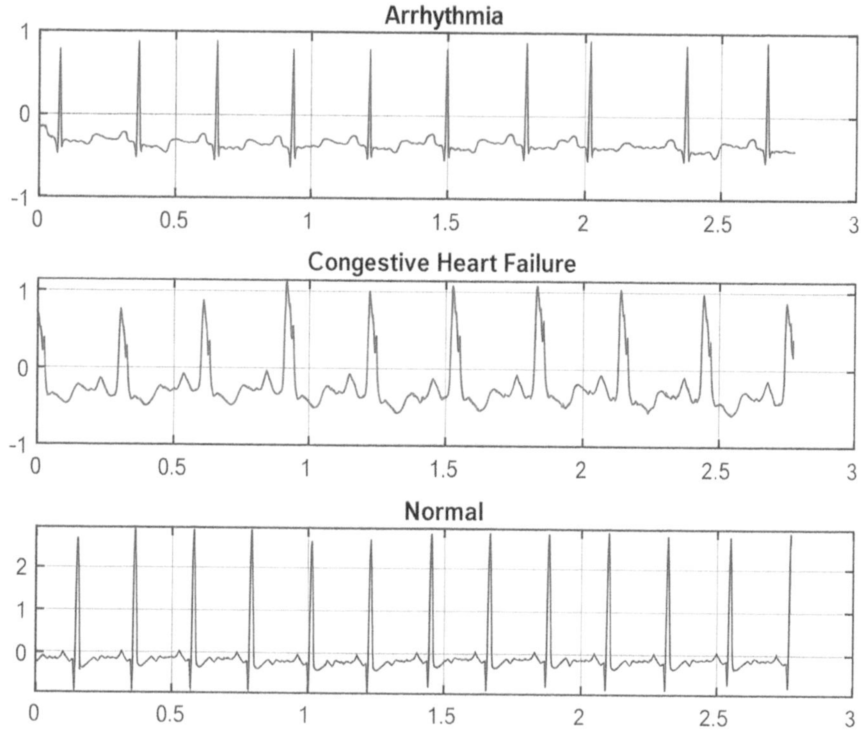

Figure 7.3 Samples from the explored dataset.

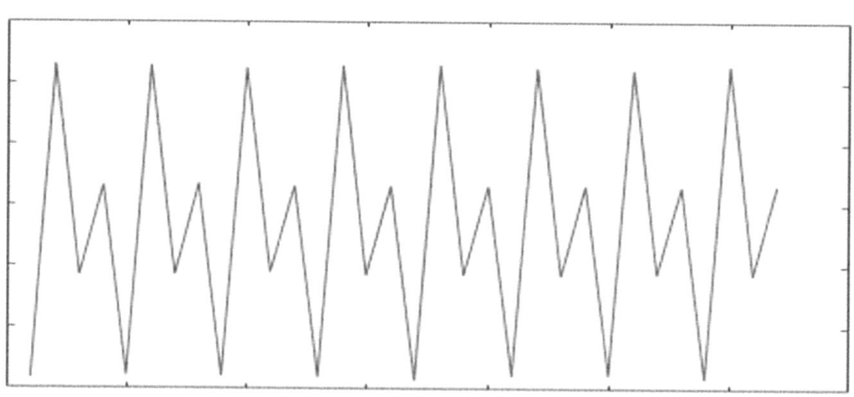

Figure 7.4 Sample of the coefficient.

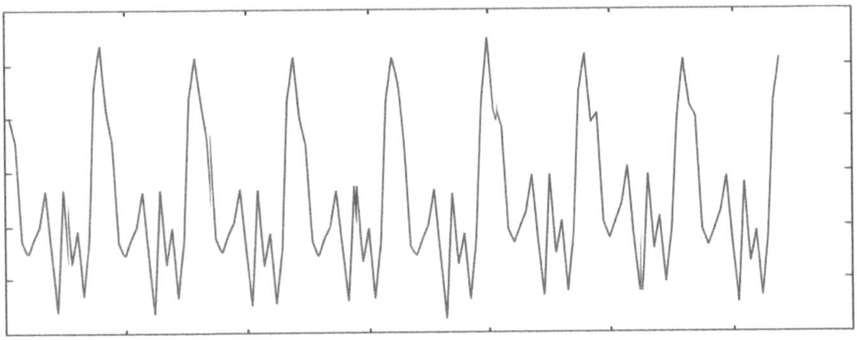

Figure 7.5 Sample of the randomness.

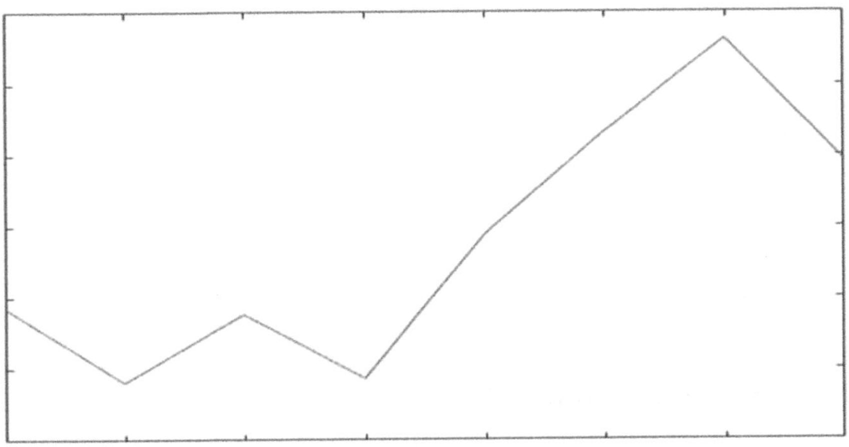

Figure 7.6 Sample of the increasing.

The last step of the feature extraction (wavelet) calculates the variance of the signal using the equation;

$$\text{Variance} = \frac{1}{N}\sum_{i=0}^{N-1} W_i^2 \tag{7.4}$$

The variance of the signal is saved as shown in Figure 7.7, and this variance may differ from one signal to another.

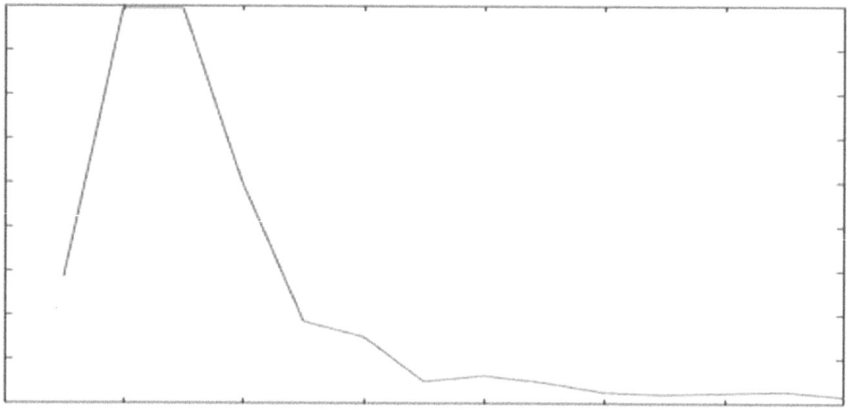

Figure 7.7 Sample of the variance for the signal.

Table 7.1 Details of the used dataset

	Number of cases		
Heart disease type	*Total*	*Training*	*Testing*
ARR	96	67	29
CHF	30	21	9
NSR	36	25	11

7.3.2 Machine learning classifier

This chapter explored a support vector machine (SVM) classifier for the classification of ECG signals. It functions using the equation for a second-degree polynomial kernel:

$$F(x)=Ax^\wedge 2+Bx+C \tag{7.5}$$

The proposed model using "Fitcecoc" is created to save the trained model and later load it to be used for classification. Decision Tree model, ~~for~~ classifies each ECG sample to their corresponding disease type (Kumaragurubaran & Jaeyalakshmi, 2024; Pandey et al., 2024; Wang et al., 2024).

7.3.2.1 Simulation

After several tests and modifications, the proposed system is modeled to a stable state and has recorded high performance. Table 7.1 depicts the

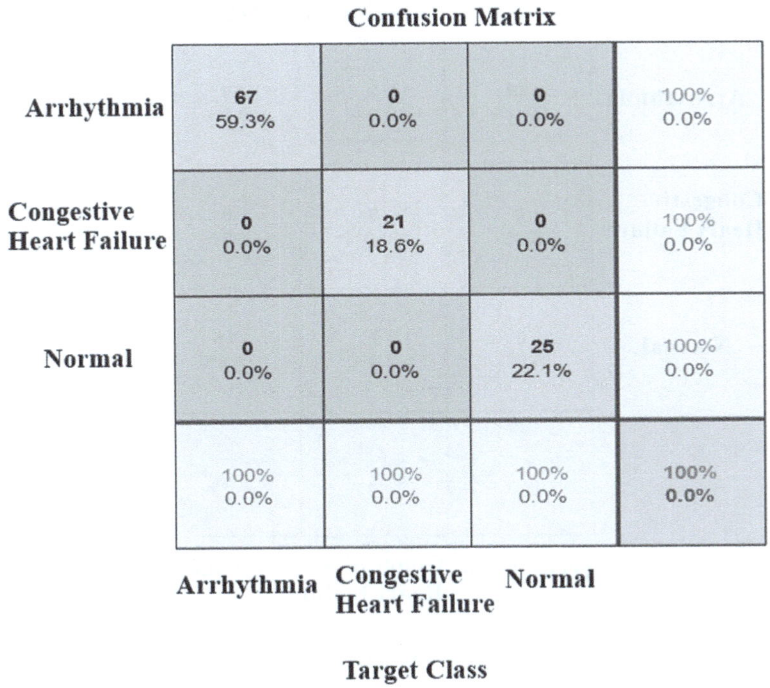

Figure 7.8 Confusion matrix (training).

summary of the utilized dataset. After feeding the dataset to the proposed system, it was able to yield an accuracy of 100.00% for training and 98.00% for testing. Figures 7.8 and 7.9 depict the confusion matrix for training and testing, respectively.

Usually, a confusion matrix for testing is utilized to measure the performance of the system. From the confusion matrix in Figure 7.8, it is proven that. There is no wrong prediction of cognitive heart failure as arrhythmia or normal sinus rhythm, resulting in a prediction of 100.00% accuracy.

- In the third row, there are 12 cases of normal sinus rhythm; 11 of those cases were predicted as normal sinus rhythm, no wrong prediction for arrhythmia, but one case was wrongly predicted as congestive heart failure. This resulted in a prediction of 91.70 % accuracy.
- On average, the system achieved 98.00% accuracy with a 2.00% error rate (Sadr et al., 2024; Shibata et al., 2024).

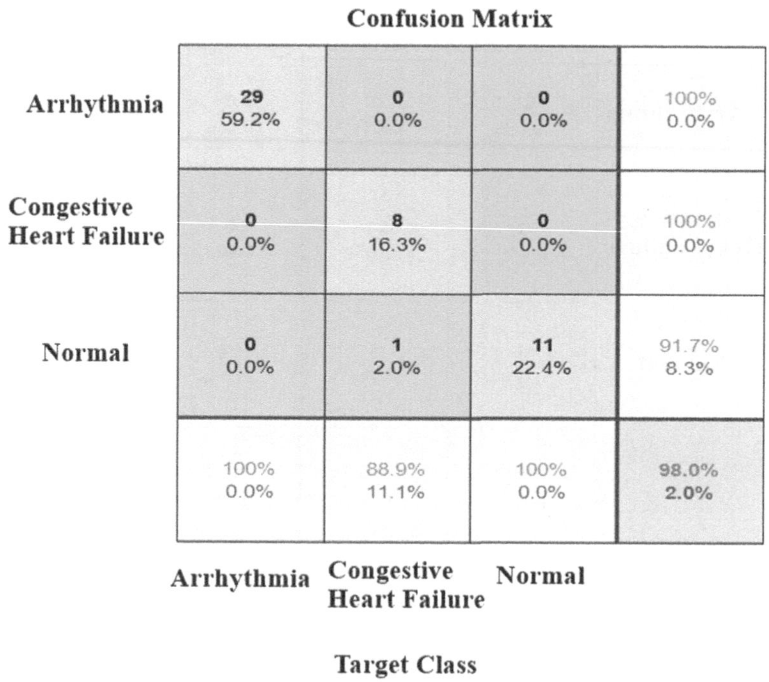

Figure 7.9 Confusion matrix (testing).

7.4 MULTIMODAL PHYSIOLOGICAL SIGNAL FUSION AND SECURE SUSTAINABLE DEPLOYMENT

Heart disease diagnosis systems are increasingly transitioning from single-modality analysis to multimodal physiological intelligence, where complementary biological signals and clinical indicators are processed together to improve prediction reliability. While the current work utilizes ECG signals as the primary diagnostic source, real-world cardiac monitoring incorporates additional parameters such as photoplethysmography (PPG), blood pressure (BP), oxygen saturation (SpO_2), heart rate variability (HRV), and demographic/clinical biomarkers. These modalities capture distinct characteristics of cardiovascular function: ECG reflects electrical cardiac activity, PPG measures blood volume variations, SpO_2 reflects oxygenation efficiency, and BP and HRV represent circulatory stress. Combining these signals enhances the differentiation between arrhythmia, congestive heart failure, and normal sinus rhythm, particularly in borderline diagnostic cases where ECG alone may be ambiguous.

To enable this pipeline, the proposed architecture can be extended to perform early-, intermediate-, or late-feature fusion. In early fusion, raw signal features from ECG and PPG are concatenated prior to training the classifier. In intermediate fusion, modality-specific feature extractors (e.g., wavelet, entropy, and AR models) feed a shared multimodal latent space to highlight correlations between oscillatory patterns of the cardiac cycle. Late fusion integrates probabilistic confidence scores from multiple models to refine classification. All three strategies are compatible with the hybrid feature extraction already implemented in this study, making multimodal expansion computationally feasible.

Because multimodal physiological data contains highly sensitive personal patterns, secure deployment is necessary for real clinical adoption. Instead of transmitting raw ECG/PPG signals to external servers for classification, privacy-preserving inference can be performed using a federated learning framework, in which model parameters—not patient data—are shared across distributed nodes. This approach enables continuous learning from hospital data without violating patient confidentiality. Blockchain-based authorization and access control can additionally guarantee traceability of data access events and prevent unauthorized modification of cardiology records. These secure strategies meet global medical standards such as HIPAA and GDPR, making the model safe for future clinical deployment.

Sustainability is also a fundamental requirement in long-term healthcare systems. Multimodal signals increase computational complexity; therefore, the system should minimize computational footprint, inference latency, RF transmission overhead, and memory usage. Running lightweight SVM inference and feature extraction on low-power wearable devices reduces the need to stream full ECG/PPG waveforms continuously. Only compact features (rather than raw signals) are transmitted to the cloud when abnormalities are detected, optimizing network energy consumption. The sustainability of the expanded system can be measured using the following KPIs:

KPI	*Description*
Computational footprint	FLOPs and processing cycles per diagnostic instance
Latency	End-to-end response time from signal capture to prediction
Power consumption	Device and cloud energy usage during inference
Resource usage	Storage/memory cost per patient and per monitoring cycle

A secure and sustainable multimodal deployment framework therefore improves:

1. classification accuracy through signal complementarity,
2. patient privacy through federated and blockchain-based access security, and
3. environmental and operational efficiency through low-power real-time inference.

These extensions position the proposed system as a clinically relevant, scalable, and long-term viable digital cardiology solution for smart hospitals and pervasive telehealth.

7.5 CONCLUSION

This chapter presents a novel system for both inexperienced and experienced doctors to making ECG-based diagnosis and obtaining immediate and accurate results. The system is built using ECG signals as a dataset. Four feature extraction methods were integrated and applied to the dataset to extract relevant features—used as input to the classifier. After rigorous training and testing, the explored classifier (SVM) was able to accurately predict the supplied classes of heart diseases. The proposed system was able to yield an accuracy of 100.00% for training and 98.00% for testing, with very low error rate. This high performance makes the system fit for recommendation and adoption in the healthcare system. Future thought of the research is propagated towards the incorporation/integration of the proposed system into ECG-based devices for fast and accurate diagnosis. This would drastically reduce the rate of death as a result of the application can be integrated for easy access.

REFERENCES

Baseer, K. K., Sivakumar, K., Veeraiah, D., Chhabra, G., Lakineni, P. K., Pasha, M. J., & Harikrishnan, G. (2024). Healthcare diagnostics with an adaptive deep learning model integrated with the Internet of medical Things (IoMT) for predicting heart disease. *Biomedical Signal Processing and Control*, 92, 105988.

Dhingra, L. S., Aminorroaya, A., Sangha, V., Pedroso, A. F., Shankar, S. V., Coppi, A., & Khera, R. (2025). Ensemble deep learning algorithm for structural heart disease screening using electrocardiographic images: PRESENT SHD. *Journal of the American College of Cardiology*, 85(12), 1302–1313.

El-Sofany, H., Bouallegue, B., & El-Latif, Y. M. A. (2024). A proposed technique for predicting heart disease using machine learning algorithms and an explainable AI method. *Scientific Reports*, 14(1), 23277.

Jha, K. M., Velaga, V., Routhu, K. K., Sadaram, G., & Boppana, S. B. (2025). Evaluating the effectiveness of machine learning for heart disease prediction in healthcare sector. *J Cardiobiol*, 9(1), 1.

Kumaragurubaran, T., & Jaeyalakshmi, M. (2024). A comparative analysis on the prediction of heart failure using machine learning algorithms. In *2024 5th International Conference on Mobile Computing and Sustainable Informatics (ICMCSI)* (pp. 206–211). IEEE.

Nasiruddin, M., Dutta, S., Sikder, R., Islam, M. R., Mukaddim, A. A., & Hider, M. A. (2024). Predicting heart failure survival with machine learning: Assessing my risk. *Journal of Computer Science and Technology Studies*, 6(3), 10–32996.

Pandey, A., Shivaji, B. A., Acharya, M., & Mohbey, K. K. (2024). Mitigating class imbalance in heart disease detection with machine learning. *Multimedia Tools and Applications*, 84, 1–26.

Petmezas, G., Papageorgiou, V. E., Vassilikos, V., Pagourelias, E., Tsaklidis, G., Katsaggelos, A. K., & Maglaveras, N. (2024). Recent advancements and applications of deep learning in heart failure: A systematic review. *Computers in Biology and Medicine*, 176, 108557.

Ramesh, B., & Lakshmanna, K. (2024). A novel early detection and prevention of coronary heart disease framework using hybrid deep learning model and neural fuzzy inference system. *IEEE Access*, 12, 26683–26695.

Rao, G. M., Ramesh, D., Sharma, V., Sinha, A., Hassan, M. M., & Gandomi, A. H. (2024). AttGRU-HMSI: Enhancing heart disease diagnosis using hybrid deep learning approach. *Scientific Reports*, 14(1), 7833.

Sadr, H., Salari, A., Ashoobi, M. T., & Nazari, M. (2024). Cardiovascular disease diagnosis: A holistic approach using the integration of machine learning and deep learning models. *European Journal of Medical Research*, 29(1), 455.

Shibata, N., Morita, Y., Ito, T., Kanzaki, Y., Watanabe, N., Yoshioka, N., & Morishima, I. (2024). A machine learning algorithm for stratification of risk of cardiovascular disease in metabolic dysfunction-associated steatotic liver disease. *European Journal of Internal Medicine*, 129, 62–70.

Türk, F. (2024). Investigation of machine learning algorithms on heart disease through dominant feature detection and feature selection. *Signal, Image and Video Processing*, 18(4), 3943–3955.

Wang, X., Rao, J., Zhang, L., Liu, X., & Zhang, Y. (2024). Identification of circadian rhythm-related gene classification patterns and immune infiltration analysis in heart failure based on machine learning. *Heliyon*, 10(6), 1–20.

Chapter 8

Multimodal intelligence for cancer management

A new dimension in healthcare applications

Jaspinder Kaur Walia, Kanan Kaura, Sita Rani, and Vikram Puri

8.1 INTRODUCTION

Despite advances made by doctors, cancer remains a difficult and widespread disease. Due to the various types of cancer, it is challenging to understand and detect them early. There are some limitations in the single-modality approaches, due to which they cannot give full information related to cancer. To solve this problem, computer and data-based technologies are used that include advanced analysis, digital health systems, and AI tools to support the existing approaches. These methods do not provide the complete solution in themselves; they collect data from different sources and combine to make systems that help the patient in accurate, ethical, and right decision-making [1, 2].

8.1.1 Overview of cancer management challenges

It is quite difficult to handle cancer due to its several interrelated challenges:

- Tumor Variations: One fixed treatment does not work the same for all patients, so doctors have to adjust the treatment according to each patient [1].
- Diagnosis Shortcoming: It is quite difficult to detect cancer at an early stage, as it has very small or unclear symptoms, and even a single type of test cannot detect it [2].
- Outcome Predictions: It is hard to detect how the cancer will grow in the future based on a single scan test [3].
- Resistance to treatment: At first, cancer may respond to the treatment, but after some time, the cancer cells learn how to adapt and stop responding, due to which doctors need to change the treatment plan [4].
- Data Combination Difficulties: In cancer treatment, the data come from different sources such as CT scans, lab tests, and it's hard to integrate all the data and to make the prediction [5].

 DOI: 10.1201/9781003665656-8

8.1.2 Role of artificial intelligence in oncology

Computer-based cancer research provides a variety of techniques such as statistics, machine learning, and AI-based models. These should be used carefully by the doctors to make the predictions. Some applications of these are depicted in Table 8.1.

Even though AI and computer tools help a lot, there are still problems and limits.

8.1.3 Emergence of multimodal intelligence in healthcare

Smart computer tools combine different patient information to help doctors make the best and safest decisions for each person [1]. Some features and ethical considerations of multimodal intelligence in healthcare are shown in Table 8.2.

8.2 FUNDAMENTALS OF MULTIMODAL INTELLIGENCE

Multimodal intelligence is a new area that unites various types of information in a single system. It assists researchers in resolving issues and interpreting biomedical data. These approaches should also be in compliance with ethical and regulatory regulations [1]. The conventional computational systems tend to process a single type of data such as images or text where multimodal methods can process numerous types of data simultaneously. Such techniques assist in providing a clear picture and also in making clinical decisions. The findings should be verified to ensure that they are right and valid [6, 7].

Table 8.1 Applications of computational and AI-assisted methods

Area of application	*Supportive contribution*	*Ethical considerations*
Diagnostics	Assist radiologists and pathologists in interpreting complex imaging and historical data	Requires human oversight, risk of dataset bias
Personalized therapy	Analyze clinical and molecular data to suggest treatment options	Must undergo clinical validation and approval
Prognostic modelling	Contribute to risk stratification and survival prediction	Interpretability and transparency are essential
Drug discovery	Facilitate the identification of potential drug targets and repurposing	Requires rigorous experimental validation

Table 8.2 Main features and ethical points of multimodal AI in healthcare

Feature/capability	*Description*	*Ethical and clinical considerations*
Full information fusion	Combines imaging, genomics, and clinical data for more accurate diagnosis	Responsible use of sensitive patient data
Improved prediction	Outperforms single-modality systems in tumor grading and treatment response	Requires validation and bias monitoring
Personalized and adaptive care	Supports real-time therapy adaptation	Must comply with clinical protocols and ensure patient safety
Technical and clinical integration	Uses ML architectures to harmonize heterogeneous data	Interpretability, transparency and regulatory compliance are critical
Implementation challenges	Data incompleteness, modality imbalance, high dimensionality, and real-time integration	Careful design and clinical validation needed

There are numerous types of data that are used in cancer care. These are radiographic and pathology pictures, genomic and molecular data, clinical documentation, and real-time data of wearable devices [1, 3, 4]. These various forms of data may be combined through multimodal computational systems. This assists doctors in making better decisions and scheduling treatment that would suit individual patients. In addition, the safety of the patients, their privacy, and ethical regulations should never be violated [2, 5, 8, 9].

This chapter describes the application of multimodal intelligence in the field of oncology. It discusses the fundamentals, the nature of the data, the ways of integrating the data, and the primary system designs.

8.2.1 Definition and core concepts

Multimodal intelligence implies processing more than one form of data simultaneously. A system is able to connect text, images, or signals. It processes the data in combination and not in isolation of each source [6].

Multimodal intelligence implies processing more than one form of data simultaneously. A system is able to connect text, images, or signals. It processes the data in combination and not in isolation from each source. Multimodal systems combine several sources. They study them as a group. This gives a clearer view of complex problems. In medicine, such systems

Table 8.3 Key concepts in multimodal intelligence

Concept	*Definition*
Complementarity	Every modality offers unique data to enable an overall understanding
Correlation	Interdependencies between modalities enhance predictive performance
Redundancy	Overlapping information increases the system's robustness and mitigates the impact of missing data
Contextual alignment	Ensuring that the timing and location of modalities align together in order to enable meaningful fusion

can track how a tumor grows, check if a treatment is working, and can also show the overall condition of a patient [3, 10].

Table 8.3 lists the key points of multimodal intelligence [6].

8.2.2 Types of modalities in cancer data

Cancer care produces many kinds of data. Each type gives useful information about the disease [1, 3]:

- **Medical imaging** includes CT, MRI, PET, ultrasound, and mammography [3]. These images show the location of the tumor. They also describe its structure. Doctors use them to track how the tumor changes during treatment [11, 12].
- **Genomic and molecular profiles** come from some lab tests. DNA tests look for changes in a patient's genes. RNA tests reveal which genes are active. Protein tests describe how proteins behave inside the tumor.
- **Electronic health records (EHRs)** are digital charts with clinical notes, lab results, treatment history, personal details, and recorded symptoms [1, 3]. EHRs help doctors by showing the full medical history of the patient [13].
- **Histopathology** involves the use of tissue samples and biopsy images [3]. These pictures validate the diagnosis. They also display the tumor grade and the disease stage [11].
- **Sensor and wearable data** monitor the heart rate and activity of a patient. They are also able to log sleep and other health information in real time [8, 14].

The various forms of data applied in multimodal cancer care are demonstrated in Figure 8.1.

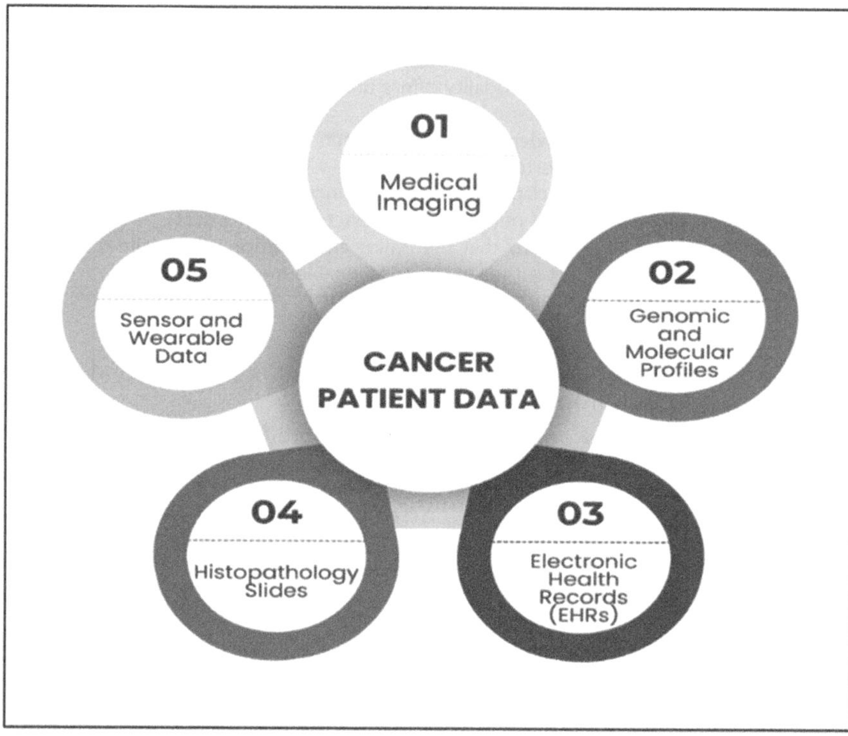

Figure 8.1 Multimodal data sources in cancer care.

8.2.3 Fusion techniques: early, late, and hybrid fusion

Fusion methods combine different types of data in multimodal systems. There are three main approaches [6, 10]:

- **Early Fusion** joins all the data at the start. The system sees everything together. This helps it find patterns across different types of data immediately. Researchers often test this fusion in experiments. It needs careful checking before using it in healthcare [6, 10].
- **Late Fusion** keeps each type of data separate at first. Each stream goes through its own model. Later, the system combines the results. This can happen by averaging, voting, or giving more weight to some results [10].
- **Hybrid Fusion** starts by processing each type of data separately. Then their features come together later in the model. This lets the system find unique patterns for each data type. It also helps understand how the data interacts before making a final decision [10].

8.2.4 Architectures and frameworks for multimodal learning

Modern multimodal systems mostly use deep learning models to handle complex biomedical data [6, 7, 14]. Each model works better with certain types of data and is suitable for specific tasks.

- **Convolutional Neural Networks or CNNs** are mainly used for images, and they are applied to medical scans and tissue slides. Doctors need to check them carefully before using them in medical facilities [3, 11].
- **Recurrent Neural Networks or RNNs** and their variants such as long short-term memory or LSTM, and gated recurrent unit or GRU work with data that comes in order. They can handle patient records over time and also process sensor readings. In healthcare, these models need careful monitoring to make sure they are applied properly [6].
- **Transformers** use self-attention to find links in long sequences of data and can spot patterns that other models might miss. They work well for multimodal learning, but in healthcare, they must follow ethical and regulatory rules [7, 15].
- **Graph Neural Networks (GNNs)** work with connected data and networks. They can model biological systems and show relationships in biomedical datasets. In cancer research, these models should be used carefully and responsibly [16].

The primary requirement of all these models is to ensure that patients are safe, and the information is confidential. They have rules to be obeyed and be sustainable. Only under these conditions, these models may be applied in cancer research and digital health. One of the ways to visualize the interaction between the models with multimodal data and handling various kinds of information is provided in Figure 8.2.

8.3 MULTIMODAL DATA SOURCES IN CANCER MANAGEMENT

The unification of the various forms of biomedical data is a revolutionary move in the contemporary cancer treatment. The data that is multimodal and includes medical imaging, genomics, clinical records, histopathology, and wearable device monitoring, which gives detailed information about the tumor biology, patient health status, and treatment response. It is believed that the combination of these heterogeneous forms of data by means of sophisticated AI and machine learning models will provide more accurate diagnoses, better risk classification, and tailored treatment plans, which will eventually result in improved patient outcomes [1–3, 5, 6]. The following

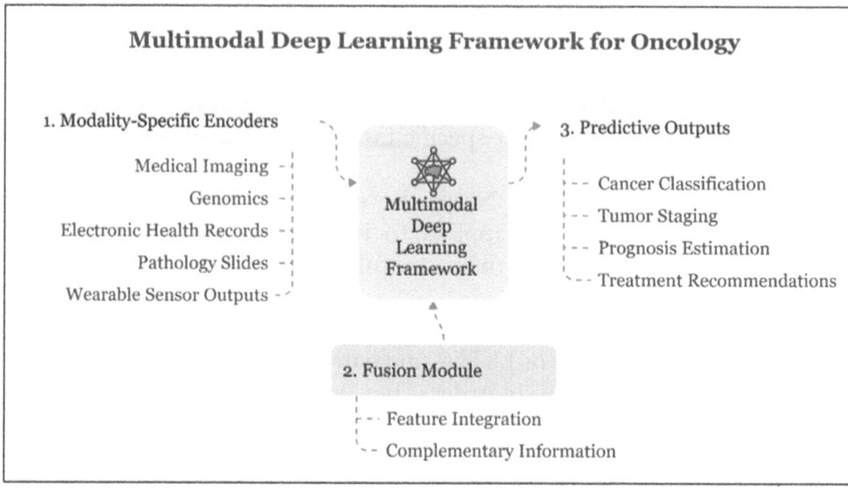

Figure 8.2 An example framework of multimodal deep learning.

section will analyze the most important sources of oncological data that have a high potential of being used in multimodal intelligence.

8.3.1 Medical imaging (CT, MRI, PET, mammograms)

Medical imaging is consistently used in the routine care of cancer patients to offer noninvasive, high-resolution data regarding the location, characteristics, and progression of the tumors. The important imaging modalities are as follows:

Computed Tomography (CT): Gives accurate anatomical detail that is necessary in locating tumors, staging, planning treatments, and evaluating responses.

- **Magnetic Resonance Imaging** (MRI): It has superior soft-tissue contrast and functional imaging, diffusion-weighted imaging (DWI), and perfusion-weighted imaging (PWI) to improve tumor characterization.
- **Positron Emission Tomography** (PET): Image of metabolic and molecular activity, which is usually used with CT (PET-CT) to associate functional tumor activity with the anatomy.
- **Mammography**: The best screening and early detection of breast cancer. These modalities and their clinical uses are discussed in Table 8.4.

Table 8.4 Imaging modalities and roles

Modality	*Primary role*	*Typical use cases*
CT	Anatomical localization	Staging, monitoring
MRI	Soft tissue, functional imaging	Brain, breast, pelvic tumors
PET	Metabolic activity	Detecting metastasis, therapy
Mammogram	Early detection	Breast cancer screening

Table 8.5 Some important genomic and molecular datatypes in cancer management

Datatype	*Key function*	*Clinical and ethical considerations*
Next-generation sequencing (NGS)	Detects mutations, CNVs, gene fusions	Therapy selection, prognosis require patient consent and regulatory compliance
Transcriptomics (RNA-seq)	Measures gene expression and molecular subtypes	Predictive modelling, risk stratification, validated and ethically used
Proteomics/ metabolomics	Profiles proteins and metabolites reflecting tumor state	Treatment response assessment, privacy safeguards and oversight required

- **Clinical Value:** Imaging information can be used to diagnose, plan surgery and radiotherapy, and monitor long-term outcomes.

Advanced AI models can extract quantitative radiomic features (e.g., intensity, shape, texture) that correlate with molecular subtypes and predict prognosis [8, 11]. Integration of imaging data with clinical, genomic, or pathological information has demonstrated improved predictive accuracy for treatment response and patient outcomes [1, 4, 12].

8.3.2 Genomic and molecular data

By studying patients' genes and molecules in their cells, it helps doctors to understand how cancer works. It also helps to plan for future care. When this information is combined with the patient's scan, test, and medical history, doctors can make treatment plans specifically for that patient. All this should be done carefully and by following ethical standards. Table 8.5 shows the main parts of patient records and the medical and ethical points to keep in mind.

8.3.3 Clinical and electronic health records

Electronic health records (EHRs) capture comprehensive longitudinal clinical trajectories that are essential for cancer patient management:

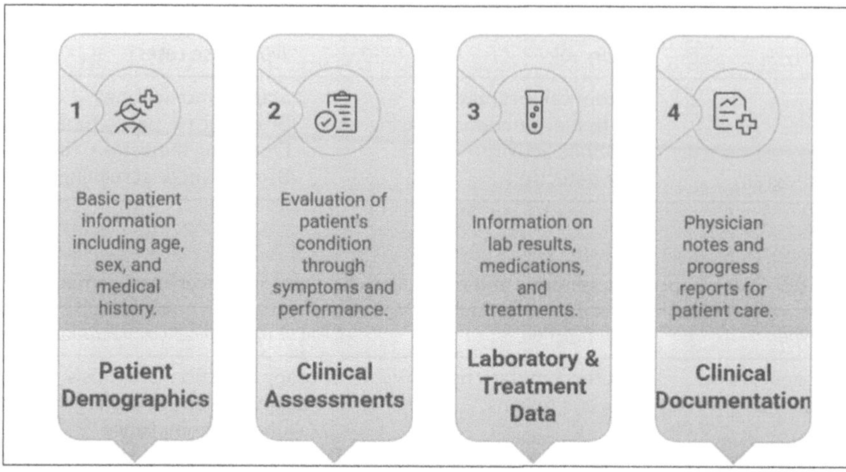

Figure 8.3 Patient health information.

EHRs are digital records of a patient's health. The records that are included in EHRs are shown in Figure 8.3.

Clinical Value: EHRs are useful for doctors. They help the doctors to understand the imaging data, such as scans, X-rays, and also genetically related data. AI tools help to make better decisions, but we must be careful about missing data, privacy, and ethical use [1, 3, 5, 8, 7, 13, 14].

8.3.4 Pathology and histopathological slides

Digital pathology converts tissue samples into digital images. These images show how the individual cells look like and how cells are organized in the tissue. This will help doctors to diagnose cancer accurately and help to identify the type of cancer. Some AI-assisted tools can be used, but they should be used only under the supervision of doctors and should be used safely and ethically [4, 8,11,12].

Figure 8.4 depicts the comprehensive cancer data integration process.

8.3.5 Sensor and wearable data

Wearable devices help to monitor the health records of patients in real time and for long durations. These wearables check some parameters like:

- Physical activity: body movement, exercise, sleep
- Body signals: heart rate, body temperature
- Patient-reported feedback: symptoms and quality of life

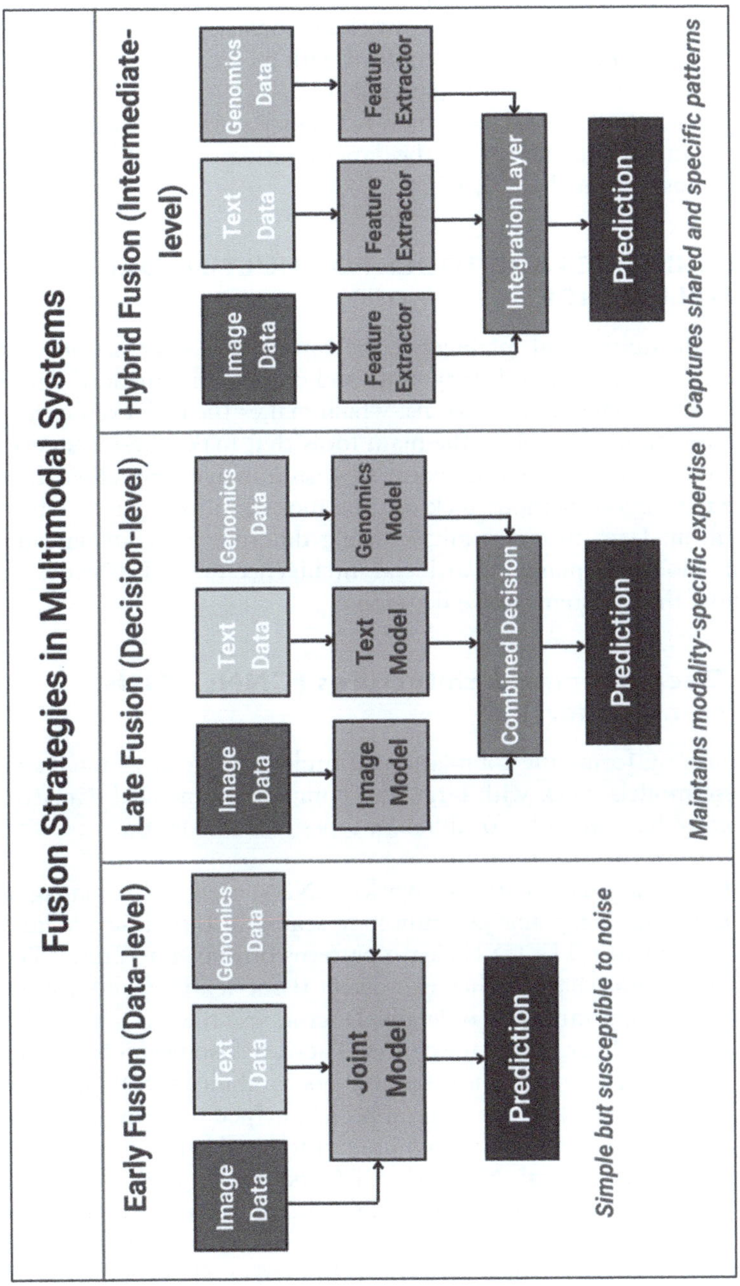

Figure 8.4 Cancer data integration.

Clinical Value: For continuous monitoring of patients, wearables are used. With these problems and complications, they can be detected. It also helps to check whether the treatment is working correctly or not [1, 5, 8]. If the data collected from devices is combined with medical data, then specialized treatments will be given to the patients [14].

Challenges: Wearable data is high-frequency data and can contain some noisy and missing data. Further, the data of patients should be kept safe and should be used ethically [10, 17].

8.4 TECHNIQUES AND TOOLS FOR MULTIMODAL CANCER INTELLIGENCE

Progress in multimodal intelligence for cancer care depends on computer methods that can deal with very large and complex biomedical data [1, 4]. The data also come in many forms, which makes the task even harder.

In this section, we look at the main tools that make these systems work. Deep learning helps in finding patterns within images and clinical records. Feature extraction methods pick out the most important signals from raw information. Data fusion strategies bring different kinds of data together into one model. Explainable artificial intelligence or XAI provides ways to show how these systems make decisions.

8.4.1 Deep learning architectures (CNNs, RNNs, transformers)

Deep learning forms the foundation of multimodal cancer intelligence [6, 7]. These models work with large and complex biomedical datasets. Each architecture has strengths for different types of information.

- **Convolutional Neural Networks** (CNNs) are good at managing spatial data. They analyze radiology scans, histopathology slides, and skin images [11]. CNNs learn patterns one layer at a time. They can find tumor shapes. They can detect tissue textures and also identify other important spatial details. Doctors use these results to diagnose patients. They help stage cancer. They are also useful for segmenting tissues [3, 18]. In a study, researchers combined CNN image analysis with genomic data, and this approach helped them in predicting how patients would respond to immunotherapy [19].
- **Recurrent Neural Networks** (RNNs) work well with data that changes with time. They study patient records, wearable device readings, and treatment histories [6]. Researchers use them to study how diseases progress and also help predict clinical outcomes [6].
- **Transformers** bring different types of data together. Vision transformers or ViTs focus on images, and BERT-based models handle

Table 8.6 Common deep learning architectures and their applications in oncology

Architecture	*Input modality*	*Application example*
CNNs	Radiology images, pathology slides, dermatology images	Tumour detection, segmentation of lesions, and grading of histopathology
RNNs	Longitudinal EHRs, time series (wearables, vitals), treatment timelines	Predicting disease progression, estimating survival curves, and monitoring therapy response
Transformers	Imaging + genomics + clinical text	Multimodal risk stratification, prognosis prediction, and integrated clinical decision support

text and genomic information [7, 13]. Multimodal transformers combine these inputs into a single, context-rich representation. Doctors use this information to support clinical decisions [15].

Table 8.6 shows the main deep learning architectures used in the treatment of cancer.

8.4.2 Feature extraction and representation learning

Turning raw multimodal data into clear and simple forms is a key step in building learning systems [9, 10]. Researchers use two main ways to prepare data for models:

- **Hand-Crafted Features:** Experts make features by hand. They use pathway analysis for molecular data. They study clinical notes using text mining and also analyze medical images with radiomic methods [3]. These features give useful knowledge and do not always find hidden patterns in the data.
- **Representation Learning (Deep Features):** Modern methods let models learn features from raw data [14]. They find patterns and connections across different types of data.
    a. **Autoencoders** reduce the size of the data and then reconstruct the original data [14].
    b. **Embedding Layers** convert large data into compact and simple forms. They keep the key information [10].
    c. **Pre-trained Models** such as ResNet for images and BioBERT for biomedical text use knowledge from large datasets. This helps models do better on specific tasks [13].

These learned features are strong and flexible. They work well for many tasks. They can combine different types of data and make them useful for research and clinical studies.

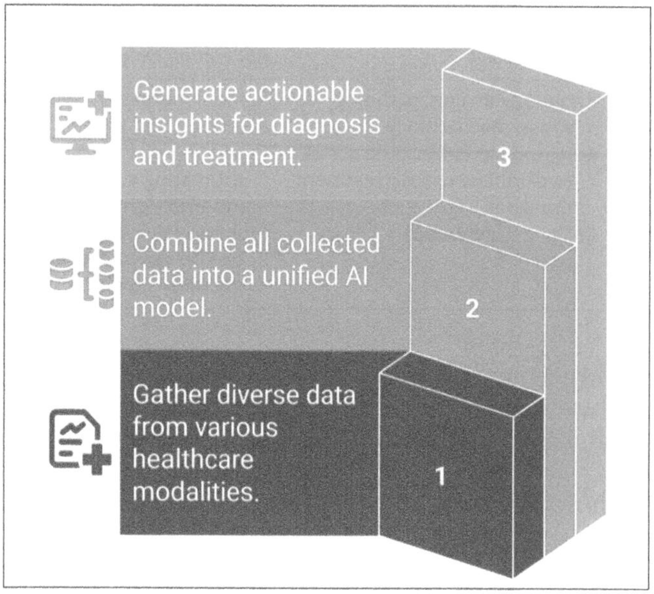

Figure 8.5 Fusion techniques in multimodal intelligence.

8.4.3 Data fusion strategies and multimodal embedding

A key part of multimodal systems is joining information from different types of data. Combining these features allows the system to consider all the information and improves its performance [10, 14]. Figure 8.5 shows how the different fusion strategies combine features in multimodal systems.

- **Early Fusion** joins raw or simple features before sending them into one model and allows the system to learn from all data at the same time [10, 14].
- **Late Fusion** lets each type of data go through its own model first and then combines the outputs using voting or ensemble methods [10, 14].
- **Hybrid Fusion** combines features from different data types at hidden layers and keeps both common and unique information for each type [10, 14].
- **Multimodal Embeddings** map different types of data into a shared space, which makes it easier to find connections and relationships [19].
- **Graph Embeddings and Attention** improve the quality of embeddings by focusing on the most important links between features [16, 20].

8.4.4 Explainable AI in multimodal systems

Multimodal models can be very effective but sometimes they are complex and hard to understand. This can reduce trust and acceptance in clinical settings [4, 18, 19]. Explainable methods help doctors understand how the models are making their predictions.

- **Saliency Maps and Heatmaps** highlight areas in an image or genetic features that had the most influence on the result.
- **SHAP and LIME** show which features in text or tabular data were most important for the decision.
- **Attention Weights Visualization** shows the attention weights in transformer-based models and indicates which data or features the model focused on the most.

These explainable methods help clinicians trust the results and also reveal hidden patterns in the data. It can reveal new features in the data and increase transparency in the results [21].

Figure 8.6 shows different methods used to make multimodal models more understandable.

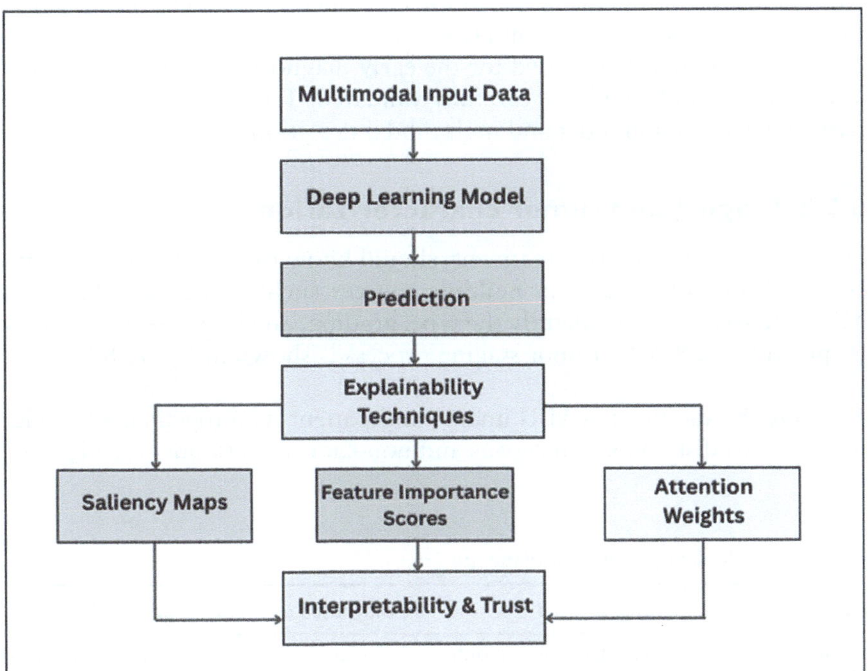

Figure 8.6 Explainability in multimodal models.

8.5 APPLICATIONS IN CANCER CARE

The implementation of multimodal intelligence in oncology has revolutionized the entire cancer care from early screening to real-time action. By integrating information across imaging, genomics, clinical records, pathology, and wearables, AI-enabled multimodal systems can support more accurate, timely, and personalized decision making in the face of the complexity and heterogeneity of cancer [1–3, 5, 8].

8.5.1 Early detection and diagnosis

Multimodal AI can assist early cancer diagnosis when clinical records, imaging, pathology, genomic, and other omics data are combined and patterns of subtle findings are detected single-modality methods might miss that [2, 4, 5, 8], e.g, the early detection of disease based upon the integration of radiological imaging (CT, MRI) with laboratory testing and human clinical notes [8, 14].

Use Case: A recent analysis shows the use of AI. They discovered a method to detect cancer symptoms, such as weight and muscle loss. In this, they combine data from multiple sources like body imaging, demographic details, lab tests, and clinical reports. The combined data was given to the AI, and a prediction was made. With this, doctors can get a personalized risk assessment of every patient [1, 4].

The multimodal model used for the early diagnosis must be transparent, interpretable, and should be carefully validated. Table 8.7 depicts the comparison between unimodal and multimodal detection.

8.5.2 Staging and tumor characterization

Doctors, before doing the treatment, should know the tumor type, size, and spread. Data collected from multiple sources such as CT scan, PET, and MRI help to accurately identify the type, grading, and how much the disease is spread [2, 5, 8, 10]. Tumor staging process is shown in Figure 8.7.

Example: By monitoring MRI images and patient data together, AI models were able to distinguish cancerous and non-cancerous tumors [8, 11, 12].

Table 8.7 Single datatype vs multi-datatype

Approach	*Datatype used*	*Diagnostic accuracy*	*Clinical utility*
Single-modality AI	Imaging or clinical only	Moderate	Limited, less robust
Multimodal AI	Imaging + clinical + omics	High	Comprehensive, adaptive

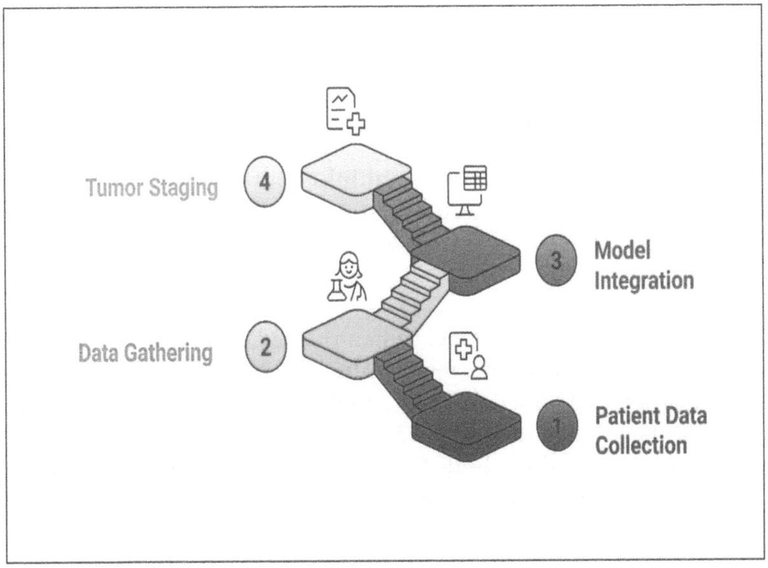

Figure 8.7 Multimodal staging workflow.

However, for real implementation, doctors must check whether correct and reliable results are given by models or not. For using this, proper government approvals should be taken, and proper care of the patient should be taken.

8.5.3 Personalized treatment planning

To plan different treatments for each patient, doctors analyse data collected from multiple sources like CT scans, MRI, and EHRs. This also helps to prevent patients from harmful side effects [2, 4, 7, 8, 10].

Data modalities used in multimodal treatment planning are summarized in Table 8.8.

Table 8.8 Modalities used in multimodal

Modality	*Contribution to planning*
Imaging	Tumor size, location, and spread
Genomics	Mutation status, drug targets
HER/clinical	Comorbidities, prior treatments
Pathology	Tumor grade, immune markers

Clinical Importance: AI tools that collect different types of data help to group patients based on risk (low-risk, high-risk) and help to choose patient-specific treatment and provide better results [1, 5, 12].

8.5.4 Prognosis and survival prediction

When an AI model is trained on multiple data sources, such as imaging, clinical information, and molecular data, then the model can predict better survival and risk rates of patients as compared to previous techniques [1, 4, 8, 10, 11].

Example: Computer-based model, when trained on CT scan data and clinical variables (age, symptoms, test results, etc), was able to accurately give risk groups (low risk, medium risk, high risk) for lung, head, and neck cancer patients. The model achieved high accuracy (AUC up to 0.85) as compared to traditional methods [4, 8, 11]. These methods should be tested and should be used in a safe and ethical way only [22].

8.5.5 Real-time monitoring and relapse detection

Continuous multimodal monitoring allows doctors to keep track of patients, and they can detect whether the same disease is again spreading and can even see other complications [1, 5, 8, 12].

Example: A model was developed by researchers that combines the data from multiple records of patients. The model was able to predict breast cancer and liver cancer patients' relapse of diseases [1, 8, 11, 12, 14].

8.6 CASE STUDIES AND REAL-WORLD IMPLEMENTATIONS

Multimodal intelligence is changing cancer care by combining information from sensors, imaging, genomics, pathology, and clinical records [1, 3, 5, 9]. The following examples show how different approaches work in practice and highlight both the strengths and the challenges of using multimodal methods in oncology.

8.6.1 Multimodal AI in breast cancer diagnosis

One of the most common cancers in the world, breast cancer can be prevented with early and precise detection. These days, multimodal AI systems integrate clinical records, pathology slides, MRI, ultrasound, and mammography to enhance diagnosis [8, 11, 12, 23].

Table 8.9 Diagnostic performance in breast cancer

Approach	*Modalities used*	*Accuracy (%)*
Radiologist	Mammogram only	85
Single-modality AI	Mammogram + AI	88
Multimodal AI	Imaging + Pathology + EHR	92

Clinical Impact

- In women with dense breast tissue, combining mammography and ultrasound leads to higher detection of cases [23].
- More accurate tumour classification is made possible by including biopsy (pathology) data [11, 24].

Example: A deep learning-based multimodal system that combined biopsy pathology reports, patient demographics, and mammograms was implemented in a recent study [11]. With a 92% diagnostic accuracy rate, this model outperformed radiologists who only used imaging [23].

The diagnostic performance of different approaches in breast cancer detection is shown in Table 8.9.

8.6.2 Integrating genomics and imaging in lung cancer management

Due to its complexity, lung cancer requires individualized treatment and an accurate diagnosis. Multimodal systems now combine CT or PET imaging with genomic profiling, for example, EGFR and ALK mutations, and a patient's clinical history to guide decisions [1, 4, 25].

Clinical Impact

- Helps group patients more effectively for targeted therapies [4].
- Predicts resistance to first-line treatments by linking imaging and genomic patterns [1, 25].

Example: A multimodal AI model that integrated genomic mutation data and CT radiomics predicted progression-free survival and therapy response with an AUC of 0.89, which outperformed models that only used one type of data [19, 25].

The overall process of integrating imaging, genomics, and clinical data in lung cancer management is illustrated in Figure 8.8.

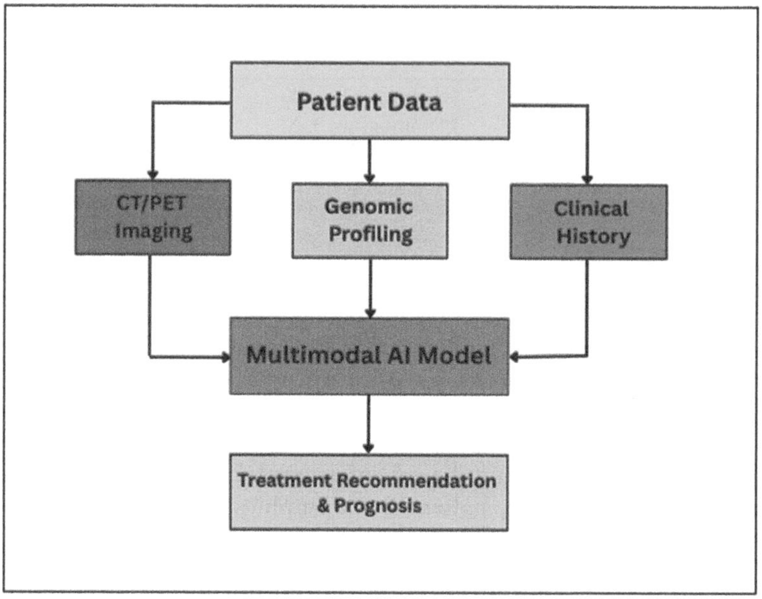

Figure 8.8 Multimodal AI workflow in lung cancer.

8.6.3 Digital pathology for colorectal cancer detection

The diagnosis of colorectal cancer (CRC) was earlier dependent on microscopic examination of tissue. Today, AI-powered digital pathology enables more accurate tumor grade assessment and cancerous area detection [3, 24].

Clinical Impact

- Reduces differences in diagnosis between pathologists [24].
- Finds subtle cell patterns linked to more serious illnesses [24].

Example: In a study, a multimodal AI model grouped CRC patients according to risk by combining digital H&E slides, immunohistochemistry markers, and EHR data. In addition to achieving 95% sensitivity, it discovered novel tissue patterns connected to unfavorable results [24].

The workflow for AI-powered digital pathology in colorectal cancer detection is shown in Figure 8.9.

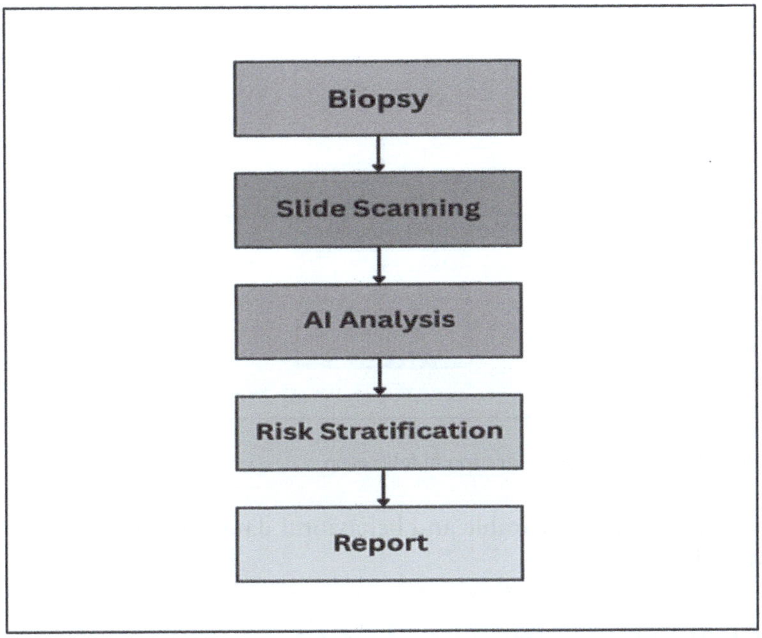

Figure 8.9 Digital pathology workflow in CRC.

8.6.4 Wearable and behavioral data for patient follow-up

Patient monitoring is important for managing side effects and identifying relapses early after the treatment. This is made possible with the help of multimodal AI systems, which provide real-time insights by integrating data from follow-up imaging and wearable sensors such as heart rate and activity, and EHRs [9, 26].

Clinical Impact

- Supports early identification of relapses or other complications [26].
- Keep a careful check on vital signs to deliver patient-specific supportive care [9, 26].

Example: In a pilot study, breast cancer survivors used activity trackers and logged daily symptoms through a mobile app. Combined with periodic scans and EHR data, a multimodal AI platform detected early signs of relapse with 80% sensitivity, allowing timely intervention [26].

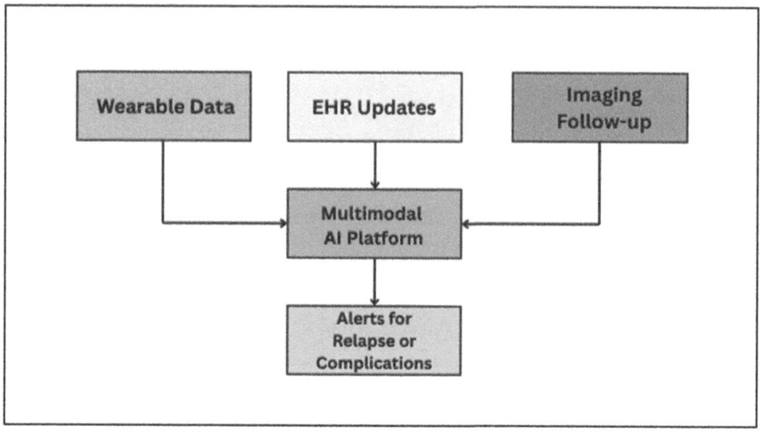

Figure 8.10 Wearable data integration in follow-up.

The integration of wearable and behavioral data for patient follow-up is shown in Figure 8.10.

8.7 CHALLENGES AND LIMITATIONS

Multimodal intelligence is becoming more common in clinical practice, at least in oncology, but there are still numerous obstacles to be overcome. These limitations are technical, clinical, and ethical in nature and need to be addressed for the safe and comprehensive application of multimodal AI systems in oncology [27].

8.7.1 Data heterogeneity and standardization

Cancer line data are intrinsically heterogeneous, which include a diverse set of datatypes (imaging, genomics, pathology images, and EHRs) with different formats, scales, and quality levels [3, 10, 14]. The between-centre diversity caused complex integration of data, training of the model, and clinical application. For instance, images are in DICOM, genomics data are high-dimensional data matrices, and clinical notes are free text [5, 7]. Heterogeneity introduced by differences in image acquisition protocols, annotation, and instrumentation across centers compounds these difficulties, resulting in variable outcomes and poor reproducibility [2, 8, 10, 28].

8.7.2 Missing or incomplete modalities

Residual missingness is common in multimodal oncology research [5, 8, 10]. Not all patients who go through all diagnostic tests or molecular tests, and some data can be missing because of technical failures, budget limitations, or low sample material quality. For example, some patients may have no available transcriptomic or proteomic data due to either poor quality of sample, resulting in sample degradation, or too little tissue, and the imaging or EHR entries may also be incomplete [3, 5].

Some of the common approaches to tackle missing modalities are:

- **Exclusions:** Patients with any missing data will be excluded, encouraging another source of bias.
- **Imputation:** Replacing absence data with statistical or deep learning-based methods, which may add biased or noisy related information.
- **Partial Prediction:** Vision models that can work in the presence of modalities only, e.g., missing-modality-aware models (e.g., MAGNET), through attention mechanisms and binary masks to focus on existing data [7, 14, 29].

Steps to handle missing modalities in multimodal AI are depicted in Figure 8.11.

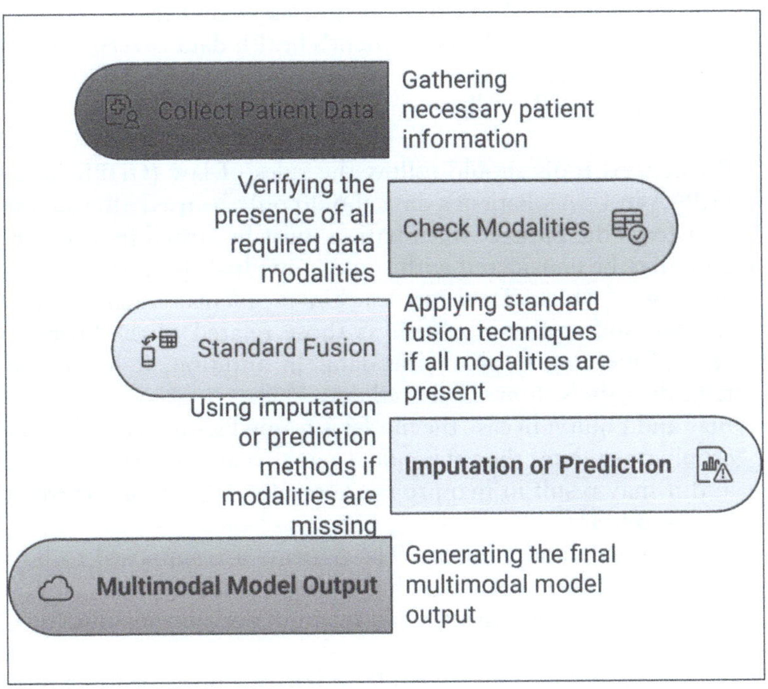

Figure 8.11 Handling missing modalities.

8.7.3 Computational and integration barriers

The comprehensive causal influence networks of big multimodal cancer data collection need to be analyzed by high computational resources and sophisticated algorithm designs [2, 4, 7, 15, 16, 28]. Deep learning, particularly transformers [15] and graph neural network-based models [16], requires specialized hardware and ML expertise.

Some Challenges include:

- Scalability: Learning from multidimensional data consumes a lot of power and time.
- Data Alignment: To match different data types according to time and location is quite difficult [5, 7].
- Model Generalization: It's quite difficult to train models, as it is difficult to say that the model works accurately for new data and patients [3, 8].
- Interpretability: Some models developed are quite difficult to understand by the doctors [4, 11, 10, 30].

8.7.4 Ethical, legal, and privacy issues

The use of multimodal AI in cancer diagnosis raises serious ethical, legal, and privacy concerns [1, 3, 8, 14]. Patient's health data is very sensitive and if leaked can cause serious issues.

Some issues include the following:

- Privacy: AI tools should follow the rules of law (GDPR in Europe, HIPAA in USA). Patient's data should only be used after taking consent from the patient. Information must be stored in a secure place and must be considered with some individuals [14, 31].
- Sharing of Data: There are certain problems associated with the sharing and ownership, such as those related to the hospitals and centers merging to share the data. In addition, it has restrictions regarding the volume of shared data [17].
- Bias and Equity: In case the model is trained with incomplete and discriminatory data, then the model might make incorrect predictions, and it may result in inappropriate results or even unfair treatments [4, 14, 30, 31].
- Transparency and Consent: The patients are supposed to be aware that their information is being utilized, and they are supposed to know that models assist the physician in decision-making [6, 13].

A compilation of these ethical and legal issues is presented in Table 8.10.

Table 8.10 Ethical and legal issues

Issue	*Description*	*Regulation/guidelines*
Privacy	Protect patient identity and health info	GDPR, HIPAA
Consent	Inform and obtain patient agreement	Informed consent laws
Data security	Prevent unauthorized access or breaches	Encryption, access control
Bias and fairness	Avoid discrimination, ensure equity	Human rights frameworks

8.8 FUTURE DIRECTIONS AND EMERGING TRENDS

Computational methods are used to gather and integrate patient information to aid physicians in disease understanding. This part examines techniques that maintain patient confidentiality, massive AI models, simulating patients, and applications of these tools in hospitals. The concepts assist in simplifying and making multimodal approaches more practical in actual healthcare [1, 2].

8.8.1 Federated and privacy-preserving multimodal learning

Hospitals do not always have the ability to share big datasets of patients since the records do include confidential and sensitive information [3, 4]. Privacy-preserving approaches have been adopted by researchers to address this issue. These approaches enable hospitals to participate in artificial intelligence research at the same time the raw data remains secure [32, 33]. Federated learning trains the models locally inside the hospitals. Only updates are sent to a central server in the system. In this manner, the model is trained on numerous datasets, and the information about the patients is not compromised [33]. Other methods apply homomorphic encryption or differential privacy. Homomorphic encryption allows computing on encrypted data. Differential privacy is a small noise to sensitive data. Such techniques are effective in genomics, medical images, and clinical records [32, 33]. Such strategies facilitate safe collaboration among hospitals. They also ensure that they meet the legal standards. Two of them are the Health Insurance Portability and Accountability Act, or HIPAA, and the General Data Protection Regulation, or GDPR [34, 35].

8.8.2 Role of large multimodal foundation models

Neural networks that are trained on massive datasets are called large foundation models. They will be able to change to various tasks and assist researchers in analyzing complex patient data [15, 36].When trained on

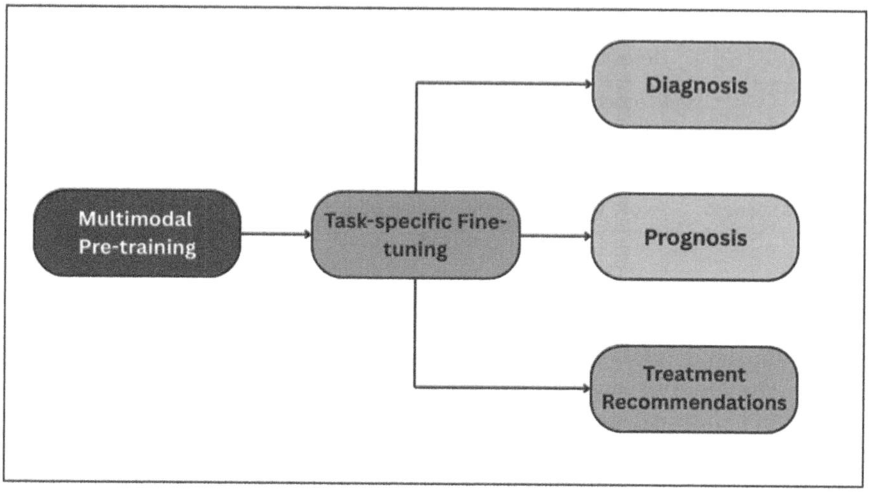

Figure 8.12 Foundation model workflow in cancer care.

several types of biomedical information, such as medical images, clinical notes, DNA and RNA data, and wearable device readings, these models can detect patterns using very little additional labeled data [1, 8, 11, 12]. They can support research on patient survival, different cancer types, and rare diseases.

These models can combine various kinds of data at the same time. This allows them to handle the complexity of cancer care and provide doctors with more thorough and helpful guidance [4, 36]. Figure 8.11 illustrates how large multimodal foundation models are applied in cancer care.

These models process many data types effectively, but their outputs only help research and decision-making. These models do not replace the judgment of a clinician. Building models specifically for oncology requires careful attention to fairness, clear reasoning, and reliability [30, 36].

Figure 8.12 shows how large foundation models process different patient data, combine the information and produce guidance for research and clinical decision-making.

8.8.3 Digital twins and virtual cancer patients

A digital twin is a computer-based model of a patient [5, 30]. It uses information from the real person and acts like a mirror of their body. Doctors and scientists look at these models to understand how an illness may grow

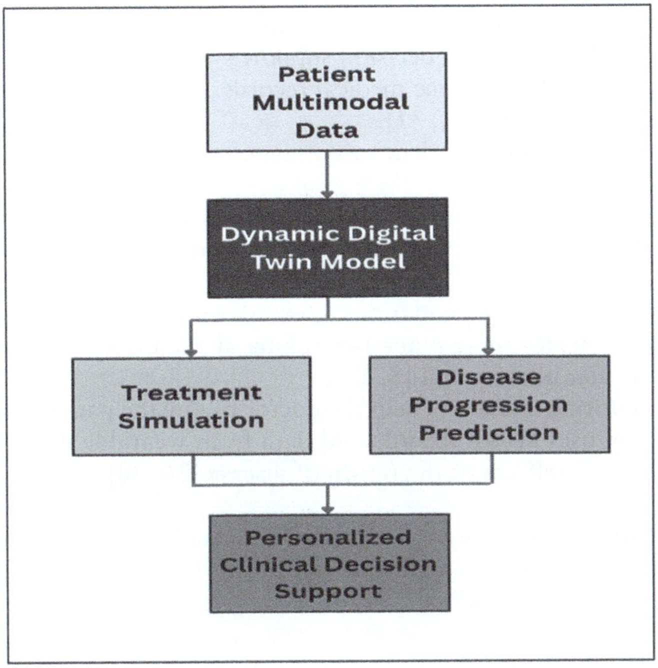

Figure 8.13 Digital twin workflow in oncology.

inside the body. They also test different treatment plans on the model first, so they can see the effect before giving the treatment to the patient [37].

The model is built from many kinds of information. Imaging, genomic data, pathology results, medical records, and even signals from wearable devices all add to it [18, 30]. When these pieces of data come together, the digital twin can give a full picture of the patient. Through such an image, physicians are able to pre-examine treatment options as well as identify issues at an earlier stage. An example is that of breast cancer. A patient with this disease can have a digital twin that can be used to test various radiation treatment regimens [38] and predict the potential reaction of the body. This concept is currently being researched in terms of lung cancer and melanoma [5, 20, 30]. Figure 8.13 shows how researchers build and use digital twins in oncology to create virtual cancer patients. Despite the advances, a digital twin cannot be easily built. The models should remain close to the actual human biology. They should also be simple enough to make them understood and relied upon by the doctors [30]. They are working on this to resolve these challenges [39].

8.8.4 Integration with clinical decision support systems

Multimodal tools should help doctors in their daily work and not add more pressure [14, 31]. A clinical decision support system (CDSS) can join multimodal insights with electronic medical records. It can then guide the doctor at the time of treatment [11, 31].

These systems support patient care in many ways:

- Risk stratification means finding patients who have a higher chance of disease. The system does this by using clinical data, genomic data, and imaging results together [1, 2].
- Treatment recommendations give advice on treatment plans. The system makes these plans by looking at the tumor features and the molecular information [8, 11].
- Monitoring and alerts help the doctor follow the patient closely. The system uses health records and data from wearable devices to warn about side effects or the return of disease [26, 30].

For doctors to trust these systems, CDSS must be clear and easy to use. They must follow accepted clinical rules. They must also protect patient safety at every step [21, 27, 30, 31, 40–42].

8.9 CONCLUSION

8.9.1 Summary of key insights

By collecting and combining data from multiple sources, such as imaging, genomics, pathology, EHRs, and wearable sensor data, doctors can get a complete idea of the patient's health. This approach provides early detection, personalized treatment, and real-time monitoring.

However, when this approach is practically used by doctors and hospitals, then some difficulties and problems arise in this process. Several issues arise, like some important data can be missed. It is difficult to understand the combined data. All this process should be done ethically, and proper rules should be followed. However, some innovations, such as federated learning, foundation models, and digital twins can help resolve difficulties. Table 8.11 shows how multimodal AI resolves the limitations of traditional methods and also highlights the challenges that are left.

8.9.2 Path forward for clinical translation

Moving multimodal AI successfully from research to practical usage in hospitals requires technology, rules, and systems that need to work well.

Table 8.11 Highlights of multimodal intelligence in oncology

Theme	*Key takeaway*
Complexity of cancer care	Cancer is genetically and clinically diverse; single-modality methods are sufficient
Advantages of multimodal AI	Improves early detection, tumor profiling, risk prediction and therapy response
Challenges and scalability	Data diversity, incomplete modalities and high computational needs are major hurdles
Ethical and legal issues	Privacy, equity and compliance (GDPR/HIPAA) are critical for patient trust
Future developments	Digital twins, federated learning, explainable AI and CDSS integration are emerging

Table 8.12 Practical approach for clinical use of multimodal AI

Strategy	*Implementation Example*
Data standardization	HL7 FHIR/DICOM for consistent data exchange across hospitals
Missing data management	Imputation models, modality-agnostic architectures
Explainability	SHAP/LIME for transparent AI decision pathways
Privacy-preserving methods	Federated learning, differential privacy, and encrypted computation
Workflow integration	Embedding AI into EMR/CDSS for real-time decision support
Continuous validation	Prospective trials and feedback-driven monitoring

Key directions include:

- To keep the data in a common format so that hospitals and systems can easily share and use the data.
- Try to reduce bias by training models on a diverse dataset and try to keep a check if any data is missing or not.
- AI should make decisions that are easy to understand so that doctors can easily get to know about.
- Try to keep the patient data safe and private.
- To test the model on big studies, to make sure that it works accurately.

Table 8.12 shows steps to safely use multimodal AI in hospitals and make it work for many patients.

In conclusion, multimodal intelligence is improving oncology by providing a framework for precise, personalized, and proactive care. Making the most of its potential and converting it into improved global patient care requires addressing present issues and rigorously evaluating new technologies.

REFERENCES

[1] Keyl, J., Keyl, P., Montavon, G., Hosch, R., Brehmer, A., Mochmann, L., Jurmeister, P., Dernbach, G., Kim, M., Koitka, S., Bauer, S., Bechrakis, N., Forsting, M., Führer-Sakel, D., Glas, M., Grünwald, V., Hadaschik, B., Haubold, J., Herrmann, K., Kasper, S., Kimmig, R., Lang, S., Rassaf, T., Roesch, A., Schadendorf, D., Siveke, J. T., Stuschke, M., Sure, U., Totzeck, M., Welt, A., Wiesweg, M., Baba, H. A., Nensa, F., Egger, J., Müller, K.-R., Schuler, M., Klauschen, F., & Kleesiek, J. (2025, January). Decoding pan-cancer treatment outcomes using multimodal real-world data and explainable artificial intelligence. *Nature Cancer*, *6*(2), 307–322, doi: 10.1038/s43018-024-00891-1.

[2] Yang, H., Yang, M., Chen, J., Yao, G., Zou, Q., & Jia, L. (2024, November). Multimodal deep learning approaches for precision oncology: a comprehensive review. *Briefings in Bioinformatics*, *26*(1), bbae699, doi: 10.1093/bib/bbae699.

[3] Van Vugt, M. A. T. M., & Parkes, E. E. (2022, March). When breaks get hot: inflammatory signaling in BRCA1/2-mutant cancers. *Trends Cancer*, *8*(3), 174–189, doi: 10.1016/j.trecan.2021.12.003.

[4] Yates, J., & Van Allen, E. M. (2025, April). New horizons at the interface of artificial intelligence and translational cancer research. *Cancer Cell*, *43*(4), 708–727, doi: 10.1016/j.ccell.2025.03.018.

[5] Waqas, A., Tripathi, A., Ramachandran, R. P., Stewart, P. A., & Rasool, G. (2024, July). Multimodal data integration for oncology in the era of deep neural networks: a review. *Frontiers in Artificial Intelligence*, *7*, 1408843, doi: 10.3389/frai.2024.1408843.

[6] Park, D. *et al.* (2025, May). Multimodal AI model for preoperative prediction of axillary lymph node metastasis in breast cancer using whole slide images. *Npj Precision Onco*logy, *9*(1), 131, doi: 10.1038/s41698-025-00914-9.

[7] Cui, C. *et al.* (2023, April). Deep multimodal fusion of image and non-image data in disease diagnosis and prognosis: a review. *Progress Biomedical Engineering*, *5*(2), 022001, doi: 10.1088/2516-1091/acc2fe.

[8] Kline, A., Wang, H., Li, Y., Dennis, S., Hutch, M., Xu, Z.,... & Luo, Y. (2022). Multimodal machine learning in precision health: a scoping review. *NPJ Digital Medicine*, *5*(1), 171

[9] Wang, Z. *et al.* (2024, May). Deep learning-based multi-modal data integration enhancing breast cancer disease-free survival prediction. *Precision Clinical Medicine*, *7*(2), pbae012, doi: 10.1093/pcmedi/pbae012.

[10] Gao, P. *et al.* (2024, December). Interpretable multi-modal artificial intelligence model for predicting gastric cancer response to neoadjuvant chemotherapy. *Cell Reports Medicine*, *5*(12), 101848, doi: 10.1016/j.xcrm.2024.101848.

[11] Xu, P., Zhu, X., & Clifton, D. A. (2023, October). Multimodal learning with transformers: a survey. *IEEE Transactions on Pattern Analysis and Machine Intelligence*, *45*(10), 12113–12132, doi: 10.1109/TPAMI.2023.3275156.

[12] Vaswani, A., Shazeer, N., Parmar, N., Uszkoreit, J., Jones, L., Gomez, A. N.,... & Polosukhin, I. (2017). Attention is all you need. *Advances in Neural Information Processing Systems*, *30*, 6000–6010.

[13] Lee, J., Yoon, W., Kim, S., Kim, D., Kim, S., So, C. H., & Kang, J. (2020). BioBERT: a pre-trained biomedical language representation model for biomedical text mining. *Bioinformatics*, *36*(4), 1234–1240.

[14] Zhou, J., Cui, G., Hu, S., Zhang, Z., Yang, C., Liu, Z.,... & Sun, M. (2020). Graph neural networks: a review of methods and applications. *AI Open*, *1*, 57–81.

[15] Chen, R. J., Lu, M. Y., Chen, T. Y., Williamson, D. F., & Mahmood, F. (2021). Synthetic data in machine learning for medicine and healthcare. *Nature Biomedical Engineering*, *5*(6), 493–497.

[16] Xia, Y., Zhou, J., Xun, X., Zhang, J., Wei, T., Gao, R.,... & Yu, Z. (2024). CT-based multimodal deep learning for non-invasive overall survival prediction in advanced hepatocellular carcinoma patients treated with immunotherapy. *Insights into Imaging*, *15*(1), 214.

[17] Singhal, A., Agrawal, K. K., Quezada, A., Aguiñaga, A. R., Jiménez, S., & Yadav, S. P. (2024). Explainable artificial intelligence (XAI) model for cancer image classification. *CMES-Computer Modeling in Engineering & Sciences*, *141*(1), 401–441.

[18] Siam, A., Alsaify, A. R., Mohammad, B., Biswas, M. R., Ali, H., & Shah, Z. (2023). Multimodal deep learning for liver cancer applications: a scoping review. *Frontiers in Artificial Intelligence*, *6*, 1247195.

[19] Tian, Y., Xu, Z., Ma, Y., Ding, W., Wang, R., Gao, Z.,... & Zhao, X. (2023). Survey on deep learning in multimodal medical imaging for cancer detection. *Neural Computing and Applications*, *37*, 1–16.

[20] Baltrusaitis, T., Ahuja, C., & Morency, L.-P. (2019, February). Multimodal machine learning: a survey and taxonomy. *IEEE Transactions on Pattern Analysis and Machine Intelligence*, *41*(2), 423–443, doi: 10.1109/TPAMI.2018.2798607.

[21] Wagner, J., Oldenburg, J., Nath, N., & Simm, S. (2025). Explainable AI model reveals informative mutational signatures for cancer-type classification. *Cancers*, *17*(11), 1731.

[22] Rosen-Zvi, M., Mullen, L., Lukas, R. J., Guindy, M., & Gabrani, M. (2023). Explainable multimodal AI in cancer patient care: how can we reduce the gap between technology and practice? *Frontiers in Medicine*, *10*, 1190429.

[23] Tabakhi, S., & Lu, H. (2025). Missing-modality-aware graph neural network for cancer classification. *arXiv preprint arXiv:2506.22901*.

[24] Aresta, G., Araújo, T., Kwok, S., Chennamsetty, S. S., Safwan, M., Alex, V.,... & Aguiar, P. (2019). Bach: grand challenge on breast cancer histology images. *Medical Image Analysis*, *56*, 122–139.

[25] Shukla, S., Rajkumar, S., Sinha, A., Esha, M., Elango, K., & Sampath, V. (2025). Federated learning with differential privacy for breast cancer

diagnosis enabling secure data sharing and model integrity. *Scientific Reports*, *15*(1), 13061.

[26] Kaissis, G. A., Makowski, M. R., Rückert, D., & Braren, R. F. (2020). Secure, privacy-preserving and federated machine learning in medical imaging. *Nature Machine Intelligence*, *2*(6), 305–311.

[27] Oh, Y., Park, S., Byun, H. K., Cho, Y., Lee, I. J., Kim, J. S., & Ye, J. C. (2024). LLM-driven multimodal target volume contouring in radiation oncology. *Nature Communications*, *15*(1), 9186.

[28] Waqas, A., Tripathi, A., Ramachandran, R. P., Stewart, P. A., & Rasool, G. (2024). Multimodal data integration for oncology in the era of deep neural networks: a review. *Frontiers in Artificial Intelligence*, *7*, 1408843.

[29] Wang, X., Zhang, X., Wang, G., He, J., Li, Z., Zhu, W.,... & Zhang, S. (2024). OpenMEDLab: an open-source platform for multi-modality foundation models in medicine. *arXiv preprint arXiv:2402.18028*.

[30] Chowdhury, A., Kassem, H., Padoy, N., Umeton, R., & Karargyris, A. (2021, September). A review of medical federated learning: Applications in oncology and cancer research. In *International MICCAI Brainlesion Workshop* (pp. 3–24). Cham: Springer International Publishing.

[31] Naveen Kumar, G. S., & Reddy, V. S. K., 2022. High performance algorithm for content-based video retrieval using multiple features. In *Intelligent Systems and Sustainable Computing: Proceedings of ICISSC 2021* (pp. 637–646). Singapore: Springer Nature Singapore.

[32] GS, N. K., Chinni, P. B. M. R., Abdul, A. B., Silamanthula, H. K., Shaik, J., & Kakumanu, V. N. (2024). Neurosynthetics: adaptive dynamic risk factor integration network architecture for cardiac risk prediction. *Telecommunications and Radio Engineering, 84*(3), 27–41.

[33] Naveen Kumar, G. S., Venkateswara Reddy, E., Siva Naga Dhipti, G., & Swathi, B. (2022, June). An Effective Automatic Facial Expression Recognition System Using Deep Neural Networks. In *International Conference on Soft Computing and Signal Processing* (pp. 665–674). Singapore: Springer Nature Singapore.

[34] Naveen Kumar, G. S., & Reddy, V. S. K. (2019). Key frame extraction using rough set theory for video retrieval. In *Soft Computing and Signal Processing: Proceedings of ICSCSP 2018, Volume 2* (pp. 751–757). Singapore: Springer Singapore.

[35] Tan, T., Rodriguez-Ruiz, A., Zhang, T., Xu, L., Beets-Tan, R. G., Shen, Y.,... & Bao, L. (2023). Multi-modal artificial intelligence for the combination of automated 3D breast ultrasound and mammograms in a population of women with predominantly dense breasts. *Insights into Imaging*, *14*(1), 10.

[36] Pham, T. (2025). Ethical and legal considerations in healthcare AI: innovation and policy for safe and fair use. *Royal Society Open Science*, *12*(5), 241873.

[37] Kumar, G. N., Reddy, V. S. K., & Srinivas Kumar, S. (2018, July). Video shot boundary detection and key frame extraction for video retrieval. In *Proceedings of the Second International Conference on Computational Intelligence and Informatics: ICCII 2017* (pp. 557–567). Singapore: Springer Singapore.

[38] Reddy, P. S., Kumar, G. N., Ritish, B., SaiSwetha, C., & Abhilash, K. B. (2013). Intelligent parking space detection system based on image segmentation. *International Journal of Scientific Development and Research*, *1*(6), 1310–1312.

[39] Ortiz, V. *et al.* (2024). Data preprocessing techniques for AI and machine learning readiness: scoping review of wearable sensor data in cancer care. *JMIR Mhealth Uhealth*, *12*, e59587. https://mhealth.jmir.org/2024/1/e59587

[40] Naveen Kumar, G. S., & Reddy, V. S. K. (2019, June). Extraction of key frames using rough set theory for video retrieval. In *International Conference on Soft Computing and Signal Processing* (pp. 761–768). Singapore: Springer Singapore.

[41] Naveen Kumar, G. S., & Reddy, V. S. K. (2020). Detection of shot boundaries and extraction of key frames for video retrieval. *International Journal of Knowledge-based and Intelligent Engineering Systems*, 24(1), 11–17.

[42] Srinivasa Naveen Kumar, G., Reddy, V. S. K., & Balivada, L. K., 2022, December. Content-Based Video Retrieval Using Deep Learning Algorithms. In *International Conference on Intelligent Systems and Sustainable Computing* (pp. 557–568). Singapore: Springer Nature Singapore.

Chapter 9

Generative multimodal framework for adaptive therapeutic game content in digital health applications

Veera Venkata Siva Prasad Balusupati, Raja Sekhar Reddy Pocha, Srilatha Pulipati, and Sarma K. S. R. K.

9.1 INTRODUCTION

Generative multimodal AI is the next wave in artificial intelligence, and one of the systems will be capable of perceiving and creating content in multiple data forms (text, pictures, audio, video, and sensor data) in a cohesive architecture. In contrast to the old unimodal systems that pay attention to one modality, multimodal AI learns common representations, which enable it to perceive and produce complex and real-world information in a better way (Buess et al., 2025). It can produce coherent and context-sensitive outputs, including (but not limited to) generating images given textual prompts, creating narratives given visual input, or generating audio-visual experiences that are synchronized: powered by models such as large language models, transformers, and diffusion architecture. This ability has allowed adaptive, immersive, and personalised applications in the fields of healthcare, education, gaming, and human–computer interaction (El Saddik et al., 2025). Multimodal AI that generates content is also generative, which increases reasoning, cross-modal retrieval, and creative generation of content, thus making the interaction more natural and intelligent (Naga Ramesh et al., 2025). With the development of the field, it will be essential to work on such aspects as the alignment of data, bias, and ethical issues to make the use of such powerful technologies responsible and effective (Qu et al., 2024).

The drive behind the incorporation of generative multimodal AI into diversified applications is that it can be used to combine and capitalize on a variety of data modalities to develop more richer, more adaptive, and context-aware solutions (El Saddik et al., 2025; Dastagiraiah et al., 2024). The real world has many complexities in terms of interactions between text, visuals, audio, and sensor information and traditional systems that are unimodal cannot fully represent such phenomena. Generative multimodal AI increases understanding and decision-making, and facilitates seamless cross-modal interactions by means of modalities combination (Kumar et al., 2024; Rani et al., 2024). It can create personalized therapeutic content in

DOI: 10.1201/9781003665656-9

healthcare, simulate the process of immersive and interactive learning in education, and spur the creation of dynamic content in the gaming and entertainment industries, and predictive modeling and automation in industry (Karthiga et al., 2025). The integration enables systems to implement intelligent changes according to the needs of various users and their environments, which promotes innovation in sectors. Additionally, it provides avenues to creative content creation, cross-domain knowledge transfer, and enhanced human–AI interaction, which creates more user-friendly applications that are effective and efficient.

9.1.1 Role of generative multimodal AI in digital health

Digital health is being revolutionized with generative multimodal AI that will combine and interpret various types of data like medical imaging, electronic health records, physiological sensor data, genomic data, and patient speech or text input to offer more comprehensive, adaptive, and intelligent healthcare solutions (Rahman & Al-Hazzaa, 2024). Compared to unimodal system, it is capable of integrating visual, textual, and physiological cues to produce more rich and context-sensitive outputs to produce better diagnostics, customized interventions, and increased engagement with the patient (S. Rani et al., 2024).

Generative multimodal models may be used in clinical practice to synthesize realistic medical data to train diagnostic algorithms, to simulate complicated patient scenarios in medical education, and to aid clinical decision-making by accurately and multimodally reasoning. In therapy, such models have the ability to produce adaptive content like custom rehabilitation exercises or custom therapeutic games that dynamically react to the progress and emotional condition of a patient (Kaur et al., 2025; K. P. Rani, G. Roja, et al., 2024).

In addition, generative multimodal AI can be used to fill data gaps, making heterogeneous health systems interoperable, and create synthetic but privacy-preserving data to conduct research and develop models. It also helps with the timely and more accurate detection of disease by the combination of speech, imaging, and biometrics, which helps detect disease at an earlier stage. In general, its integrating and generative potential allows changing the inert and monolithic digital health solutions to smart, adaptive, and patient-centric healthcare systems (Ghebrehiwet et al., 2024).

9.1.2 Objectives and scope

This chapter of the book is aimed at discussing the development and use of generative multimodal artificial intelligence models to generate adaptive therapeutic game content based on the needs of individual patients in the field of digital health. It also seeks to explore how the combination of modalities, including speech, vision, physiological data, and clinical records can improve personalization, engagement, and outcomes of the therapy. The areas involved in the scope are the examination of existing multimodal generative methods, framework architectures, strategies of adaptive game design and clinical integration, privacy of data, and real-time responsiveness. Also, it discusses issues and the future in the implementation of such intelligent systems in various health care settings (Srinivasa et al., 2022).

9.2 THERAPEUTIC GAME DESIGN AND MULTIMODAL DATA

Therapeutic game design leverages multimodal data such as physiological signals, motion tracking, speech, and clinical records to create personalized, adaptive, and engaging interventions. By integrating diverse data streams, these games dynamically adjust difficulty, feedback, and content to match patient needs, enhancing rehabilitation effectiveness, motivation, and real-time therapeutic responsiveness (Mader et al., 2016).

9.2.1 Principles of therapeutic game design

The principles of therapeutic game design focus on creating engaging, effective, and safe interventions for health improvement. Key principles include (Rodrigues et al., 2018):

- **Personalization** – Tailoring game mechanics and content to individual patient needs, abilities, and progress.
- **Adaptivity** – Dynamically adjusting difficulty and challenges based on real-time performance and feedback.
- **Engagement and Motivation** – Incorporating rewards, storytelling, and interactive elements to sustain participation.
- **Clinical Relevance** – Aligning gameplay tasks with therapeutic goals and evidence-based practices.
- **Multimodal Data Integration** – Using inputs like physiological signals, motion tracking, and cognitive assessments to guide interventions.
- **Accessibility** – Designing for diverse ages, abilities, and cognitive or physical limitations.
- **Feedback and Reinforcement** – Providing immediate, meaningful feedback to support learning and improvement.
- **Safety and Ethics** – Ensuring patient privacy, data security, and ethical deployment in healthcare contexts.

These principles collectively ensure that therapeutic games are not only engaging but also effective and clinically meaningful.

9.2.2 Personalization and adaptivity in health contexts

Personalization in digital health refers to the process of customizing interventions, therapies, or content based on unique attributes of an individual, including age, medical history, cognitive or physical capabilities, and preferences. This will make healthcare solutions relevant, effective, and patient-centered.

Adaptivity means the capacity of the system to change its behavior or contents dynamically in real-time depending on patient responses, performance, or physiological responses. As an illustration, adaptive therapeutic games have the ability to change the difficulty, pace, or feedback based on the level of progress or fatigue that a user may have (Dastagiraiah, 2024; Grua et al., 2022).

A combination of personalization and adaptivity increases the level of engagement, facilitates treatment outcomes, and provides care that is patient-centric. Digital health applications can deliver responsive, continuous, and optimized interventions to assist patients in rehabilitation, managing diseases, and preventive care by using patient-specific information and smart algorithms.

9.2.3 Types of multimodal data

Figure 9.1 illustrates that multimodal data in digital health combines various sources to have a comprehensive perspective of patient health to tailor and responsive interventions. Signals that are emitted by physiology like heart rate, blood pressure, EEG, EMG, and oxygen saturation give information about the real-time state of the body. Medical imaging MRI, CT, X-ray, and ultrasound can provide both structural and functional data that is essential in diagnosis and follow-up. Electronic health records, clinical notes, prescriptions, and patient-reported outcomes provide textual

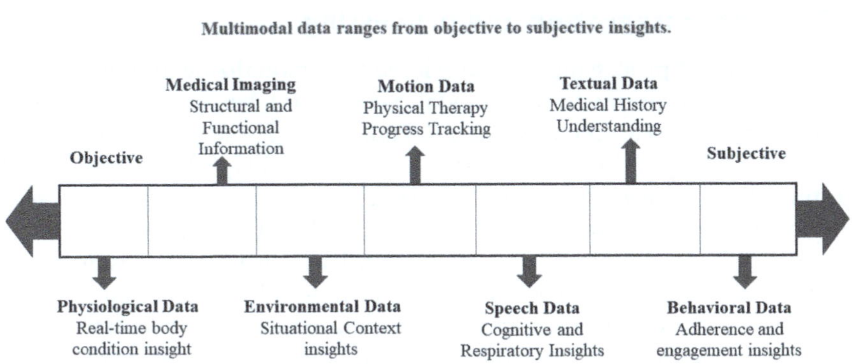

Figure 9.1 Multimodal data in digital health.

Table 9.1 Multimodal data, sources, and applications in digital health

Data type	*Source/example*	*Application*	*Purpose/benefit*
Physiological data	Heart rate, EEG, EMG, blood pressure	Stress monitoring, biofeedback, rehabilitation	Tracks physical or emotional states for adaptive interventions
Behavioral data	Gameplay actions, response times, choices	Cognitive training, engagement tracking	Assesses performance and adapts difficulty or content
Visual/motion data	Facial expressions, body movements, gestures	Physical therapy, emotion recognition	Supports motor skill training and emotional state detection
Audio/voice data	Speech, tone, verbal responses	Mental health monitoring, cognitive exercises	Detects emotional states, provides feedback or guidance

information that adds value to the comprehension of medical history and patient treatment. Voice, respiratory sounds, and verbal reactions are captured under speech and audio data, and they are helpful in both mental and respiratory testing. Accelerator, gyroscopes, and motion capture devices record motion and gesture information used to monitor physical therapy development and mobility (Cai et al., 2019). Situational data includes environmental and contextual data including ambient sensors and location tracking. Finally, adherence, engagement, and therapeutic effectiveness are informed by behavioral data, such as interaction patterns and game performance (Dastagiraiah & Reddy, 2022; Sudhakar et al., 2024). The combination of these modalities will allow providing all-encompassing, dynamic and patient-centred health solutions (Chaabene et al., 2025).

Various types of multimodal data, along with sources and applications, are summarized in Table 9.1.

9.2.4 Data integration and processing

Integration and processing of data related to personalizing and dynamically adjusting interventions to multimodal patient data are essential in adaptive therapeutic games as demonstrated in Figure 9.2. These games amass a variety of inputs (physiological signals heart rate, EEG, EMG), motion and gesture data, speech, behavioral metrics, and contextual data of sensors or gameplay interactions (Abdullah et al., 2023). Preprocessing is used to remove noise and normalize scales as well as ensuring consistency, and aligning data over time to allow it to be meaningfully interpreted.

The feature extraction processes raw data into descriptive actions, like accuracy of movement, exhaustion, or patterns of engagement. Fusion methods bring together these properties to form a comprehensive picture

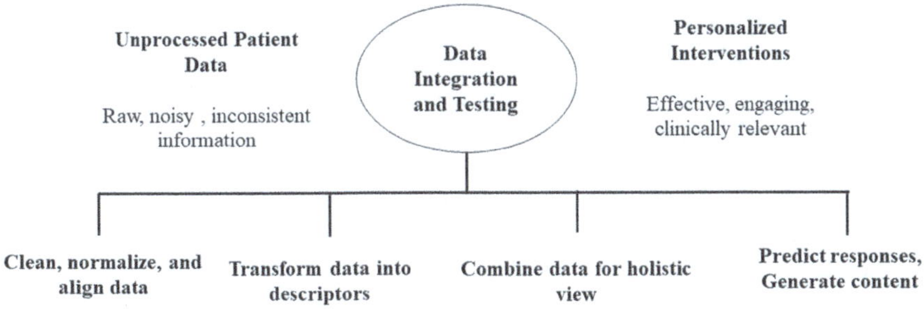

Figure 9.2 Data integration and preprocessing for adaptive therapeutic games.

of the condition of the patient: early fusion combines raw streams, intermediate fusion combines extracted features, and late fusion combines model outputs. Generative multimodal AI also improves processing by learning cross-modal associations and patient responses, as well as creating game contents that are adaptive to therapeutic goals (Zhan et al., 2023).

By means of effective integration and processing, therapeutic games may change dynamically in terms of difficulty, feedback, or exercise patterns, and they can accurately track progress. This will make interventions personalized, engaging, and clinically effective to make the rehabilitation outcome as well as patient motivation as high as possible.

9.3 GENERATIVE FRAMEWORK AND ADAPTIVE CONTENT

The adaptive therapeutic game based on the generative multimodal framework allows the development of tailored and dynamic content through the combination of various sources of patient data (Rani et al., 2024). This model takes physiological indicators, movement data, speech, behavioral measurements, and clinical history to make sense of the present physical and mental condition of the patient. With the assistance of generative AI models, the system can create new game conditions, exercises, or feedback that match the capabilities of the patient and his or her therapeutic requirements (Balaraju et al., 2024; Núñez V et al., 2025).

The adaptive content is created on the fly, and difficulty, pacing, and rewards are modified according to the level of performance, engagement, and fatigue. For example, when a patient has a specific motor task that he or she cannot cope with, the game can make the task easier, or may offer more feedback with the progressively more difficult task being given as the progress occurs. The strategy makes therapeutic interventions individualized, inspiring, and successful. In general, the generative framework adds to patient engagement, facilitates persistent monitoring, and provides adaptive therapy based on data in the context of digital health applications.

9.3.1 System architecture

The system architecture has a main orchestration engine that controls the flow of data and commands among various modules. These modules have their assigned tasks, including user profiling, content generation, adaptation logic, and game engine integration (Rahman & Al-Hazzaa, 2024). The architecture allows input of multimodes such as user behavior, physiological, and self-report information to give a complete picture of the user condition as depicted by Figure 9.3.

The architectural system includes the following major elements:

- **User Profiling Module:** This module is charged with the task of creating and maintaining user profiles depending on a number of sources of data. It gathers and processes user information such as demographics, medical history, behavioral patterns, and performance in the games. The module uses machine learning to determine groups of users and forecasts on a case-by-case basis individual needs and preferences.
- **Content Generation Module:** The content generation module is based on generative AI models to generate game content, including narratives, characters, challenges, and rewards. It uses natural language processing (NLP) and computer vision to create interesting and meaningful information that is relevant to the profile of the user and therapeutic outcomes.

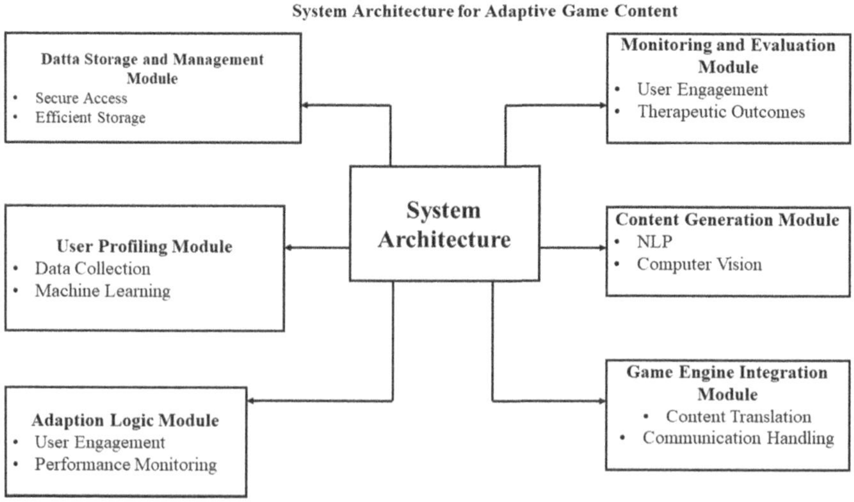

Figure 9.3 System architecture. Adaptive game content for multimodal healthcare data.

- **Adaptation Logic Module:** This module is a module that applies the rules and algorithms that control how the content of the games adapts according to user feedback and performance. It also tracks engagement, progress, and emotional response of the user to dynamically modify the complexity, speed, and content of the game.
- **Game Engine Integration Module:** This component gives an interface between the generative framework and the game engine. It converts the content and adaptation instructions generated into game-specific commands and events. It is also involved in the communication of the game engine with the other modules of the framework.
- **Data Storage and Management Module:** The module handles the storage and management of all the information in the system such as user profiles, game content, adaptation rules, and performance measurements. It offers safe and effective accessibility to information across modules in the framework.
- **Monitoring and Evaluation Module:** This module is a continuous monitor of the system performance and measures how effective the produced content and methods of adapting to changes are. It gathers user engagement, therapeutic results, and efficiency of a system to determine the areas that need improvement.

9.3.2 Generative models for game content

Transformative generative models are used to generate dynamic and personalized game content in digital health applications. These models can be used to produce adaptive game scenarios, narratives, and interactive content, autonomously, using methods like generative adversarial networks (GANs), variational autoencoders (VAEs) and transformer-based models, to meet therapeutic objectives. This type of content creation allows personalization in real time, making changes to the difficulty, feedback, and visual or audio stimuli depending on the user data and progress. Such flexibility improves involvement and retention of the user, as well as fostering personalized treatment processes. In rehabilitation games, generative models can be used to adapt movement-based tasks to the motor capabilities of the patient, whereas in mental health they can be used to dynamically create supportive environments or stories to control emotion. Designing health-oriented games with the inclusion of generative AI, the developers will be able to make them immersive, flexible, and clinically meaningful, surpassing tangible content, and deliver greater therapeutic value and patient outcomes (Avanaki et al., 2020).

9.3.3 Adaptive feedback and real-time personalization

One of the factors contributing to the effectiveness of digital health games is adaptive feedback, as well as real-time personalization. Adaptive feedback, also known as dynamic adjusting of responses in the game, e.g. visualization, rewards, or the game difficulty, is based on the behavior and performance of the user and physiological or emotional conditions. Real-time personalization uses real-time streams of data, such as sensor readings, gameplay statistics, and user profile data, to adjust gameplay and content to a specific person in real time. It is a strategy where the difficulty of therapeutic tasks is not overwhelmingly high, but at the same time is not so low as to disengage the user and demotivate them. Rehabilitation games may also serve as an example, with difficulty increasing or decreasing in response to the motor ability of a patient, and mental health applications may also adapt environments or tones of feedback in response to mood. Using AI-based models and adaptive algorithms, digital health games are able to provide highly responsive, personal experiences in order to promote a variety of therapeutic objectives. This eventually results in meaningful interaction, lifelong engagement, and better clinical outcomes among users (Jimenez et al., 2023).

9.3.4 Privacy, ethics, and security considerations

The design and implementation of generative and adaptive game content in digital health applications is the most important when it comes to privacy, ethics, and security. This is because often these systems handle sensitive personal, behavioral, and physiological data that needs to be well safeguarded in terms of privacy. Ethical considerations encompass making sure that there is an informed consent, transparency in the use of data and to make sure that game designs are not manipulative or biased towards a negative effect on the users. To avoid the unauthorized use or breach, security mechanisms, including encryption, secure authentication, and controlled data access, are required. Also, the generative models need to be supervised to prevent the creation of inappropriate, harmful, or misleading content, especially among vulnerable groups, such as children or patients undergoing therapy. Regulatory frameworks such as GDPR or HIPAA are supposed to be followed by the developers, privacy-saving mechanisms, such as anonymization or federated learning, are expected to be utilized, and regular audits are to be conducted to sustain trust. A holistic approach to these issues will make digital health games safe, ethical, and respectful of user rights and will provide them with therapeutic advantages (Shafik, 2025).

9.4 APPLICATIONS AND EVALUATION

Examples of generative game-based content applications in digital health are rehabilitation, cognitive, mental health, and personalized therapy, as shown in Table 9.2. The process of evaluation includes the evaluation of clinical effectiveness, user engagement, adaptability, and data security using user

Table 9.2 Summarization of the applications of generative game content in digital health

Application area	*Purpose*	*Example*
Mental health	Stress reduction, anxiety, and depression management	Games that generate calming environments and supportive narratives
Cognitive therapy	Memory, attention, and problem-solving improvement	Adaptive tasks that adjust difficulty based on performance
Physical rehabilitation	Motor skills training, mobility, and strength	Movement-based games that personalize exercises to patient ability

studies, performance metrics, and standardized health outcomes (Shafik, 2025). Strict validation will provide reliability, ethical conformance, and significant therapeutic effect.

9.4.1 Mental health and cognitive therapy

Content of the generative games can be useful when it comes to the mental health and cognitive therapy because, in this case, therapeutic experiences can be customized and tailored. Games may also be designed to support the user in scenarios that cause stress, anxiety, and depression by creating calming environments and supportive narratives and focus on emotion and interaction. In the case of cognitive therapy, the generative models are able to generate and adapt to the users performance real-time tasks, which induce training and development of problem-solving, attention, and memory. This is the adjustment in tasks in real-time to concentrate on goals, which assist in motivating and provide effective therapeutic results. In addition to this, games can be modified to give feedback throughout a session, feedback on progress, and individual goals on outcomes and objectives. By embedding the clinical methods modified with the generative technologies, digital health games will offer users a valuable tool in the form of a portable and versatile product that offers cognitive and mental health benefits to the user.

9.4.2 Physical rehabilitation and motor skills training

The creation of self-generating content game tech can assist in motor skill development and physical rehabilitation. These interactive exercises can be tailored to each individual's capacity and progressively increase in challenge as the patient's strength or mobility improves. For instance, sensor-based movement capture games can adjust the range and difficulty of the movement to match the player, thus gamifying the physical rehabilitation process. This increases the enjoyment of the activities and thus the motivation of the rehabilitation patients to engage in their exercises daily, which is crucial in the healing process.

Such systems can enhance the effectiveness of therapy and rehabilitation by automatically adjusting varying exercises to avoid monotony and tediousness. The integration of fun gameplay that adapts to a patient's rehabilitation progress makes the process of physical rehabilitation more convenient and achievable.

9.4.3 Evaluation metrics and validation methods

Researchers evaluate the effectiveness and safety of health-related generative technology games using various methodologies. They evaluate user engagement metrics, task completion rates, adaptability, and accuracy of personalizations, and symptom or functional improvements attributable to the games.

Self-reported and system use metrics inform user experience assessments. Health goal attainment is ascertained through clinical validation, including controlled clinical trials and small pilot studies. Further, analyses of risk to user data, ethics, and privacy oversight provide evidence of compliance with data protection laws and user data privacy. Through the amalgamation of quantitative, qualitative, and clinical feedback, developers assess the efficacy of the system. This ensures that these health games are enjoyable and effective in real-world healthcare.

9.4.4 Clinical and user-centered assessments

Evaluating how generative game content functions in real healthcare contexts requires performing both clinical and user-centered assessments. Clinical evaluations determine the therapy's effectiveness through medical and psychological assessments, such as whether patients experience symptom relief, gain function in daily activities, or improve during recovery. Clinical evaluations are usually described in clinical trials, small pilot projects, or expert opinion files (Kumar & Reddy, 2019; Kumar & Reddy, 2022).

User-centered assessments, in contrast, concentrate on the players' feelings and interactions with the game. They evaluate aspects such as ease of use, enjoyment, motivation, and overall user satisfaction. To assess the experience of the user, researchers may conduct surveys, perform interviews, or analyze player activity from logging tools (GS et al., 2024).

Integrating both evaluations allows developers to guarantee that the technology is clinically useful and that the other aspects are psychologically engaging, motivating, and appropriate for human use. Such a duality is crucial for the adoption and effectiveness of tools of digital health.

9.5 CHALLENGES AND FUTURE DIRECTIONS

Although the current state of affairs has come a long way, certain aspects of creating generative multimodal frameworks of the clinical game contents need to be addressed (El Saddik et al., 2025). Ensuring privacy of the data, clinical accuracy, handling the real-time personalization, and monitoring therapeutic outcomes are some of the most important issues. Future trends are aimed to incorporate the latest AI, ethical safeguards, and interprofessional cooperation so as to increase efficacy and scalability.

9.5.1 Technical and clinical challenges

It is not easy to make smart computer models to develop therapeutic computer games. Many technical and medical problems should be addressed. These models consume a lot of computing power and specialized skills as they must be able to handle an array of different types of data, such as images, audio, text, and sensor signals. The system is not well-positioned to comply with changes instantaneously. It should also be able to act swiftly in matters related to user behavior, physical indicators, and performance levels among other things and keep the game running smoothly.

Another serious issue is to add those intelligent models to cases where they are safe, and on the other hand, they should protect the privacy of people. Moreover, it is difficult to design a game that could be fun to play and at the same time helpful in therapy. It is critical to have the right balance between the goals and fun in games in relation to fitness. Medically, establishing whether such games are helpful or not is a wall since every patient is different. Their responses may depend on their age, wellness, and the degree of motivation. We must make sure that these therapy games are safe and do not violate certain rules.

It is also difficult to measure the results that will be consistent in different forms of treatment, including both mental and physical health. To be accepted by doctors, such games have to undergo extensive tests and evaluation, which is a lengthy and cumbersome process. We need to solve all these problems to develop digital therapy games that people can trust and consider easy to use.

9.5.2 Scalability and integration with health ecosystems

To be effective in digital healthcare, generative multimodal systems must be capable of expanding and collaborating effectively with the existing health systems. Scalability refers to ensuring the ability of adaptive therapeutic games to assist a significant number of people without compromising quality, personalization, or safety. This is possible through cloud-based systems, machine-intensive AI systems, and effective data systems capable of producing content on demand and monitoring users.

These tools have to be readily interconnected with electronic health records (EHRs), wearable devices, telemedicine services, and clinical support tools to fit into medical systems. It is thanks to this connection that individual care could be offered based on the most recent medical information. Physicians have an opportunity to trace the progress of patients, modify treatments, and ensure continuity of care.

The reliance on the standard data format, secure APIs, and adherence to healthcare regulations such as HIPAA and GDPR are the items that contribute to trust and data safety. When the issues of scaling up and integrating with other systems are resolved using digital health games, these games can become more than stand-alone applications and become integral components of the treatment. This will ease their usage, enhance their usefulness, and durability in most medical institutions.

9.5.3 Emerging research opportunities

The possibilities of how we can make use of generative AI to improve therapy games are exciting and offer new opportunities to explore. One of the aims is to develop AI models, which comprehend how individuals act, how they feel, and what type of treatment they require to make the games instantly adjust to an individual. Through various forms of information, such as body language, facial expression, tone, and ability of an individual to play, the games can be made more precise, interesting, and helpful. An additional prospective concept is to introduce virtual reality (VR) and augmented reality (AR) and create immersive worlds that will adapt to the skills and progress of the player. Ethics and privacy should also be carefully considered by the researchers, who should ensure that the games are fair to all, that personal data is secure, and that the process of how the content is created is also described.

It will be significant to conduct long-term clinical trials to test the effectiveness of such systems and their safety among various types of persons. Through collaboration, AI experts, medical practitioners, game developers, and patients can develop more accessible, more customized, and more effective therapy games in most types of treatments.

9.5.4 Concluding remarks

The development of generative multimodal adaptive therapeutic game content is a good indication of the future of artificial intelligence, game development, and digital health. Such systems generate dynamic content that varies according to the needs of the individual user and his or her therapeutic objectives, which makes it possible to deliver personalised content, dynamic, and clinically relevant interventions. They can be used in the treatment of mentally ill individuals, cognitive training, physical rehabilitation, and other forms of therapy. They provide the users with dynamic and compelling experiences. Although the potential is high, the issues related to such aspects as real-time personalization, clinical validation, data privacy, ethical compliance and seamless integration with healthcare ecosystems still exist. The solution to these issues is to collaborate across disciplines with the help of AI researchers, doctors, game designers, and policymakers. Digital health games can be more effective, accessible, and scalable by focusing research in the future on advanced AI models, immersive experiences, high-quality evaluation, and other ethical considerations. Overall, generative systems can do much to transform therapeutic interventions and make healthcare more interactive, personalized, and patient-centred.

REFERENCES

Abdullah, Z. H., Ismail, W., Zakaria, L. Q., Ismail, S., & Abdullah, A. (2022). Classification of Exercise Game Data for Rehabilitation Using Machine Learning Algorithms. In Wah, Y.B., Berry, M.W., Mohamed, A., Al-Jumeily, D. (eds) *Data Science and Emerging Technologies*. DaSET 2022. Lecture Notes on Data Engineering and Communications Technologies, vol 165. Springer, Singapore. https://doi.org/10.1007/978-981-99-0741-0_21

Avanaki, N. J., Zadtootaghaj, S., Barman, N., Schmidt, S., Martini, M. G., & Möller, S. (2020). Quality Enhancement of Gaming Content using Generative Adversarial Networks. In *2020 Twelfth International Conference on Quality of Multimedia Experience (QoMEX)*, Athlone, Ireland, IEEE, pp. 1-6, doi: 10.1109/QoMEX48832.2020.9123074.

Balaraju, J., Kumar, A. V., & Dastagiraiah, C. (2024). Ethereum Blockchain-Based KYC Verification. In Reddy, V.S., Prasad, V.K., Wang, J., Rao Dasari, N.M. (eds) *Intelligent Systems and Sustainable Computing*. ICISSC 2024. Smart Innovation, Systems and Technologies, vol 417. Springer, Singapore. https://doi.org/10.1007/978-981-97-8355-7_30

Buess, L., Keicher, M., Navab, N., Maier, A., & Tayebi Arasteh, S. (2025). From Large Language Models to Multimodal AI: A Scoping Review on the Potential of Generative AI in Medicine. *Biomedical Engineering Letters*, 15, 1–19.

Cai, Q., Wang, H., Li, Z., & Liu, X. (2019). A Survey on Multimodal Data-Driven Smart Healthcare Systems: Approaches and Applications. *IEEE Access*, 7, 133583–133599.

Chaabene, S., Boudaya, A., Bouaziz, B., & Chaari, L. (2025). An Overview of Methods and Techniques in Multimodal Data Fusion with Application to Healthcare. *International Journal of Data Science and Analytics*, *20*, 3093–3117. https://doi.org/10.1007/s41060-025-00715-0.

Dastagiraiah, C., & Reddy, V. K. (2022). Novel Machine Learning Methodology in Resource Provisioning for Forecasting of Workload in Distributed Cloud Environment. *Journal of Theoretical and Applied Information Technology*, *100*(10), 3319–3327.

Dastagiraiah, C., Reddy, V. K., Rani, K. P., & Veeranna, T. (2024). Optimizing Load Balancing Using Deep Learning in a Cloud Environment. In *2024 11th International Conference on Computing for Sustainable Global Development (INDIACom)*, New Delhi, India, IEEE, 1374–1380, doi: 10.23919/INDIACom61295.2024.10498539.

Dastagiraiah, D. (2024). A System for Analysing Call Drop Dynamics in the Telecom industry using Machine Learning and Feature Selection. *Journal of Theoretical and Applied Information Technology*, *102*(22), 8034–8049.

El Saddik, A., Ahmad, J., Khan, M., Abouzahir, S., & Gueaieb, W. (2025). Unleashing Creativity in the Metaverse: Generative AI and Multimodal Content. *ACM Transactions on Multimedia Computing, Communications and Applications*, *21*(7), 1–43.

Ghebrehiwet, I., Zaki, N., Damseh, R., & Mohamad, M. S. (2024). Revolutionizing Personalized Medicine with Generative AI: A Systematic Review. *Artificial Intelligence Review*, *57*(5), 128.

Grua, E. M., De Sanctis, M., Malavolta, I., Hoogendoorn, M., & Lago, P. (2022). An Evaluation of the Effectiveness of Personalization and Self-Adaptation for e-Health Apps. *Information and Software Technology*, *146*, 106841.

GS, N. K., Chinni, P. B. M. R., Abdul, A. B., Silamanthula, H. K., Shaik, J., & Kakumanu, V. N. (2024). Neurosynthetics: Adaptive Dynamic Risk Factor Integration Network Architecture for Cardiac Risk Prediction. *Telecommunications and Radio Engineering, 84*(3), 27–41.

Jimenez, J., Del Rio, A., Berman, A. N., & Grande, M. (2023). Personalizing Digital Health: Adapting Health Technology Systems to Meet the Needs of Different Older Populations. *Healthcare*, *11*, 1–14.

Karthiga, M., Abirami, S., Arunkumar, B., & Sheba, M. V. (2025). Entertainment Analysis in Gaming Model for Business Management with Decision Making and Machine Learning Model. *Entertainment Computing*, *52*, 100725.

Kaur, D., Singh, B., & Rani, S. (2025). Machine Learning for Internet of Medical Things Applications: Framework, Developments, and Challenges. In Arun Kumar Rana, Vishnu Sharma, Sanjeev Kumar Rana, Vijay Shanker Chaudhary (Eds.) *Evolution of Machine Learning and Internet of Things Applications in Biomedical Engineering* (pp. 18–40). CRC Press.

Kumar, S., Rani, S., Sharma, S., & Min, H. (2024). Multimodality Fusion Aspects of Medical Diagnosis: A Comprehensive Review. *Bioengineering*, *11*(12), 1233.

Mader, S., Levieux, G., & Natkin, S. (2016). A Game Design Method for Therapeutic Games. In *2016 8th International Conference on Games and Virtual Worlds for Serious Applications (VS-GAMES)*, Barcelona, Spain, IEEE, pp. 1-8, doi: 10.1109/VS-GAMES.2016.7590333

Naga Ramesh, J. V., Dastagiraiah, C., Mubeen, S., Priya, W. D., Rao, M. K., & Kumar, B. B. (2025). Butterfly Magnetoreception based Neighbour Awareness Strategy Protocol for Autonomous Aerial Vehicles. *Scientific Reports*, *15*(1), 12814.

Naveen Kumar, G. S., & Reddy, V. S. K. (2019, June). Extraction of key frames using rough set theory for video retrieval. In *International Conference on Soft Computing and Signal Processing* (pp. 761–768). Springer Singapore.

Naveen Kumar, G. S., & Reddy, V. S. K. (2022). High Performance Algorithm for Content-based Video Retrieval using Multiple Features. In *Intelligent Systems and Sustainable Computing: Proceedings of ICISSC 2021* (pp. 637–646). Springer Nature Singapore.

Núñez V, J. M., Munar, L. S., Arias Sánchez, C. L., Vargas, V. L., & De la Prieta, F. (2025). Framework for Adaptive and Creative Learning Based on Generative Artificial Intelligence in Higher Education. In Progress in Artificial Intelligence: 24th EPIA Conference on Artificial Intelligence, EPIA 2025, Faro, Portugal, October 1–3, 2025, Proceedings, Part II. Springer-Verlag, Berlin, Heidelberg, 368–381. https://doi.org/10.1007/978-3-032-05179-0_28

Qu, Y., Nathaniel, J., Li, S., & Gentine, P. (2024). Deep Generative Data Assimilation in Multimodal Setting. *2024 IEEE/CVF Conference on Computer Vision and Pattern Recognition Workshops (CVPRW)*, Seattle, WA, USA, IEEE, pp. 449-459, doi: 10.1109/CVPRW63382.2024.00050.

Rahman, M. A., & Al-Hazzaa, S. (2024). Next-Generation Virtual Hospital: Integrating Discriminative and Large Multi-Modal Generative AI for Personalized Healthcare. *GLOBECOM 2024 - 2024 IEEE Global Communications Conference*, Cape Town, South Africa, 2024, pp. 3509-3514, doi: 10.1109/GLOBECOM52923.2024.10901624.

Rani, K. P., Roja, G., Lalitha, E., Deepika, B., Dastagiriah, C., & Arshad, M. (2024). Sentiment Analysis of Online Reviews in the Field of Tourism for Hyderabad Popular Places. *2024 International Conference on Advancements in Smart, Secure and Intelligent Computing (ASSIC)*, Bhubaneswar, India, IEEE, pp. 1-4, doi: 10.1109/ASSIC60049.2024.10508009.

Rani, K. P., Sreedevi, P., Dastagiriah, C., Rao, K. S., Subbaraju, G., & Padmavathi, J. (2024). Land Cover Extraction from Satellite Imagery using U-Net Model. *2024 11th International Conference on Computing for Sustainable Global Development (INDIACom)*, IEEE.

Rani, S., Kumar, S., Kataria, A., & Min, H. (2024). SmartHealth: An Intelligent Framework to Secure IoMT Service Applications using Machine Learning. *ICT Express*, *10*(2), 425–430.

Rodrigues, K. R., Conrado, D. B., & Neris, V. P. (2018). Lessons Learned in Designing a Digital Therapeutic Game to Support the Treatment and Well-being of Children with Cancer. In: Marcus, A., Wang, W. (eds) Design, User Experience, and Usability: Users, Contexts and Case Studies. DUXU 2018. Lecture Notes in Computer Science, vol 10920. Springer, Cham. https://doi.org/10.1007/978-3-319-91806-8_18

Shafik, W. (2025). Generative Adversarial Networks: Security, Privacy, and Ethical Considerations. In Narasimha Rao Vajjhala, Sanjiban Sekhar Roy, Burak Taşcı, Muhammad Enamul Hoque Chowdhury (Eds.) *Generative Artificial Intelligence (AI) Approaches for Industrial Applications* (pp. 93–117). Springer.

Srinivasa Naveen Kumar, G., Reddy, V. S. K., & Balivada, L. K. (2022, December). Content-Based Video Retrieval Using Deep Learning Algorithms. In *International Conference on Intelligent Systems and Sustainable Computing* (pp. 557–568). Springer Nature Singapore.

Sudhakar, R. V., Dastagiraiah, C., Pattem, S., & Bhukya, S. (2024). Multi-Objective Reinforcement Learning Based Algorithm for Dynamic Workflow Scheduling in Cloud Computing. *Indonesian Journal of Electrical Engineering and Informatics (IJEEI)*, *12*(3), 640–649.

Zhan, F., Yu, Y., Wu, R., Zhang, J., Lu, S., Liu, L., Kortylewski, A., Theobalt, C., & Xing, E. (2023). Multimodal Image Synthesis and Editing: The Generative AI Era. *IEEE Transactions on Pattern Analysis and Machine Intelligence*, *45*(12), 15098–15119.

Chapter 10

Healthcare and assistive technologies

Multimodal AI for rehabilitation, monitoring, and patient independence

Debarpita Santra and Indraneel Mukhopadhyay

10.1 INTRODUCTION

In the digital era, rapid advances are seen in communication, computing, and biomedical engineering. These rapid advances have changed the healthcare delivery model, enabling a new generation of assistive technologies. Integration of telecommunication and intelligent devices in modern healthcare enhances the access, diagnosis, and self-management of patients. For instance, wearable sensors are for continuous monitoring of vital signs, telehealth platforms are there for connecting patients and physicians remotely, and machine learning (ML) algorithms are there for analysis of complex health data. This kind of transformation in healthcare domain was envisioned back in 1879 when speculation on telephonic medical consultations was done by *The Lancet* and by 1925, discussion started on remote video examinations [1]. The space program initiated by NASA later advanced remote physiological monitoring (for example, astronaut telemetry), and the STARPAHC project enhanced the pilot telehealth for indigenous communities [1]. The current healthcare ecosystem is built on such kinds of innovation done over decades.

The primary domains of healthcare and assistive technologies include the following:

i) Internet-based telemedicine/telehealth, which uses networks for offering remote clinical care
ii) Smart sensors and wearable devices to track the health status continuously
iii) Disease detection from images or signals by using artificial intelligence (AI) or machine learning (ML), especially the deep neural networks
iv) Surgical robots (for example, da Vinci systems) and socially assistive robots as well as exoskeletons
v) Internet-of-Things (IoT) systems for smart home and ambient tech to monitor and support people in their living environments

DOI: 10.1201/9781003665656-10

vi) Rehabilitation technologies that include virtual reality (VR) rehabilitation platforms and robotic therapy devices
vii) Use of digital therapeutics, software-based interventions like mobile apps for delivering evidence-based treatment like cognitive behavioral therapy for addiction

The current study explores each of the above-mentioned domains in technical depth, summarizing the historical background, current capabilities, clinical evidence, and the challenges faced. The study also includes case studies on telestroke networks in rural areas [2], studies on monitoring through wearable devices, as well as specific devices that are FDA-approved. At the end of the study, discussion has been done on various cross-cutting issues like regulatory constraints, data privacy, interoperability, etc. and the future trends of the field of healthcare assistive technology that involve 5G/6G connectivity, brain–computer interfaces, precision medicine, and so on.

10.2 BACKGROUND AND HISTORICAL CONTEXT

Healthcare technology has hand-shaken with the advances in communications and electronics long time back. The concept of remote care in telemedicine got introduced before the Internet. In 1879, a *Lancet* article proposed the use of telephone to perform a preliminary assessment of patients for determining any urgency, and a video diagnosis mechanism was envisioned back in 1925 [1]. Pioneering experiments included Willem Einthoven's 1906 "telecardiogram" (transmitting ECGs by telephone) and WWII radar technology repurposed for health monitoring. In the 1960s, NASA's telemetry systems were adapted for patient monitoring and rural care (e.g. the Papago project) [1].

Robot-assisted therapy also began decades ago. The concept of telesurgery emerged in the 1980s (e.g. DARPA's remote operation experiments), culminating in clinical platforms like the da Vinci Surgical System (approved in 2000) for minimally invasive surgery. Similarly, the first functional neuroprosthetic and exoskeleton devices appeared in the late 20th century. The field of digital health has broadly matured with the proliferation of personal computing and smartphones. Wearable biomedical devices began with simple heart rate monitors and evolved into smartwatches and implantable sensors.

Regulatory and professional interest has accelerated recently. For instance, a National Academy of Medicine workshop in 2012 explicitly called for telehealth to be central in redesigning care delivery (e.g. overcoming rural specialist shortages) [1]. Chronic disease management, which traditionally relied on infrequent office visits, has benefited from home monitoring: remote care management programs (e.g. the U.S. Veterans Affairs system) showed reduced hospitalizations and costs through at-home data collection [1]. Nowadays, the efforts for integration put emphasis on device portability and interoperability, anticipating that the future wearables would be combined with accelerometry, ECG, and other sensors into single small platforms [1].

In spite of this long history, varied adoption has been seen. Telehealth was considered as a niche until there was a dramatic change in policy during the COVID-19 pandemic that caused widespread reimbursement for virtual visits. Recent survey results show that 60% of physicians started believing that telehealth enables high-quality care, with 80% finding it as a platform for increased patient access [3]. However, this rapid expansion exposes telehealth to great privacy and security gaps [3]. The insights gained from COVID-19 conclude that though there are many clinically mature technologies, the integration at a large scale requires lots of research work.

10.3 TELEMEDICINE AND TELEHEALTH

Telemedicine or telehealth is described as a mode for offering clinical care at a distance via telecommunications that involve real-time video visits, remote monitoring of vital signs, store-and-forward image consultation, and asynchronous messaging. Typical architecture includes patient endpoints (e.g. home computers, tablets, kiosks with cameras/sensors) communicating with provider systems (video conferencing hardware, integrated electronic health records (EHRs), and clinical dashboards). Key enabling technologies are broadband Internet, secure video platforms (VoIP), medical peripherals (digital stethoscopes, otoscopes), and software for data sharing.

Telemedicine applications are diverse. Synchronous video visits allow remote history-taking and even limited examinations, particularly effective in dermatology, psychiatry, and chronic disease follow-ups. Remote patient monitoring uses home sensors (blood pressure cuffs, pulse oximeters, glucometers) to send longitudinal data to clinicians. For instance, when patients with heart failure are discharged from the hospital, they need measurement of body weight and blood pressure on daily basis, and that readings should be streamed to care teams. The store-and-forward technique is often used for specialty consultations—for example, radiologic images like X-rays or CT scans as well as pathology slides can be sent to specialists for interpreting remotely. Moreover, better care can be provided through emergent telemedicine (for example, ambulance-to-hospital stroke triage): neurologists are connected with rural emergency departments through *telestroke* networks, enabling thrombolysis even without the physical presence of specialists at the site. The rural stroke outcomes have been found to be improved with the emergence of *telestroke*, which helps experts to respond promptly [2].

Benefits of telemedicine have been well documented. Telehealth systems, while integrated with AI diagnostic tools and EHRs, can perform continuous patient tracking and decision support. Telemedicine helps physicians diagnose and manage patients more effectively as monitoring of patients is done in real time and the care plans can be adjusted without geographic limitations [4]. As a result, more patients can be treated by providers even if the number of staffs is limited. Through continuous data flow, telemedicine helps clinicians track patients in real time and modify care plans. Therefore, the travel time of the patients gets reduced, the number of missed workdays gets reduced, and the access to specialists becomes faster. For instance, remote consultation can reduce the expense of air transfer of critically ill neonates or cuts down the need for aged patients to board trains for routine follow-ups [4].

The impact of telemedicine is illustrated using important case studies. In the USA, through a telehealth program named the Veterans Affairs (VA), millions of veterans are connected for receiving remote care, thereby reducing rehospitalizations. In India, through a telemedicine portal named eSanjeevani, more than 100 million virtual consultations were done during a period of 3 years from 2021 to 2024, significantly expanding access to rural healthcare. During COVID-19 pandemic, hundred times increase in video visits were reported by the major health systems overnight. China and Western countries take the help of telemonitoring for chronic disease programs like COPD or diabetes. A trial has shown that patients who are using home monitoring of blood pressure or glucose have better control and less no. of admissions compared to the standard care.

As a result of telemedicine, provider–provider collaboration has improved. The clinics at rural areas where specialists are unavailable can send images or video to urban centers. For example, in Alaska, community health helps in performing exams like audiometry or otoscopy and in sending data to Anchorage specialists [1]. A tele-dermatology consult may help in sending skin lesion photos to a dermatologist for having faster opinion. These workflows mitigate delays and duplication as a physician can receive a second opinion from anywhere so that repeated tests can be avoided.

But telemedicine has a number of significant limitations. Due to a lack of reliable high-speed internet, a number of rural and low-income areas face issues of poor video quality for video visits. Though there exists network connectivity, there exist privacy concerns. As per a systematic review of telehealth, three broad risk categories in telemedicine include environmental risk, technological risk, and operational risk. Environmental risk implies a lack of private space for patients at home; technological risk involved data security, vulnerability, and unreliable networks; operational risk implies licensing issues, reimbursement policies, and training gaps [3]. For instance, a clinician cannot easily do the physical exams like auscultation or palpation at a distance, thereby questioning clinical adequacy. Also there are regulatory hurdles involving licensing and credentialing across state or national lines. Additionally, a number of patients, especially the elderly patients, initially face problems to use telehealth platforms [4].

Privacy and security are big concerns in telehealth. The surge of telehealth in recent days poses cybersecurity threats. The videoconference links used during telehealth consultations may be insecure. There is also fear that sensitive patient data might be leaked. A study shows that most of the physicians are concerned about the security of data with virtual care [3]. As a result, there are a number of major organizations that now offer security enhancements to the telehealth systems for increasing patient privacy and decreasing cybersecurity threats to patient data [3]. For achieving this, strong encryption, multifactor authentication, and compliance with health-data regulations like GDPR and HIPAA are required. Lack of privacy at home (for example, family overhearing sessions) prevents the patients from being open.

As a whole, the telemedicine technology that is integrated in diverse healthcare sectors like simple mobile apps for use at home or tele-ICU suits has proven its significance in improving access and also reducing healthcare costs [4]. Better productivity as well as more patient engagement have been shown to be offered by the tele-tools. Research is going on to design the standards and protocols for telehealth. For instance, now-a-days, a number of organizations are offering tele-exam techniques and interoperable systems for linking telemonitoring data with the EHRs at different hospitals. In future, the use of 5G networks in telehealth for supporting high-resolution video and real-time streaming of sensor data, as well as the use of augmented reality tools would definitely allow the remote specialist physicians to guide the procedures in a better way.

10.4 WEARABLE AND SENSOR DEVICES

Wearable devices and implants enable continuous, at-home health monitoring and feedback. These include wristbands, patches, smart clothing, and ingestible or implantable sensors. Common measures are heart rate, blood oxygen (SpO_2), activity/motion (via accelerometers), glucose, blood pressure, and more specialized signals such as ECG or EEG. Technically, modern wearables integrate miniaturized sensors, low-power microcontrollers, and wireless transmitters (Bluetooth, Wi-Fi, or cellular) to send data to phones or cloud servers. Advances in materials science (e.g. stretchable electronics) and battery technology have enabled comfortable, long-term monitoring.

Wearables are used for both wellness and clinical purposes. For example, smartwatches are now widely used by consumers and have demonstrated clear medical utility. A recent review notes that "smartwatches are the most commonly used wearable devices" for health monitoring [5]. In fact, some smartwatches have FDA clearance for ECG rhythm detection.

Clinical studies like the Apple Heart Study (NEJM 2019) have shown that a smartwatch irregular-pulse notification can identify atrial fibrillation with a high positive predictive value (0.84) in a large cohort of hundreds of thousands [5]. Wearables have also detected other conditions: the Annual Review of Medicine highlights that continuous tracking enabled COVID-19 detection (via subtle temperature/respiration changes), as well as alerts for arrhythmias, inflammation, or even Lyme disease symptoms [5].

Beyond watches, specialized wearables include chest-straps for ECG, patches for heart rhythm or respiratory monitoring, and off-body networks (environmental sensors plus wearables). The wearable medical device market in the USA is growing exponentially in the next decade [6]. More than 50% of the home-based medical device usage is due to wearables. Remote patient monitoring devices account for 18% of the wearable health market [6].

The number of evidences that show clinical benefits of wearables is growing day by day. Enabling longitudinal data collection leads to early detection of personalized interventions and deteriorations. In the case of chronic disease management, continuous glucose monitors and activity trackers can enhance outcomes and adherence. In a 2024 scoping review, it was stated that 53% students used wearable activity trackers in interventional studies for diabetes and other chronic conditions [7]. In the case of diabetes, continuous glucose monitors have developed self-management. In the case of cardiac care, the traditional method for Holter monitors might miss intermittent arrhythmias that can be captured by the wearable ECG monitors. There are wearable accelerometer devices that can detect changes or falls in gait, thereby helping to manage Parkinson's disease or frailty.

However, there exist challenges related to accuracy or user acceptance of wearables. Though the devices are highly engineered devices, the quality of data may vary (for example, sensor drift, motion artifacts). Only those devices that are regulatory-compliant by FDA or CE offer strict accuracy standards. While using the wearbles, user comfort and battery life must be taken care of, as a wearable needs to be comfortable for long wear. In a 2024 patient-centred review, general positive satisfaction and usability with wearables were found, which was mixed with comfort [6]. Wrist-worn devices have been found to be cumbersome for older adults who also worry about the data. There is another issue on how to ingest streams of wearable data and present the relevant summaries in a clinically acceptable form to the doctors.

When these wearable devices effectively work as integrated analytical units [5], significant engineering efforts need to put for ensuring security and interoperability. As wearables frequently transmit health-related metrics through wireless protocols, maintaining data privacy is critical always. Though efforts like the Continua Alliance encourage maintaining standards for device-to-cloud communication, wearables generate amplitude of data (big data). As a result, there is a requirement for robust analytics and ML for the derivation of actionable digital biomarkers. Research is now going on to formalize digital biomarkers. For example, in a 2024 study on digital biomarkers, raw wearable data such as step counts and heart rate variability can be converted to metrics of disease states such as fatigue and gait stability with the help of careful modeling and validation [8]. This conversion also requires calibration of measurements to clinical benchmarks and validation of the calibrated measurements via trials. There is guidance issued by the FDA on how to use wearable-derived measures in drug trials and clinical practice.

Case Example

Incorporation of wearable sensor data in the USA and UK National Institutes of Health's Biobank projects has been started. A wearable ECG study shows that more than 16% of the patients generated alerts for atrial fibrillation, and these findings were validated by cardiologists. In consumer health, population studies were done using Fitbit's millions of users, in which heart rate patterns capturing early disease signals were linked. These examples show the potential for wearables for enabling precision medicine: individualized baselines allow detecting subtle changes. For instance, a typical signature of an elderly person's gait could be tracked; any kind of deviation may indicate dementia onset or risk of fall.

If we look forward, wearables would become more advanced and ubiquitous. The continuing research involves flexible skin patches with numerous biosensors, dresses embedded with sensing fibers, and minimally invasive implants like sensor capsules. Once wearables are combined with AI, a new closed-loop system will be generated. For instance, the dose of a smart insulin pump is decided based on continuous glucose monitoring; smart pacemakers adapt to arrhythmias. However, concerns regarding the accuracy and lack of bias exist there. Though there is biomedical validation, there exist hurdles for clinical translation, data security and privacy issues, data standardization, and regulatory approval [5]. If these issues are addressed using data encryption on-device, a federated learning technique to preserve privacy, the future of wearables in health will be in good shape.

10.5 AI-DRIVEN DIAGNOSTICS AND DECISION SUPPORT

AI, especially ML, is quickly changing the medical diagnostics. AI in healthcare is described as data-driven computational algorithms that help in interpreting patient data. The supervised ML models learn patterns from labeled data. There exist unsupervised ML algorithms for identifying patterns from unlabelled data. Deep learning (DL), which is a subset of ML, uses multilayer neural networks for automatic extraction of complex features from raw data. Convolutional neural networks (CNNs) are widely used in practice for analysing images [9]. In the same way, there exist recurrent neural networks (RNNs) and transformers for analysing sequential data such as clinical text or ECGs.

AI has been applied on a wide scale for imaging diagnostics. AI-based detection of pathologies on X-rays, CT, and MRI scans is gaining much attention of researchers and clinicians day by day. A review of modern radiology notes that DL "accelerates MRI scanning" and "automates triage" of chest X-rays, dramatically reducing interpretation times (one report cited a reduction from 11.2 to 2.7 days) [9]. AI-enhanced CT and PET reconstruction can improve image quality or lower the required radiation dose. The MDPI review reports that radiology (a field early to digitize) has used AI-driven computer-aided detection (CAD) for decades, and sees AI now "redefining" radiology workflows by refining CAD performance, streamlining reporting, and enabling integrated diagnostics [9].

Pathology and other domains also benefit from AI. In digital pathology, whole-slide imaging allows AI to quantify tumor cell counts, grade tissue samples, and highlight suspect regions that a human pathologist can review. Algorithms in pathology have shown accuracies rivaling experts for tasks like classifying cancers or detecting metastases. Beyond images, AI is used in genomics (variant interpretation), cardiology (ECG arrhythmia detection), and ophthalmology (retinopathy screening). For instance, some AI systems can analyze retinal fundus photos for diabetic eye disease, and have earned FDA clearance (e.g. IDx-DR system). Similarly, AI algorithms analyze lung function data, sound (cough detection), and speech patterns for respiratory diseases.

Numerous case examples, as given below, illustrate success.

An AI model detecting diabetic retinopathy from retinal images achieved ~90% sensitivity and specificity in trials, enabling primary care clinics to screen patients (FDA approved in 2018).

Deep CNNs have been validated on thousands of X-rays to identify pneumonia, tuberculosis, and bone fractures.

Wearable AI: smart watches run on-device ML to notify users of atrial fibrillation or low oxygen levels in real time.

In genomics, AI-driven variant callers sift through whole-genome data to find rare pathogenic mutations.

Application of AI is enhancing the efficiency and consistency of diagnosis. AI algorithms can find patterns from data like subtle imaging textures, multi-dimensional lab data associations that are invisible to human experts. AI can detect diseases easily and rapidly through the quick processing of big data streams. For example, after analyzing EHRs, AI algorithms can indicate whether a patient is at high risk for sepsis much before the appearance of clinical signs. This enables the treating physicians to take decisions on earlier intervention.

However, the application of AI in real clinical practice has several challenges. There is a need for rigorous clinical validation of the AI algorithms with clinical data of the intended population of real patients. Existence of bias may pose as a constraint, as an AI algorithm trained on one demographic data might perform poorly on different demographic data. For example, there is a chance of misdiagnosis of skin cancer in darker-skinned patients by AI algorithms that have been trained on data of fair-skinned patients. Explainability is also a key ethical and technical challenge in the use of AI in healthcare. The DL algorithms used for disease diagnosis act as "black box" without explaining the reason behind reaching to particular clinical decisions, thereby making the clinicians uncertain about the diagnosis. Achieving true transparency in the findings of AI diagnostic algorithms is difficult, though efforts are being put on for offering interpretability (for example, saliency maps to highlight image regions). AI systems that are trained on representative data need to be grounded in explainability, transparency, and interpretability for gaining trust in real clinical practice [10].

AI's regulatory frameworks are evolving. The FDA has already started classification of AI/ML-based devices based on their efficacy and safety. A recent study states that from 1995 to 2024, 882 AI-based medical devices such as imaging tools, remote monitoring apps, in vitro diagnostics, etc. have obtained regulatory clearance.

Ensuring data privacy is also very important. To apply AI in healthcare domain, large annotated datasets are required. An investigation is going on to find some secure computation techniques like Federated learning, so that the AI models can be trained on the patient data without sharing

Data privacy is also critical. AI in healthcare relies on large annotated datasets. Federated learning and secure computation are being explored to train models without sharing raw patient data. But for this, patient anonymity and patient consent should be maintained properly. As AI depends on huge datasets that can have conflicts with privacy rights, there may be unique privacy challenges in using AI [10]. Patient trust can be ensured only after addressing these concerns and challenges.

Though there are numerous challenges, there exists enormous potential in the use of AI in healthcare. There is a rapid surge in interdisciplinary collaborations among physicians, engineers, and data scientists. In the near future, AI-based diagnostics are expected to be integrated into routine clinical care. For example, there is a possibility that before a radiologist reviews a radiology scan, it would be promptly pre-screened by AI; also, constant monitoring of ICU data can be done by AI for predicting deterioration in prior. Research is going on to offer holistic diagnosis by using multimodal AI that combines imaging, wearable data, and genomics. Also, the development of closed-loop systems is underway, which will suggest interventions alongside diagnosis. Researchers are also continuing their work on robustness, ethics, and clinical trials to ensure fast and wide transformation of diagnosis with the help of AI.

10.6 ROBOTIC AND ASSISTIVE SYSTEMS

Robotics in healthcare is an emerging field of research that spans from surgical robots to rehabilitation/assistive robots, and socially assistive robots (SARs).

10.6.1 Surgical robots

One of the most prominent examples of surgical robot is da Vinci surgical system (Intuitive Surgical), which has over 6,000 installations globally. This kind of robot offers a master–slave platform for minimally invasive procedures in the domain of general surgery, gynecology, urology, etc. The micro-movements of robot arms holding instruments are done according to the surgeon's hand movements. The surgeries done by the surgical robots offer high precision and dexterity in confined spaces, leading to reduced blood loss, pain, and recovery time of the patients in comparison with open surgery. But its benefit over conventional laparoscopy is mixed. Recent updates include the emergence of micro-robots like magnet-guided capsules for endoscopy and autonomous telemonitoring robots. Use of surgical robots needs strict engineering controls, which include sterilizable materials, FDA regulation, and real-time fail-safes.

10.6.2 Rehabilitation robots

These kinds of robots help patients who are receiving therapy after an illness or injury. Powered exoskeletons like EksoNR, HAL, ReWalk are examples of rehabilitation robots that assist paraplegic patients stand and walk. Lokomat is another example of rehabilitation robot that is integrated with treadmill. This robot supports bodyweight to retrain gait in stroke patients. There are upper-limb rehab robots named MIT-Manus, Armeo, ReoGo, which permit repetitive arm exercises at different assistance levels. A recent study claims that motor outcomes can be improved with robotic therapy. As evidence, it provided a review of 54 post-stroke trials (n = 2744) where robotic upper-limb therapy helped patients gain a small yet significant arm capacity in comparison with the conventional rehabilitation (standardized mean difference approx. 0.14) [11]. Another study highlighted that specific design features of a device like varying degrees of freedom, multi-joint mobilization, as well as adjustable assistance might lead to produce better outcomes [11]. Despite this, robotic therapy is yet to significantly change activities-of-daily-living scores or sustain long-term improvements, implying that robotics is not a panacea—rather it's an adjunct [11].

10.6.3 Socially assistive robots (SARs)

These kinds of robots act as companions for elderly people or children living with disabilities. For instance, Paro is a SAR used for dementia care that is capable of reducing agitation and loneliness through interactions. There is a home robot called Pepper that can remind individuals of medication or exercises, facilitate video calls, or detect falls (if any) by using cameras and sensors. Though research in this domain is at embryonic stage, SARs have enormous potential in the enhancement of patient engagement and adherence to care plans.

10.6.3.1 Case study

Robotics in elderly care is an emerging research area. There are some studies that have deployed mobile robots in offering senior facilities like navigating hallways, delivering items, and calling staff. A Japanese nursing home takes the help of an assistive robot for lifting patients safely from bed, mitigating the risk of staff injuries. There exists a concept of robotic telepresence, which is a wheeled device with a video screen that permits remote family members or physicians to have a virtual walk in the patient's room.

The main technical components embedded in these kinds of systems are sensors (depth cameras, vision, force/torque), actuators (pneumatics, electric motors), and control algorithms. As safety is a main concern in using these kinds of robots, an instruction to reliably stop or change the course, as the robot encounters an obstacle or force anomalies, should always be integrated in the software of the robots. The human–robot interaction aspect also plays a vital role, especially in case of SARs. The robot's behavior, speech, and user interface must be comforting and intuitive.

As a whole, the role of robots in healthcare is to amplify human care. The surgeon capabilities are extended by the surgical robots; the patient efforts are amplified by the rehab robots; the human shortage is compensated by the assistive robots. However, use of robotics in healthcare has multiple constraints including high costs (for instance, expense of da Vinci exceeds $1), training needs, adaptations to unpredictable human behavior, and longer regulatory path as most of the robotic systems must have FDA approval to be used as a medical device. In spite of all these limitations, there is a need for introducing more number of semi-autonomous and patient-tailored robots in clinical practice to offer better care to patients and families.

10.7 SMART HOME AND AMBIENT-ASSISTED TECHNOLOGIES

Monitoring and assisting individuals, especially the elderly and the patients having chronic illness, at residential setups are done by using IoT devices. These IoT devices deploy a network of different sensors like pressure mats, door/window contacts, pressure mats, actuators like lights or smart locks, and various types of wearables—connected via home wireless networks or hubs. The goal of this kind of technology, called the smart home technology or more specifically Ambient Assisted Living (AAL) is to offer independence in living through automatic detection of emergencies or any kinds of needs and through generating alerts/reminders.

In smart homes, continuous behavioral monitoring is performed. For instance, detection of an inactivity might be an indicator of a fall; cognitive decline can be inferred by tracking mobility patterns. Daily routines can also be managed by smart homes. For example, automated pill dispensers generate an alert to the patients for taking medications; voice assistants remind users to make appointments. A study finds that smart home tech has five prime roles such as daily monitoring, assisted living activities, life reminders, functional movement, and emotional companionship, which get translated into concrete outcomes like increased independence, enhanced cognitive function, better self-managemnet, increased mobility, enhanced social engagement, and reduced caregiver burden [12]. When individuals have increased independence, they can stay at home for longer time; persons with better self-management can track diet or exercise in a better way; persons with enhanced social engagement can make video calls through the installed devices at smart homes. As a whole, the smart home technology offers better overall quality of lives to the residents.

For example, sensor arrays embedded on furniture are able to detect the sitting or standing patterns of an individual and identify the falls or abnormal posture. Gait speed, an early indicator of frailty, can be tracked by floor pressure sensors. There are smart speakers like Amazon Alexa that can monitor conversation patterns as a symbol of loneliness. There exist smart thermostats and smart lighting for adjusting home environments so that the comfort of a patient can be ensured. For instance, bedroom of a patient suffering from Parkinson's dyskinesia remains warmer to ensure comfort of the patient. There is also an emergence of telehealth integration so that the vital-sign wearables (for example, blood pressure cuffs) can be connected to smart home hubs for sending the readings to the clinicians automatically.

Smart home technologies improve the independence of elderly peoples' lives by reducing the dependence on the caregivers and promoting home-based care for older adults [12]. It has been observed that the homes having this technology have less number of chronic heart failure patients. In case of dementia care, wearable GPS and motion sensors can detect wandering risk so that timely interventions can be taken. In a pilot project conducted in Europe and North America, the proofs-of-concepts are being tested in real home environments to confirm that the older users get habituated in the well-designed home environments and usually respond with high satisfaction to the smart home aids [12].

The technologies that are used in the smart home environments include low-power wireless like Z-wave or Zigbee for sensors, edge devices like smartphones or home gateways, cloud platforms for data analysis, as well as ML algorithms for transforming raw data into alerts. Passive infrared motion detectors acted as the primary data sources in most of the home health monitoring studies [13]. Wearable trackers as well as cameras also play major roles in smart home monitoring. Data analysis helps to detect anomalies. For instance, if a patient's nighttime bathroom trips get increased (which is identified by unsupervised clustering), a health checkup will be initiated.

The major changes in smart home technology involve interoperability (different devices from different vendors often have communication issues in-between), multi-occupant differentiation (the resident triggering a sensor needs to be identified), as well as security/privacy issues. There is a strong need of secure Wi-Fi network and strong data encryption technique. The individuals, especially the elderly users, residing at the smart home might worry about the "spying" devices. The designers should ensure privacy in the design and also permit opt-in controls. Moreover, as per an IoT scoping review, most of the recent researches in this domain are technology-driven; but there is a need to do research on making the design as user-centric as possible so that people can actually have interactions with the smart home systems [13].

Tele-rehabilitation is another aspect in this context, in which gamified therapy and VR are offered through home consoles. For instance, a Kinect-based system can be used by a stroke patient for practicing arm exercises guided by virtual tasks. In the early field deployment and trials, home VR rehab along with tele-monitoring by therapists has shown improvements in compliance and some other functional outcomes.

In summary, smart homes and ambient tech extend the healthcare continuum into the patient's living space. By 2025, we can expect increasing deployment of such systems, with even common appliances (toilets, beds, kitchens) embedded with health sensors. Edge computing and 5G will allow real-time processing, and integration with telehealth platforms will enable clinicians to "see" into patients' homes for monitoring. Ensuring usability, especially for cognitively impaired users, and establishing evidence-based standards are important frontiers.

10.8 REHABILITATION TECHNOLOGIES

Rehabilitation devices aim to restore or compensate for lost function. Beyond robotic systems (discussed above), there are many tools:

- Prosthetics and Orthotics: Modern prosthetic limbs (for amputees) often use myoelectric sensors to detect muscle signals and actuate the limb. Advanced devices provide multi-joint movement and even haptic feedback. Osseointegration (direct bone anchoring of prostheses) is an emerging technique. Orthotic exoskeletons (e.g. spinal braces with actuators) help patients with weakness stand or walk.

- Sensory rehabilitation: Vision and hearing aids have benefited from digital tech. Cochlear implants and advanced hearing aids use signal processing (and in some cases AI noise reduction) to improve function. Similarly, low-vision aids include electronic magnifiers and retinal implants.
- Virtual reality (VR) and augmented reality (AR): Immersive environments can make rehabilitation engaging. A 2024 meta-review concluded that VR, as an adjunct to conventional therapy, is "safe and effective" in stroke recovery, improving upper/lower limb, gait, and balance outcomes [14]. VR systems (like the Nintendo Wii or dedicated rehab games) encourage repetitive, task-specific training. AR systems can overlay guidance on real-world tasks (e.g. a display guiding a hemiplegic patient in arm movement). VR is also used for pain management (e.g. burn wound care distraction) and for cognitive rehab (e.g. memory and attention games for TBI patients).
- Therapeutic devices: Neurostimulation devices (TENS units, functional electrical stimulation) help in pain relief and muscle activation. Brain–computer interfaces (BCIs) are experimental assistive tech for severe paralysis.

10.9 DIGITAL THERAPEUTICS

Digital therapeutics (DTx) are software interventions designed to prevent, manage, or treat diseases. Unlike general health apps, DTx products undergo clinical testing and often regulatory clearance. They typically deliver evidence-based therapies, like cognitive behavioral therapy (CBT) or exercise programs, via mobile or web platforms. For example, prescription DTx must demonstrate efficacy in randomized trials similar to drugs.

Examples of FDA-authorized DTx (as of 2025) include – *reSET* and *reSET-O* (Pear Therapeutics): mobile apps delivering CBT modules for substance use disorder and opioid use disorder, respectively [15]. These act as an adjunct to counseling as the patients receive engaging lessons, and patient adherence is tracked. – *EndeavorRx* (Akili): a video game approved for improving attention in children with ADHD [15]. It's the first FDA-cleared digital treatment for ADHD. – *BlueStar* (WellDoc): a coaching app for type 2 diabetes, giving personalized feedback on glucose, diet, and medication [15]. – *Daylight* and *Sleepio* (Big Health): CBT-based programs for anxiety and insomnia. – *Kaia COPD*, *Somryst* (insomnia), *MyCognition Pro* (cognitive health for various conditions), among others [15].

Clinical trials underpin these approvals. For example, the efficacy of reSET was shown in trials where participants had higher abstinence and program adherence than controls. End-users generally find these apps accessible, but adherence in "real-world" use can wane. Therefore, outcomes research (real-world evidence) for DTx is a growing field [15].

DTx can bridge gaps in access (therapies delivered anywhere via smartphone). They enable frequent, personalized interaction (e.g. a diabetic patient gets real-time feedback on logged meals). They can also collect outcomes passively and adapt to patient response. In mental health, for instance, digital CBT programs have shown symptom reduction comparable to in-person therapy in some studies.

Digital interventions face unique regulatory and reimbursement issues. Healthcare systems must learn how to prescribe and pay for software. But there exist constraints on digital literacy and barriers in engagement, which might lead the patients refrain from using the app. There is an evolving need of integrating the technology with clinical care (e.g., sharing of DTx data with providers). Privacy poses as a serious concern as DTx often handles sensitive personal medical data.

There is a growing need for implementation of tele-rehabilitation (remote rehabilitation therapy for video/AI guidance) and digital behavior-change programs (for example, weight loss, smoking cessation). Personalized DTx might modify content depending on the genetics and social determinants. With the improvement of mobile sensing technology, DTx can adjust intervention intensity dynamically depending on the state of the patient. For example, there is a stress management app for the deployment of coping exercises when anxiety patterns are detected by wearable sensors.

Table 10.1 provides a summary of the key assistive technologies as stated here along with their technical specifications like algorithms, sensors, device types, connectivity standards, and therapeutic mechanisms. Clinical applications of the assistive technologies have also been highlighted.

10.10 DISCUSSION AND CHALLENGES

While individually each technology holds promise, integrating them into a coherent healthcare system is nontrivial. Some common themes and challenges emerge:

- *Interoperability*: Disparate systems (EHRs, device data platforms, telehealth apps) often cannot easily share data. Open standards (e.g. HL7 FHIR for health data, IEEE 11073 for device metrics) are being adopted to connect sensors, apps, and records. Without interoperability, clinicians risk “alert fatigue” from siloed dashboards, and patients may need to re-enter data.
- *Data Security and Privacy*: All these technologies generate sensitive data (vital signs, images, speech). Strong encryption and access controls are mandatory. For AI in particular, one ethical principle is that patients should understand (at least generally) how AI is used in their care. As discussed, healthcare AI must be developed with “transparency, explainability, and interpretability” to build trust

Table 10.1 Summary of the key assistive technologies with their technical specifications and clinical applications

Technology	*Technical Specifications*	*Clinical Applications*
Telemedicine systems	**Communication**: Encrypted video conferencing (e.g., WebRTC), real-time data streaming **Integration**: HL7/FHIR interoperability with EHRs **Devices**: Peripheral diagnostic tools (digital stethoscopes, dermatoscopes, pulse oximeters) **Security**: HIPAA-compliant platforms with end-to-end AES-256 encryption	- Remote consultation and diagnostics for underserved populations - Chronic disease monitoring (e.g., hypertension, CHF) via integrated vitals platforms - Virtual ICUs for real-time clinician oversight in emergency care settings - Behavioral health interventions through tele-mental health platforms
Wearable physiological sensors	**Types**: ECG (dry/wet electrodes), PPG, accelerometers, gyroscopes, GSR, optical SpO_2, temperature, EMG **Data Transmission**: Bluetooth Low Energy (BLE), Zigbee, Wi-Fi **Power**: Rechargeable Li-polymer batteries with low-power firmware **Software**: On-device signal processing (FFT, peak detection), anomaly detection via embedded microcontrollers (e.g., ARM Cortex-M)	- Ambulatory ECG for arrhythmia detection (e.g., AFib) - Continuous glucose monitoring (CGM) via enzymatic electrochemical sensors for diabetics - Fall detection in geriatrics via accelerometer fusion algorithms - Physical activity profiling and rehabilitation feedback in post-stroke care
AI-driven diagnostic platforms	**Algorithms**: CNNs for image classification (e.g., ResNet, DenseNet), LSTMs for time-series biosignals, ensemble methods for tabular EHR data **Data Sources**: MRI/CT, ultrasound, fundus imaging, ECG/EEG, structured EHR data **Toolkits**: TensorFlow, PyTorch, OpenCV for preprocessing and inference **Output**: Heatmaps, classification scores, diagnostic predictions with confidence intervals	- Automated radiological screening (e.g., lung nodules, breast masses) - Diabetic retinopathy staging from retinal images - Early detection of cardiac ischemia from multi-lead ECG analysis - Sepsis and readmission prediction in ICU via multimodal EHR analytics
Robotic and assistive devices	**Types**: Surgical robots (e.g., da Vinci), exoskeletons (e.g., ReWalk), prosthetic limbs (myoelectric or BCI-driven) **Sensors**: Force/torque sensors, IMUs, EMG electrodes, proximity sensors	- Precision-enhanced minimally invasive surgeries (MIS) using tremor-filtered robotic manipulators - Gait rehabilitation with powered lower-limb exoskeletons post spinal cord injury or stroke

Smart Home and ambient assisted living (AAL)	**Actuators**: Servo motors, hydraulic/pneumatic cylinders **Control**: PID controllers, model predictive control (MPC), neural controllers **Interfaces**: Haptic feedback, brain-machine interface (EEG/ECoG) **Sensors**: PIR motion detectors, pressure mats, door/window sensors, smart pillboxes, ambient light/temp/humidity sensors **Connectivity**: IoT protocols (MQTT, Zigbee, Z-Wave), edge computing via local gateways **AI Integration**: Activity recognition via HMMs, Bayesian networks **Interfacing**: Voice assistants (e.g., Alexa, Google Home), mobile dashboards for caregivers	- Prosthetic arm control via surface EMG signals or cortical implants - Service robots for medication dispensing and mobility support in eldercare facilities - Behavioral monitoring in dementia and Alzheimer's patients (e.g., night wandering, ADL compliance) - Emergency detection (e.g., unresponsiveness, stove left on) - Automated lighting, fall prevention via predictive gait assessment - Medication adherence tracking through smart dispensers and SMS alerts
Rehabilitation engineering systems	**Technologies**: Robotic therapy arms (e.g., MIT-Manus), sensorized gloves, VR/AR-based biofeedback modules **Motion Capture**: Inertial sensors, depth cameras (e.g., Kinect, Intel RealSense), EMG **Control**: Adaptive impedance controllers, trajectory planning algorithms **Feedback**: Real-time haptic, visual, auditory feedback loops	- Motor function retraining for hemiparesis using force-adaptive therapy robots - VR-based balance rehabilitation in vestibular disorder patients - EMG-triggered hand therapy for post-stroke upper-limb rehab - Dual-task gait training with AR overlays for Parkinson's disease
Digital therapeutics (DTx)	**Delivery**: Mobile apps (Android/iOS), web platforms **Content**: CBT modules, interactive games, behavioral coaching, reinforcement learning models **Compliance**: FDA/CE regulation, HIPAA/GDPR-compliant data handling **Tracking**: Patient-reported outcomes (PROs), ecological momentary assessment (EMA), gamification metrics	- Prescription DTx for ADHD (e.g., EndeavorRx, FDA-approved) - Digital CBT for anxiety, insomnia, PTSD (e.g., Sleepio, reSET-O) - Behavioral modification in chronic pain or obesity management - Substance use disorder relapse prevention via just-in-time adaptive interventions (JITAI)

[10]. Privacy-preserving ML (federated learning, de-identification) is a hot research area.

- *Regulation and Reimbursement*: The pace of tech often outstrips policy. For instance, telehealth licensing was relaxed during a public health emergency, but permanent rules are still solidifying. Reimbursement codes for digital health (DTx or telemonitoring) are under development. Regulatory bodies are crafting new frameworks: the FDA's Digital Health Innovation Action Plan and Europe's MDR for medical devices now cover software as a medical device (SaMD). For meeting these requirements, developers must plan for evidence generation.
- *Equity and Access*: Potential risk of increasing healthcare disparities exists if only those having the means can benefit from assistive technology. High costs of surgical robots or AI platforms mean wealthier hospitals can afford them first. Similarly, rural areas may lack broadband for telehealth, and older or low-income patients may lack smartphones for DTx. Policymakers and designers must prioritize accessibility, such as low-cost devices and inclusive UI design.
- *Clinical Validation and Acceptance*: Engineers and clinicians sometimes speak different languages. Translational research is needed to test technologies in real-world clinical settings. For example, while AI diagnostics may work on curated image datasets, their performance in busy clinics (with low-quality images and diverse populations) must be proven. Engaging clinicians early in design (human-centered design) improves adoption; a smart home system must not just be technically sound, but also acceptable to residents (perceived as helpful, not intrusive).
- *Education and Training*: Healthcare professionals need training to use new tools. Telemedicine requires learning "webside manner". Interpreting wearable-generated data or AI reports needs new competencies. Some institutions now include informatics or digital health in medical curricula.

10.11 CONCLUSION AND FUTURE DIRECTIONS

The convergence of healthcare with ICT and robotics is creating a qualitatively new care paradigm. This chapter has surveyed how telemedicine, wearables, AI, robotics, smart homes, rehab devices, and digital therapeutics are reshaping prevention, diagnosis, and treatment. Historically, we see a trajectory from telephone and radio links to today's AI-enhanced, cloud-connected systems. Evidences like systematic reviews or case studies claim substantial clinical promise of assistive technology such as patient satisfaction, improved access, and in some cases improved health outcomes.

In spite of all these, there exist limitations that would be addressed through further research. In near future, telemedicine will be done through integrating the home-based sensors and predictive analytics for preemption of crises. Wearables will be upgraded to multimodal, unobstrusive sensors, potentially including genetic and biochemical markers. AI-based diagnostics would become better through the integration of "explainable AI" with decision support, as the models would not only detect disease but also offer personalized treatment options. Research is going on to incorporate more autonomy to robots with human oversight so that the robots can offer better natural interaction. Smart homes will be empowered with more adaptivity so that the technology can learn individual habits. The rehabilitation tech will amalgamate the virtual reality with physiological sensing for offering fully remote therapy. As evidence accumulates, digital therapeutics will expand to provide therapeutics in new fields of medicine like autoimmunity, cardiology, etc.

Achieving these visions requires interdisciplinary collaboration among clinicians, engineers, and patients. The technology must be developed in such a way that it ensures effectiveness, robustness, and safety. Policymakers and the payers need to come forward for creating incentives/mandates for adoption without violating the safety features. Moreover, proper ethical considerations should be there ensuring equitable access, upholding patient privacy, and maintaining the primacy of human judgment in care.

As a whole, the field of healthcare and assistive technologies is ever-expanding and holds enormous potential for the enhancement of quality of lives. However, the challenges regarding security and bias need to be addressed properly to introduce the technology-driven revolution in the domain of healthcare.

REFERENCES

[1] Lustig, T. A. (2012). *The role of telehealth in an evolving health care environment: workshop summary*. National Academies Press.

[2] Kulcsar, M., Gilchrist, S., & George, M. G. (2014). Improving stroke outcomes in rural areas through telestroke programs: an examination of barriers, facilitators, and state policies. *Telemedicine and e-Health*, *20*(1), 3–10.

[3] Houser, S. H., Flite, C. A., & Foster, S. L. (2023). Privacy and security risk factors related to telehealth services–a systematic review. *Perspectives in Health Information Management*, *20*(1), 1f.

[4] Haleem, A., Javaid, M., Singh, R. P., & Suman, R. (2021). Telemedicine for healthcare: capabilities, features, barriers, and applications. *Sensors International*, *2*, 100117.

[5] Babu, M., Lautman, Z., Lin, X., Sobota, M. H., & Snyder, M. P. (2024). Wearable devices: implications for precision medicine and the future of health care. *Annual Review of Medicine*, *75*(1), 401–415.

[6] Hoff, T., Kitsakos, A., & Silva, J. (2024). A scoping review of the patient experience with wearable technology. *Digital Health*, *10*, 20552076241308439.

[7] Gagnon, M. P., Ouellet, S., Attisso, E., Supper, W., Amil, S., Rhéaume, C.,... & Sasseville, M. (2024). Wearable devices for supporting chronic disease self-management: scoping review. *Interactive Journal of Medical Research*, *13*(1), e55925.

[8] Daniore, P., Nittas, V., Haag, C., Bernard, J., Gonzenbach, R., & von Wyl, V. (2024). From wearable sensor data to digital biomarker development: ten lessons learned and a framework proposal. *NPJ Digital Medicine*, *7*(1), 161.

[9] Najjar, R. (2023). Redefining radiology: a review of artificial intelligence integration in medical imaging. *Diagnostics*, *13*(17), 2760.

[10] Weiner, E. B., Dankwa-Mullan, I., Nelson, W. A., & Hassanpour, S. (2025). Ethical challenges and evolving strategies in the integration of artificial intelligence into clinical practice. *PLOS Digital Health*, *4*(4), e0000810.

[11] Boardsworth, K., Rashid, U., Olsen, S., Rodriguez-Ramirez, E., Browne, W., Alder, G., & Signal, N. (2025). Upper limb robotic rehabilitation following stroke: a systematic review and meta-analysis investigating efficacy and the influence of device features and program parameters. *Journal of NeuroEngineering and Rehabilitation*, *22*(1), 164.

[12] Wang, Y., Sun, H., Xu, S., Xia, Q., Ge, S., Li, M., & Tang, X. (2025). Smart home technologies for enhancing independence of living and reducing care dependence in older adults: a systematic review. *Journal of Advanced Nursing*, *81*(6), 2885–2912.

[13] Morita, P. P., Sahu, K. S., & Oetomo, A. (2023). Health monitoring using smart home technologies: scoping review. *JMIR mHealth and uHealth*, *11*, e37347.

[14] Khan, A., Imam, Y. Z., Muneer, M., Al Jerdi, S., & Gill, S. K. (2024). Virtual reality in stroke recovery: a meta-review of systematic reviews. *Bioelectronic Medicine*, *10*(1), 23.

[15] Hong, J. S., Wasden, C., & Han, D. H. (2021). Introduction of digital therapeutics. *Computer Methods and Programs in Biomedicine*, *209*, 106319.

Chapter 11

AI-powered smart hospitals and digital twin healthcare systems

Amandeep Kaur and Upinder Kaur

11.1 INTRODUCTION

Digital twin technology, which can transform patient results and expedite healthcare operations, is becoming more and more popular in the healthcare sector [3]. By making it possible to develop virtual representations of patients, medical devices, and healthcare methods, digital twin technology revolutionized development in the management and delivery of healthcare. This cutting-edge technology creates dynamic simulations of real-world healthcare entities by combining real data collection, historical analysis, and sophisticated machine learning algorithms. From the integration to the application layer, the architectural layer implementation is enabled through patient monitoring, predictive diagnosis, and customized therapy optimization. Medical device management, increasing operational efficiency, and improving patient outcomes are transformed by the healthcare digital twins with the advanced security protocols and scalable infrastructures [4]. Figure 11.1 shows how the utilization of Digital Twin technology is increasingly prevalent within the healthcare field by connecting the Digital Space (virtual models, decision support, personalized care, medical research, and training) with the Physical Space (real-world patient data, diagnosis, treatment, clinical parameters, and real-time information) [15]. The two areas are connected via real-time data flow, which enables ongoing observation, individualized care, and enhanced clinical results via insights derived from data.

Digital twin technology is the combination of three systems: the physical, virtual, and connective link layer. It serves as a duplicate, and it offers the virtual representation of actual physical objects. Gaps to overcome the difficulties of creating intelligent healthcare ecosystems are revealed by a schematic review of the state of digital twins in the healthcare field today. With the help of many technologies, digital twins in healthcare offer new features and capabilities with a wide range of uses [5]. The current status, technical implementations, uses, difficulties, and prospects of AI-powered smart

DOI: 10.1201/9781003665656-11

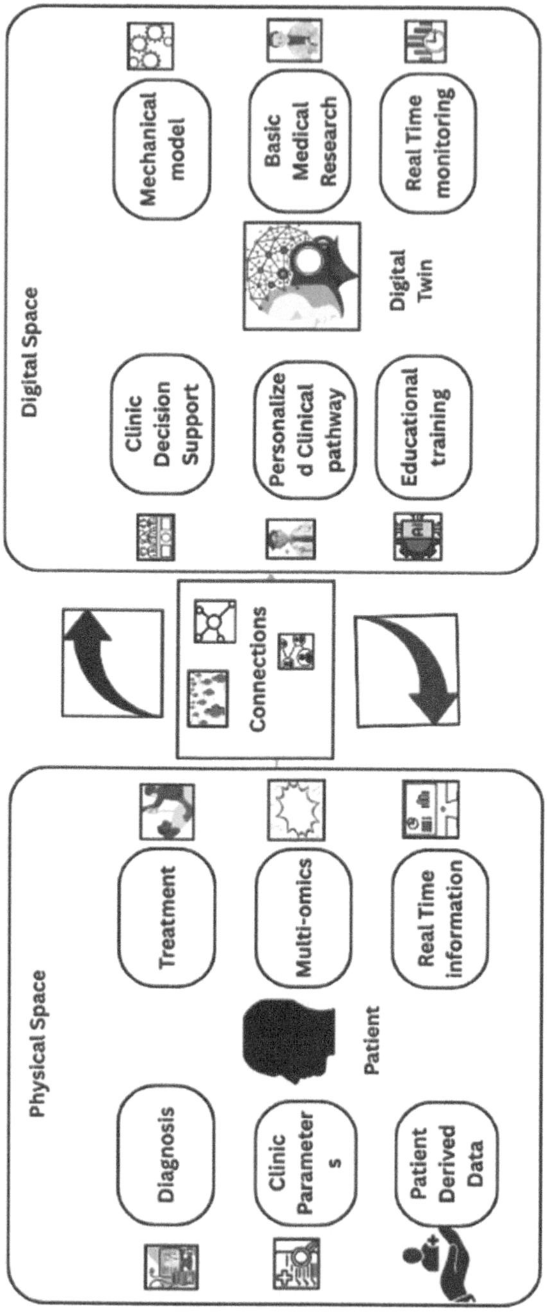

Figure 11.1 Digital twin.

hospitals and digital twin healthcare systems are all thoroughly examined in this review of the literature.

11.1.1 Evolution of digital twin in healthcare

Major developments in the creation of DT technologies for the healthcare sector have been made in recent years. In recent years, patient-specific, precise diagnosis and treatment have become essential to improve efficiency in the healthcare sector [6]. The Digital Twin (DT) is one technology that exemplifies the Industry 4.0 Revolution. In addition to the manufacturing and automotive sectors, DTs are also emerging in the healthcare industry [11]. COVID-19 has accelerated a broad focus on smart hospital development. However, there isn't a single, agreed-upon definition of what a smart hospital is. Rare hospitals have become "smart," mainly due to a lack of system integration and consideration of all potential consequences. With the aid of 5G apps, cloud computing, IoT, and AI, hospitals can achieve intelligence. Figure 11.2 illustrates the evolution of medical services from traditional, offline methods to a more advanced, individualized healthcare system. Traditional medicine initially required follow-up care, diagnosis, treatment, and payment to be done in person [7]. With the introduction of technology, healthcare shifted into a networked paradigm embracing telemedicine, enabling remote diagnosis, consultation, monitoring, and education. Precision medicine started in 2019 with the combination of digital and intelligent technology. In this stage, genetic testing, individualized prevention, customized treatments, and all-encompassing personal health management are combined with traditional medicine and telemedicine. Although the exact future of medical services is still up in the air, it is anticipated that advances in digital health technologies will drive efforts to increase continuity of care and individualization.as depicted in Figure 11.2. At the same time, medical models are changing from the evidence-based medicine mode of contemporary medicine to the precision medicine mode of person-specific targeted medications, which is based on cloud computing, big data, IoT, and mobile internet. Targeting the illness before it manifests itself is a key objective of precision medicine, which makes use of technologies like genetics, genomics, and intelligent medical monitoring systems [5]. If the disease cannot be prevented, therapy will be tailored to the patient rather than being administered to the whole public as was previously the case. Moreover, smart healthcare is driven by data for precision medicine, encompassing a range of data, including patient data. This technology creates a digital replica of the human body, its organs, and their associated processes, which can be utilized for various purposes, including drug discovery, treatment planning, and medical research. with the development of AI, Big Data, IOT digital twin, it can replicate complex processes and facilitate customized

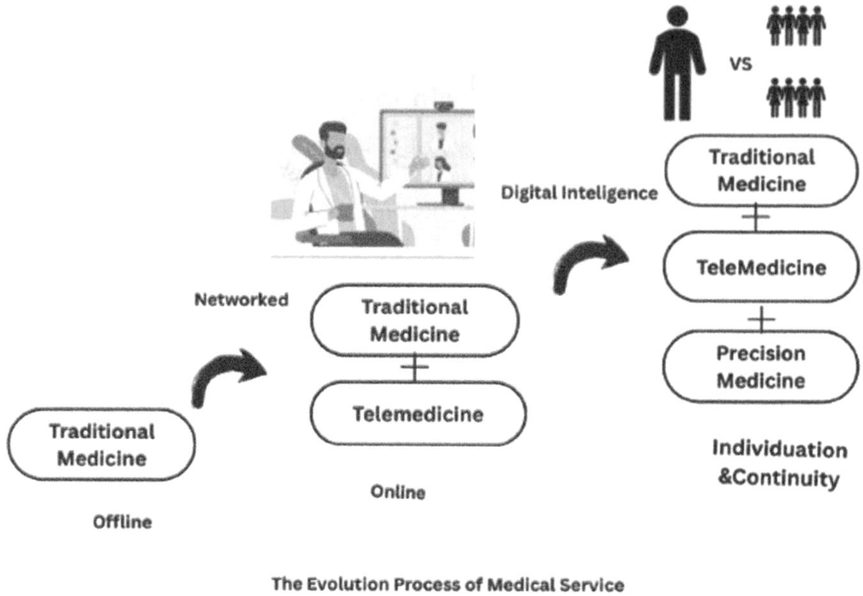

Figure 11.2 The evolution process of medical service.

healthcare solutions for the patient's needs [11]. The current studies explore the potential and ramifications of Digital twin technology in the healthcare.

11.1.2 Implementation of digital twins in healthcare

A structured framework known as "digital twin layered architecture," this architecture links virtual and physical medical systems and provides intelligent, real-time healthcare [6]. The foremost layer in Figure 11.3 is the physical layer, which consists of individuals, tools used in medical field and clinical settings which collects the health data which consists of individuals, medical tools, and clinical settings that collect health data [12]. The layer that gathers and integrates the data from various sources that involve wearables, sensors, and ESR is the data acquisition layer [15]. Further, the modelling layer makes use of artificial intelligence and computational simulation to raise virtual genre of people and systems with the aim of assessment as well as prognosticating health issues [22]. The application layer assists in making clinical decisions for remote monitoring, along with the customization of treatments with the help of these models. Eventually, the digital twin uses user-friendly interfaces that are laid out by a user interaction layer that can be accessed and engaged by the medical professional and patients. These layers work in collaboration to support [28].

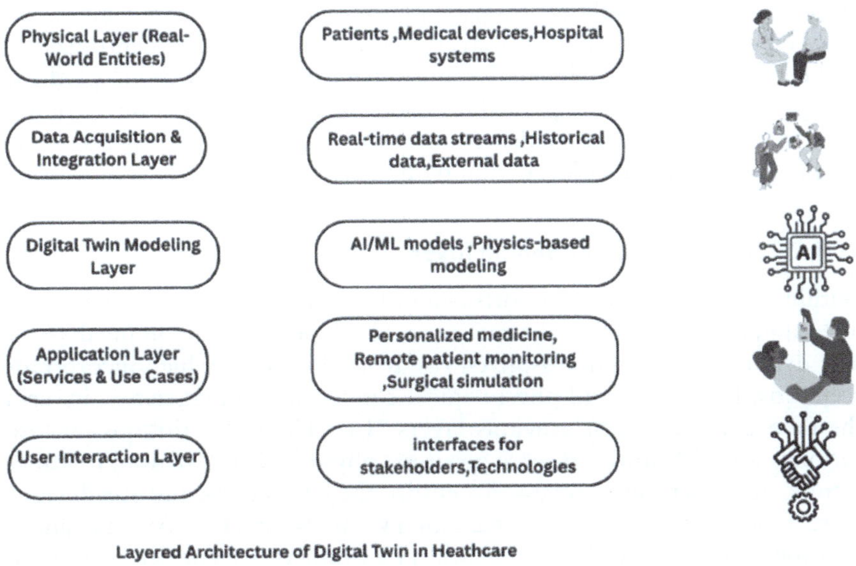

Figure 11.3 Architecture of the digital twin.

11.1.2.1 Physical layer

The physical layer acts as a stand-in for the tangible systems and bodies that are reflected by the digital twin, circumscribed patients, medical tools, wearable computing, and medical settings [12]. The creation of real-time done by these strata via utilizing sensors and medical apparatus such as glucose monitoring, MRI, ECG machines, as well as the tools that are used in diagnosis and cure [6]. The operational and physiological data are perpetually assembled by these components that is passed on to the digital twin in subsequence in the view of the fact layer aids in the establishment of framework of monitoring modelling, replication, and advanced analytics within the twin frame. It makes an effort to put a significant impact on the accurate as well as reliable outcomes of the digital twin [16].

11.1.2.2 Data acquisition and integration layer

On the domain of medical digital twin, this clinical layer acts as a mediator between the digital replica and the tangible reality [6]. The primary work is to collect, aggregate, merge, and organize the data that is obtained from a multitude of origins, medical tools, and surrounding wearable sensors, EHR lab infrastructure and medical monitors [8]. The strata have a capability to collect and convert the data efficiently in a standardized framework that suits the analytical investigations, not of systematics [12, 13]. It is a temporal sequence or organizational framework for the well-organized interaction between efficient. The physical layer and its replica, data synchronization, authentication, and amalgamation are supervised across varying platforms and protocols [20]. This procedure makes sure the pre-severing, comprehensive, and contemporary depiction of the patent or healthcare system is confined within the medical digital twin [22].

11.1.2.3 Digital twin modelling layer

Within this layer, the digital portrayal of tangible entities for patients, medical equipment's or clinical practice is developed and maintained [6, 8]. The dynamic presentation is given rise to in this layer, which incorporates scenarios, behaviors, and physiological conditions. Concurrently, by using the data gathered from previous layers [14]. These descriptions enclosed the anatomical features, disease progress, physiological function, treatment results, and operation process. To ensure the correctness and steadiness of these models, state-of-the-art technology involving [15]. AI and simulation tools are employed. The medical practitioners are entitled to replicate various treatment protocols, envision medical scenarios, as well as build up medical practice via this stratum. This is the core mechanism of a digital twin [18].

11.1.2.4 Application layer in a digital twin

The improvement of real-world decision-making and operational processes is done in this application layer[6]. With the help of the manipulation of knowledge that is withdrawn from the digital model, the strata assist in interaction between practitioners, clinicians, and patients by its tools and interface [12]. This strata includes different functionalities such as diagnostic help, treatment strategy development, and many more [14]. In addition, it gives support to the prognosis of results, operational streamlining, and scenario analysis [17]. The dashboard notification and visualization mechanisms are utilized in the modification of integrated data and model outcomes into practical insights [23]. Finally, this model brings concrete merits by supplementing the quality of patient care and the decision-making process [22].

11.1.2.5 User integration layer

The integration layer acts as an intermediary between the digital twin and varying end users within the medical field, such as administrators, patients, doctors, and nurses [12]. The significant role is to communicate with users and interact with the data in the system via the website healthcare software, mobile app, and various platforms [12]. The user satisfaction is improved by this layer by giving precise roles with privileges, a safe communication channel, and an individual interface [6]. Not only is the shareholders' engagement smoothed due to the persistence of the collaborative attempts amongst the users for an upgraded care cooperation as well as a joint decision-making process. A conversant decision is made with integration of communication with the digital twins, thereby explicating the information and replicating it into understandable and practical insights. By putting this technology to good use, the patient results are improved, and the medical care facilities are modified [15].

11.1.3 Technology integrated in digital twin

Sensor-driven digital twin technology has enormous transformational potential for improving healthcare delivery in smart surroundings. With an emphasis on their effects on healthcare goals and results, this entails integrating sensor technology, digital health abilities, and location-based services with smart surroundings. The core technologies that support the features of smart environments include machine learning (ML), the Internet of Things (IoT), artificial intelligence (AI), and the Internet of Medical Things (IoMT) [15]. In Figure 11.4, the different technologies used in digital twins are shown.

Digital twins (DTs) are essential to healthcare, but their use in real-time patient monitoring is still constrained by difficulties in obtaining low-latency telemetry transmission and effective resource management. Innovative cloud-based digital twin frameworks that maximize real-time healthcare monitoring have been introduced, offering prompt resolutions for urgent medical issues. These frameworks use dynamic optimization models, which have been demonstrated to outperform current systems by lowering telemetry latency and improving response time. Proactive health interventions are made possible by these systems, which continually monitor vital physiological parameters, heart rate, and body temperature using inexpensive, low-latency multimodal sensors [16]. Through real-time remote monitoring, digital twin (DT) technology has been acknowledged as a crucial tool for improving patient care in the healthcare industry. However, the use of the Internet of Things in remote healthcare has brought up issues with data security, work offloading, and risk prediction [15]. There are new approaches that integrate advanced cybersecurity solutions with edge computing. A great deal of physiological and environmental information has been acquired, enabling a comprehensive comprehension of the patients. Secure communication, certificate-based authentication, Merkle Tree verification, threat prediction, and hybrid encryption have all been included in systems. Platforms such as the ESP32-Azure IoT Kit and Azure Cloud have been used to assess the viability of these ideas and determine how

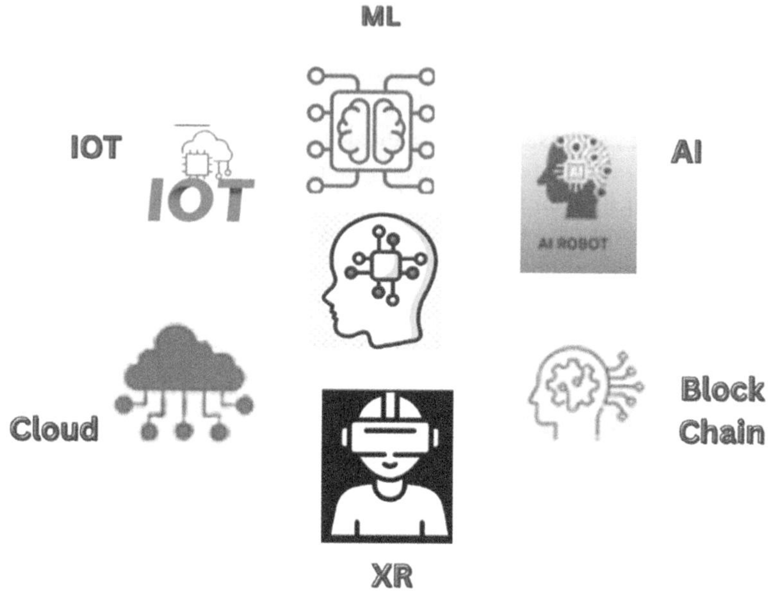

Figure 11.4 Technologies used in digital twin.

well the system can transmit patient data to stakeholders and healthcare organizations. Health monitoring systems (HMS), which are a representation of healthcare systems, are progressively emerging as a significant component of future medical technology thanks to sensing networks and edge computing. Although resource-constrained Internet of Things nodes and the topology of heterogeneous networks make data protection more challenging, HMS has been progressively implemented in actual scenarios. Since HMS anomalies frequently result in significant losses, even to human safety, prompt anomaly prediction techniques are seen to be important for ensuring HMS data protection. The majority of current solutions rely on past logs, which makes it challenging to find new issues and readily creates serious security risks. To address this issue, cloud-edge collaboration-based abnormal prediction techniques augmented by distributed digital twins (DT) have been developed to increase the availability and data protection as seen in Table 11.1.

The healthcare industry has seen a major revolution in the new year due to the combination of digital twins (DT) and artificial intelligence (AI). By combining a variety of genetic and nongenetic data with sophisticated AI models and computing techniques, precision medical methods can help researchers and clinical physicians make more accurate decisions. The system can reason and learn from data and algorithms. According to research, AI

Table 11.1 Various technologies used in DT

References	*1*	*2*	*3*	*4*	*5*	*6*	*7*	*Results*	*Limitations*
[1]	√	×	√	×	×	×	√	Improves decision-making and patient care	Privacy Cost Interoperability
[2]	√	×	√	×	×	×	√	Enables real time and personalized healthcare	Complexity
[3]	√	√	√	×	×	×	√	Patient management and reshapes workflows	Integration issues and standards
[4]	√	×	√	×	√	×	√	Enhances treatment planning and diagnosis	High resources, skill needs, and data accuracy
[5]	√	×	√	√	×	×	×	Precision and personalized medicine	Reliability, dataset quality
[6]	√	×	√	×	×	×	√	Lack of practical validation	–
[7]	√	×	√	√	×	×	√	Implementation barriers	–
[8]	√	√	×	√	×	×	√	Data man agement challenges, high simulation complexity	Supports predictive care
[9]	√	√	√	×	×	×	×	Requires high-quality biological samples, limited scalability,	Demonstrates DT potential for individual profiling and precision health
[10]	√	√	√	√	√	√	√	regional disparities, infrastructural, and policy challenges	–
[11]	√	×	√	×	×	×	√	High adoption barriers	DT progress
[12]	√	×	√	√	×	×	√	Cost, data security, and Integration challenges	Proposes a model for smart hospitals
[13]	√	√	√	√	×	×	×	Implementation difficulty	DT with Industry 4.0 for efficiency
[14]	√	×	√	×	×	×	×	Data accuracy issues	Enables real-time monitoring and predictive simulation in hospitals
[15]	√	×	√	×	×	×	×	Sensor reliability, and it needs infrastructure	Shows DT's role in enhancing monitoring, diagnostics, and smart care
[16]	√	×	×	√	×	×	√	Still conceptual, limited clinical validation	Offers a predictive framework for neurological complications
[17]	√	×	×	×	×	√	×	Hardware dependency, issues of real-time accuracy	Enhances healthcare with augmented vision
[18]	√	×	√	×	×	×	√	Ethical risks, data integration challenges	AI-driven cardiac care

(continued)

Table 11.1 (*Cont.*)

References	*1*	*2*	*3*	*4*	*5*	*6*	*7*	*Results*	*Limitations*
[19]	√	×	×	√	×	×	√	Data quality, continuous monitoring difficulty	It provides efficient tracking and treatment of chronic wounds
[20]	√	×	√	×	×	×	√	Urban infrastructure limits	Integrates AI and DT for healthcare management in smart cities
[21]	√	×	×	√	×	×	×	Integration complexity	Enhances robotic healthcare with patient interaction
[22]	√	×	×	√	×	×	×	Security	Enables remote patient monitoring with security
[23]	√	×	√	√	×	×	√	Technical challenges	Supports the future surgical sector with robotics
[24]	×	×	√	×	×	×	√	Data sharing and scalability issues	–
[25]	√	×	×	×	×	×	×	Legal uncertainty and risk	Analyses all the policies. Legal and social challenges of DT adoption
[26]	√	×	×	×	×	×	×	Lack of standardized methods	–
[27]	√	×	√	×	×	×	√	Technical, ethical, legal, and societal challenges	Highlights risks and safeguards; promotes safer DT
[28]	√	×	√	√	×	×	√	Implementation barriers, lack of frameworks	–

1. DT, 2.ML, 3.AI, 4. IoT, 5. Block chain, 6. XR, 7. Cloud.

and DT have demonstrated a vast technological application space in a variety of fields, including molecular imaging, clinical cancer treatment, and genomics [30]. However, they may also encounter obstacles, including system bias, correlation restrictions, algorithm black boxes, and unfairness. To create a precise medical intelligent system, this calls for the application of AI and DT transformations which Combining digital twin technology with robotic systems has been one way to enhance individualized healthcare in the wake of COVID-19, with a focus on decreased physical interaction and increased safety in healthcare institutions. By using the Internet of Robotic Things (IoRT) to collect health data in a secure and nonintrusive way, research signals a change [30]. These systems, as opposed to Internet of Things (IoT) methods, use robots to go around hospitals, gather patient health data via monitoring devices and safely update this data on local servers. This strategy addresses privacy issues frequently connected to IoT healthcare technologies and gives priority to data protection. This makes it easier to simulate and analyze treatment by collecting a representation of a patient's condition within the hospital. This digital duplicate, medical personnel experience physical and mental stress from the long work shifts, constant observation, and skin-to-skin contact required by traditional patient monitoring techniques. A very close attention is paid by the medical practitioners to the patients to lower the risk of infection and stress with the help of wearable sensors. RPM a virtual twin is created which helps in the collection of sensors data from the physical twin while it works to copy its behavior. Autonomous controlled has been integrated into the digital twin's base IORT. To monitor the patient with severe health problems remotely, PTs can autonomously navigate to patients' rooms, gather and send health data, and return to base stations thanks to decision-making algorithms. Digital twins and the Internet of Robotic Things (IoRT) are expected to revolutionize digital healthcare in ways that have never been seen before [30]. Digital twins are computer-based models or real or virtual machines that can "twine" or replicate the lives of real things like people, things, or characteristics associated with people. The globe has quickly incorporated a number of technologies into healthcare since the emergence of digital and smart healthcare to promote better patient care, increase life expectancy, and reduce healthcare costs. Two promising technologies that mark significant advancements in this area are digital twins. The surgical community has become interested in these ideas in recent years. The ideal method is to ensure that data is seamlessly integrated in both directions between physical and virtual devices. The introduction of artificial intelligence (AI) has greatly hastened the shift in healthcare organizations during the last 20 years, which saw them move from the initial phases of digitization and making digital to a more thorough process of digital transformation. Therefore, the formation of the modern patient digital twin (PDT) requires the progress of high-quality clinical data warehouses and is enhanced with multidomain data, including genomics, proteomics, and Internet of Things (IoT) information. This strategy is essential for utilizing AI in the changing clinical practice environment to improve the outcome of patients and advance personalized healthcare.

11.2 APPLICATIONS OF DIGITAL TWIN

Digital twin technology has three primary applications in healthcare: specialized medical care, smart hospitals, and patient monitoring with the integration of IoT, AI, and cloud computing. Digital twins help personalize treatments for patient monitoring with real-time data [2]. The main advantage of this system is for the elderly with remote patient monitoring the virtual care. An example of this technology is Duke Health, a smart hospital that uses digital twins with IoT sensors and AI to improve resource allocation and disease surveillance. In specialist medicine, digital twins help surgeons with AR-integrated real-time anatomical models, enhance cardiovascular treatment with patient-specific simulations, and support precision oncology by forecasting neurological problems in cancer patients [11]. Additionally, the system has potential for managing chronic wounds, where AI-powered digital twins monitor. India's focus on healthcare has greatly increased since COVID, and digital twin technology is now a major innovation driver. In order to lay the groundwork for upcoming digital twin applications, the government's Ayushman Bharat Digital Mission is developing a digital health ecosystem with distinct Health IDs and electronic health data. Adoption is being accelerated by programs like NITI Aayog's "AI for All" initiative and PM-ABHIM's ₹64,180 crore investment in AI-driven health infrastructure. While private companies like Wipro, GE, and TCS are testing 5 G-enabled hospital administration systems, academic institutions like AIIMS and IITs are creating digital twins specialized to the heart and other organs. AI-based prediction models that resemble early-stage digital twins are being developed by health tech businesses for the treatment of chronic diseases and radiography. Although there are still obstacles, these initiatives support the SDGs for innovation and health fairness.

Through real-time, data-driven solutions for expert medicine, hospital administration, and patient care, digital twins are transforming the healthcare industry. Through the creation of virtual copies, they make it possible to use IoT, AI, and cloud computing to provide individualized treatment plans, predictive diagnoses, and ongoing remote monitoring, particularly for elderly and rural patients. To improve operations, resource allocation, and infection control, smart hospitals use digital twins in conjunction with 5G and IoT. The technology improves surgery (AR-guided surgeries), cardiology (patient-specific cardiac simulations), [18]and oncology (cancer progression modelling) in specialized treatment. Although encouraging, issues with clinical validation, system compatibility, and data privacy still exist. These obstacles might be removed by future developments in federated learning and quantum computing, which would put digital twins in a position to change healthcare from reactive to proactive, precision medicine. UN has 17 goals for the future, and some of the Sustainable Goals will be met. [11] Major developments in digital twin technology have made it possible to create detailed real-time models that aid in clinical decision-making, facility management, and personalized treatment. From the past research, the healthcare delivery system has completely changed from the traditional framework with the advanced AI and IoT technology [2]. The digital twins enhance the outcome of patient and operational efficiency. It will be the pillar of future healthcare innovations. The concept of the implementation of DT is explored in the literature. By creating intelligent hospital twins, it could predict the neurological problems [25]. The framework represents the progression in healthcare monitoring and offers a responsive and scalable solution to latency and constraints of resources in real-time applications.

Future research could explore the advanced ML models and sensors to expand the impact of healthcare applications [16]. From Table 11.2, it is clear that the digital twin is used for various diseases of the heart, oncology, neurology, etc.

11.3 IMPACT OF DIGITAL TWIN IN SUSTAINABLE HEALTHCARE

11.3.1 Economic sustainability

Because DT allows exact resource allocation and service tailoring, which can minimize the interventions. Digital twins reduce unnecessary treatments and hospital stays and also lower the expenses of healthcare. Digital twins enhance the equipment maintenance, hospital operation, and supply chain which resulting in the saving of cost and efficient use of healthcare resources [36]. With the help of healthcare organizations, manage rising demand without correspondingly raising spending; these cost-effective methods encourage sustainable financial practices [32]. The monitoring benefits coincide with the medical care policy goals, which put emphasis on a valuable care delivery framework by the prioritization of results and efficiency, wherein the twin technology has a significant role as an enabler.

11.3.2 Environmental sustainability

The data-centric energy and resource management practices are entitled to develop the environmental sustainability within medical amenities. With the help of a digital twin, these advanced tools identify the ineffectiveness and provide useful insights to divide the footprints by simulating building energy, the functioning workflow, and materials used [32]. The dangerous medical waste volume is lower, and the disposal process is upgraded by developing and evaluating effective waste management strategies. Additionally, the sustainable supply chain management is supported by these replicas with the help of enhancing precise demand to reduce material excess as well as overproduction, which a consequently plays a pivotal role in the advancement of eco-friendly medical care initiatives by encapsulating sustainability principles into the domain of healthcare digitalization. This unification lines up with the united nation sustainable goals (SDGS) particularly SDG 12 SDG 13 bestowing the worldwide agenda for supportable advancements.

11.3.3 Sustainability in social and ethical domains

The unification of DTs in sustainable medical care encircles socio-economic dimensions, which include the management of patient data in an ethical way and the delivery of superior medical care services. It broadens

Table 11.2 Various types of applications of DT in healthcare

Application area	*Year*	*Technology*	*References*	*Summary*
General healthcare overview and transformation	2022, 2023, 2024, 2025	DT, AI	[1, 3, 4, 5, 6, 7, 11, 28]	An overall understanding of DT adoption, benefits, and challenges provides frameworks for transforming healthcare services
Smart cities management	2024	DT, AI, IoT	[10, 20]	Improves healthcare management through precision medical models in smart city health infrastructure
Simulation and predictive modeling	2022, 2025	DT	[8, 14]	Uses simulation for predictive analytics and real-time healthcare optimization
Smart hospitals	2022, 2024	DT, IoT, AI	[12, 13]	Establishes intelligent hospital twins and smart healthcare systems integrated with IoT and Industry 4.0 technologies
Remote patient monitoring, health	2022, 2023, 2024, 2025	DT, IoT, Sensors, IoRT	[2, 8, 15, 19, 21, 22, 23]	Enables continuous patient tracking, early intervention, and connected care via IoT and robotic systems
Surgery and augmented vision systems	2022, 2024	DT, IoRT, AR/VR	[17, 23]	Enhances surgical precision and collaboration with AR/VR and robotic systems
Cardiovascular care	2024	DT, AI	[18]	DT supports diagnosis, treatment planning, and patient-specific cardiovascular interventions
Chronic disease management	2022, 2023, 2024	DT, Sensors, AI	[16, 19, 27]	Uses DT for personalized care, early detection, and chronic disease management
Personalized medicine	2024	DT	[9]	Creates individual health profiles using advanced metabolomics data and DT
Healthcare training and education	2024	DT	[26]	Reviews DT use in health education and skill development for medical professionals
Public health, ethics, and legal challenges	2022, 2024	DT	[25, 27]	Addresses privacy, ethical, and legal barriers for DT adoption in healthcare

healthcare access by facilitating the amenities and facilities among geographically isolated populations [32], thereby diminishing the medical care excess differences. Continual attention is warranted, which includes information protection, patient privacy, and informed consent, even social sustainability is upgraded by performing staff's being and optimizing the care delivery process that aims to ameliorate the exhaustion of medical professionals

11.4 CHALLENGES AND LIMITATIONS

There are many legal obstacles to overcome before digital twin technology can be used in public health. Digital twins are sophisticated computer simulations designed to mimic biological processes and the functioning of human organs. [36] Their objective is to make it possible to simulate the full human body and to customize the results using the health information of each unique patient. Digital twin technology has potential for bridging the gap between precision public health and individualized care. [2] However, there are serious flaws in the laws governing data privacy, and there is a chance that health insurance systems may monitor people more, which could result in human rights abuses. [1] The usage of digital twins in public health would necessitate the worldwide study of private data, which would raise further concerns regarding the safe processing, transfer, and storage of such data. Existing legal structures. In Figure 11.5, the challenges of healthcare are shown.

11.4.1 Clinical limitations

Digital twin is not easy to implement because of its model accuracy and implementation barriers, and also has a limitation of trust of patients in these technologies.

11.4.2 Technical limitations

Digital twin has Inaccurate, incomplete, or inconsistent EHR, imaging, and wearable data that can undermine model reliability [15]. Healthcare data often exists in siloed formats, making integration across systems challenging [36].

11.4.3 Privacy and security

Protecting the sensitive data of patients that underpin digital twins is a top concern. Data leaks or breaches can have serious legal and ethical ramifications, especially when considering frameworks such as GDPR or HIPAA. The use of cloud storage and third-party systems further complicates

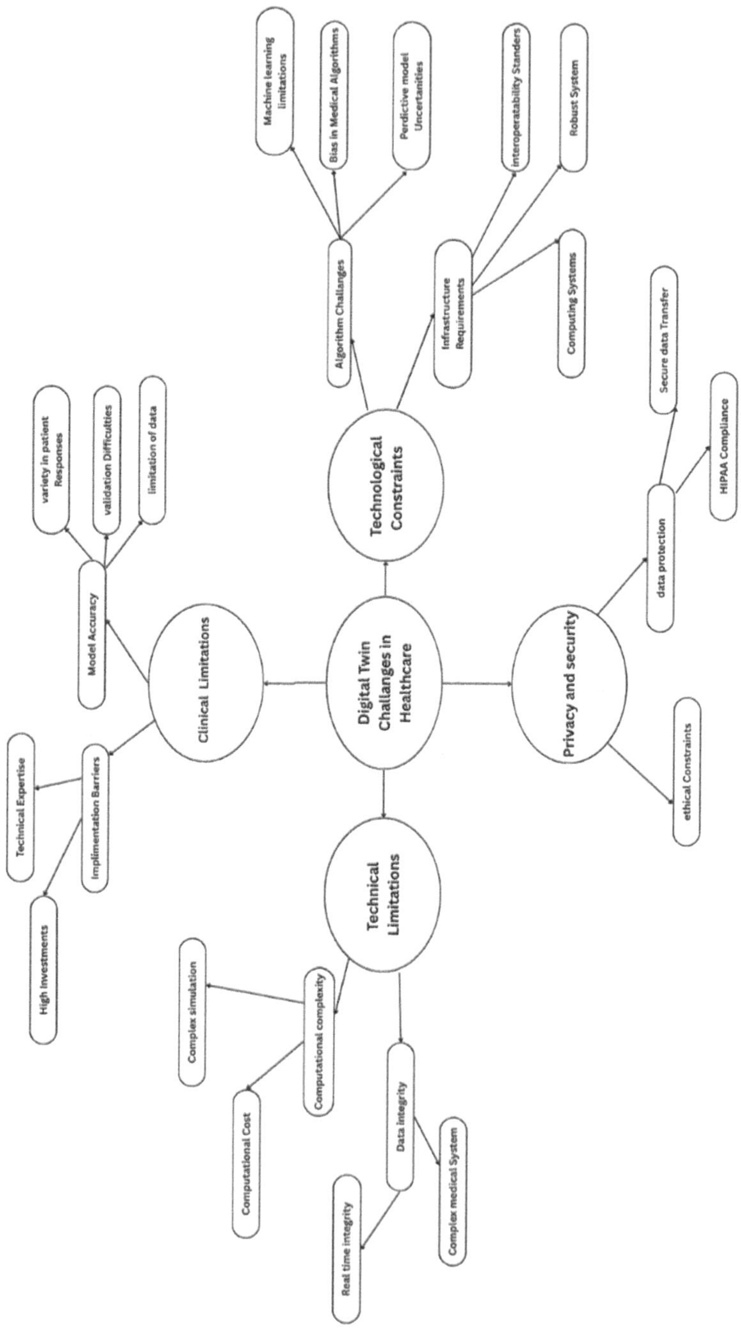

Figure 11.5 Challenges of healthcare.

the requirement for advanced cryptography, security, blockchain, and real-time audit trails.

11.4.4 Technological constraints

Modelling human physiology and disease progression is incredibly complex due to the dynamic, multi-scale nature of biological systems [15]. Many DTs remain "conceptual" rather than fully validated against real clinical outcomes, which limits trust and adoption of digital twins [2]. Digital twin technologies are untested at scale in live healthcare environments. There are concerns about reliability, robustness, and the transparency of results from pilot projects to widespread use.

11.5 FUTURE DIRECTIONS

For a number of reasons, digital twins' predictive capabilities need to be enhanced. Digital twins of hospital patient paths are created using new techniques termed Digital twin, which make use of DES and IoT devices. The two real-time models that make up these DTs are the DT for monitoring (DTM) and the DT for predicting (DTP). Before connecting to actual hospitals, methods can be validated on experimental platforms that have emulators of actual hospitals. In the DTP, near-term predictive simulations can be carried out using "dynamic" empirical distributions. To enhance the suggested DT models, further characteristics and machine learning techniques would be required in subsequent studies [14]. Through telemedicine, data exchange, and remote patient monitoring, smart homes and smart hospitals are likely to completely transform healthcare delivery. Sensor-driven digital twins can be used in innovative solution frameworks to meet user and healthcare needs. These frameworks include digital twin proof-of-concept applications, health devices, and AI-driven health analytics. The potential of location-based services (LBSs) to improve emergency response capabilities and individualized healthcare interventions is highlighted by their involvement in smart environments. The development of Digital twin in healthcare changes the traditional healthcare system to a smart environment. This new development has opportunities as well as limitations, which emphasize the study to fully grasp patient care and healthcare delivery. To creatively design precision medical smart systems in smart cities, real-world data should be built from information system data and medical knowledge data from different hospitals, along with the roles of real-world evidence (RWE), randomized clinical trials, genetic research, and AI technology in precision medicine [29]. In conclusion, untargeted metabolomics, sophisticated machine learning methods, and the application of digital twins in healthcare have the potential to completely transform the process of healthcare delivery. New horizons in customized and preventive medicine are made possible by the focus on uniqueness, dynamic metabolic profiles, and precision in patient management.

11.6 CONCLUSION

Healthcare workers' approaches to patient care, treatment planning, and facility management are evolving as a result of the digital twin revolution. Digital twins provide virtual representations of patients, medical devices, and healthcare systems to enable real-time monitoring and individualized treatment. Digital twins enable better resource management and help firms save waste and expenses by providing insights into energy use, material use, and other critical factors. As reviewed from various research studies, digital twins cover the diagnosis and investigation, cardiology and oncology. In the literature study, implementation, applications, challenges, and future discussions are covered. Digital technology shifts the paradigm of Healthcare delivery, management, and optimization in healthcare. Digital twin research aims to alter the healthcare system by providing innovative medical procedures and better care for patients. The new era is expected with digital twin technology. Digital twins provide effective and robust hospital operations, while virtual twins transfer the real-time monitoring and precision care in the complex issues of healthcare. With the development of industry, the digital twin technology, integrated with IoT, cloud computing, and advanced analytics, has the potential to revolutionize healthcare delivery, boost effectiveness, and improve the health of patients and medical institutions. This review focuses on the Digital twins' implementations in healthcare and points out opportunities as well as difficulties. Possibly, healthcare is improved in numerous ways like patient health monitors. Future research should focus on resolving the legal, moral, and technological issues, while also developing the use of digital twin in healthcare. By the review, we analyze the digital twin is used in various fields of healthcare, but it is lacking in stroke, ENT, and ophthalmology. Mostly work is done in the field of cardiology, oncology, medicine, and patient monitoring.

REFERENCES

[1] Sun, Tianze, He, Xiwang, and Li, Zhonghai. 2023. "Digital Twin in Healthcare: Recent Updates and Challenges". *Digital Health*. Pp. 1-13, vol 1https://doi.org/10.1177/20552076221149651

[2] Chen, Jiayuan, Shi, You, Yi, Changyan, Du, Hongyang, Kang, Jiawen, and Niyato, Dusist. 2024. "Generative-AI-Driven Human Digital Twin in IoT Healthcare: A Comprehensive Survey". *IEEE Internet of Things Journal*, vol. 11, no. 21, pp. 34749-34773, 1 Nov.1, 2024, doi: 10.1109/JIOT.2024.3421918

[3] Sharma, Bhanu, Kaushal, Deepak, Joshi, Sudhanshu, Sharma, Manu, and Bafila, Suhani. 2023. "Transforming Healthcare: Exploring the

Impact and Potential of Digital Twin Technology". In *2023 1st DMIHER International Conference on Artificial Intelligence in Education and Industry 4.0 (IDICAIEI)*. Wardha, India, IEEE, pp. 1-6, doi: 10.1109/IDICAIEI58380.2023.10406632

[4] Vuggumudi, Jaswanth Kumar. 2025. "Digital Twin Technology: Revolutionizing Modern Healthcare Systems". *International Journal of Scientific Research in Computer Science Engineering and Information Technology*. Vol 11, pp. 2947-294 https://doi.org/10.32628/cseit251112312

[5] Sun, T., He, X., Song, X. and Li Z. 2022. "The Digital Twin in Medicine: A Key to the Future of Healthcare?" *Front Med (Lausanne)*. Vol 9, pp. 1-8 www.frontiersin.org/journals/medicine/articles/10.3389/fmed.2022.907066/

[6] Pellegrino, Giulia, Gervasi, Massimiliano, Angelelli, Mario, and Corallo, Angelo. 2024. "A Conceptual Framework for Digital Twin in Healthcare: Evidence from a Systematic Meta-Review". *Information Systems Frontiers*. Volume 27, pages 7–32 https://doi.org/10.1007/s10796-024-10536-4

[7] Subashini, Dr. R., Kanishghasriee, M., Grace, S., Shifa, C., Fatima, Sidhiq, Sankar, Anupama, Rifa, C., and Fathima, Sidhik. 2024. "Digital Twin – An Innovative Strategy in Healthcare Transformation: An Extensive Review". Vol 3, pp 7-19, *Journal for Research in Applied Sciences and Biotechnology*. https://doi.org/10.55544/jrasb.3.6.2

[8] Nadeem, Mubaris, Kostic, Sascha, Dornhöfer, Mareike, Weber, Christian, and Fathi, M. 2025. "A Comprehensive Review of Digital Twin in Healthcare in the Scope of Simulative Health-Monitoring". *Digital Health*. Vol.11, pp. 1-25, https://doi.org/10.1177/20552076241304078

[9] Fradin, Manon, Noël, Louis-Philippe, Talbot-Lachance, Gabriel, Snell, Pierre, Voyer, Keven, and Rhéaume, Caroline. 2024. "Human Digital Twin Technology for Individual Profiling using LC-MS Untargeted Metabolomics Analysis of Dried Blood Spot Samples". *Digital Twin*. Vol 4, pp.1-26, https://doi.org/10.12688/digitaltwin.17936.1

[10] Shao, Yinjie. 2024. "Investigating the Possible Impact of Chinese Digital Twin Technology and AI in Facilitating Healthcare and Medical Systems in Belt and Road Regions: A Case Study on Smart Cities in the Middle East". *Journal of World Economy*. Vol 3, pp.130-145, https://doi.org/10.56397/jwe.2024.12.16

[11] Roopa, M. S. 2023. "A Systematic Review: Digital Twin in Healthcare". *International Journal for Research in Applied Science and Engineering Technology*. Vol.11, pp. 4818-4825, https://doi.org/10.22214/ijraset.2023.52792

[12] Cheng, Weibin, Lian, Wanmin, and Tian, Junzhang. 2022. "Building the Hospital Intelligent Twins for All-Scenario Intelligence Health Care". *Digital Health*.Vol 8, pp.1-4 https://doi.org/10.1177/20552076221107894

[13] Jena, M. C., Mishra, Sarat, and Moharana, H. S. 2024. "Application of Industry 4.0 and Digital Twin in the Field of Smart Healthcare". *Insight – Automatic Control*.Vol 7,pp. 1-5, https://doi.org/10.18282/iac.v7i1.606

[14] Karakra, A., Fontanili, F., Lamine, E., and Lamothe, J. 2022. "A Discrete Event Simulation-Based Methodology for Building a Digital Twin of Patient

Pathways in the Hospital for Near Real-Time Monitoring and Predictive Simulation". *Digital Twin.*, vol 2, pp. 1-24, https://doi.org/10.12688/digitaltwin.17454.1

[15] Adibi, S., Rajabifard, Abbas, Shojaei, D., and Wickramasinghe, Nilmini. 2024. "Enhancing Healthcare through Sensor-Enabled Digital Twins in Smart Environments: A Comprehensive Analysis". *Italian National Conference on Sensors*.vol 24, pp. 1-30, https://doi.org/10.3390/s24092793

[16] Thiong'o, Grace M., and Rutka, J. 2022. "Digital Twin Technology: The Future of Predicting Neurological Complications of Pediatric Cancers and Their Treatment". *Frontiers in Oncology*. Vol 11. Pp. 1-10 https://doi.org/10.3389/fonc.2021.781499

[17] Kaliappan, Dr. S., and Logesh, S. 2024. "Digital Twin-Driven Augmented Vision System for Healthcare". *2024 9th International Conference on Communication and Electronics Systems (ICCES)*, Coimbatore, India, IEEE, pp. 842-847, doi: 10.1109/ICCES63552.2024.1085981.

[18] Thangaraj, P., Benson, Sean H., Oikonomou, E., Asselbergs, F., and Khera, R. 2024. "Cardiovascular Care with Digital Twin Technology in the Era of Generative Artificial Intelligence.". *European Heart Journal*. Vol. 45, pp.4808-4821, https://doi.org/10.1093/eurheartj/ehae619

[19] Sarp, S., Kuzlu, M., Zhao, Y., and Gueler, O. 2023. "Digital Twin in Healthcare: A Study for Chronic Wound Management". *IEEE Journal of Biomedical and Health Informatics*. vol. 27, pp. 5634-5643 https://doi.org/10.1109/JBHI.2023.3299028

[20] Ahmed, Atique, Shoukat, Khadija, Muneeb, Muhammad Ahmad, Qasem, Doaa Abdo Othman All, Shahzad, Muhammad Adeel, Nissa, Laraib Ul, Amir, Rabia, Zubair, Muhammad, Younas, Muhammad Waqas, and Ali, Asad. 2024. "AI and Digital Twin Transforms in the Construction of Precision Medical Model: Healthcare Management in Smart Cities". *European Journal of Medical and Health Research*.Vol 2, pp.36-42, https://doi.org/10.59324/ejmhr.2024.2(1).05

[21] Rajurkar, Chanda, Murugan, B., and Namasivayam, G. 2024. "Design and Integration of IoRT-Enabled Robotic Systems with Wearable Devices in a Digital Twin Framework". *2024 9th International Conference on Control and Robotics Engineering (ICCRE)*, Osaka, Japan, IEEE, pp. 45-49, doi: 10.1109/ICCRE61448.2024.10589845

[22] Khan, Sangeen, Ullah, Sehat, Ullah, Khalil, Almutairi, S., and Aftan, Sulaiman. 2024. "Implementing Autonomous Control in the Digital-Twins-Based Internet of Robotic Things for Remote Patient Monitoring". *Italian National Conference on Sensors*. Vol 24, pp.1-20, https://doi.org/10.3390/s24175840

[23] Das, Chetana, Mumu, Anika Anis, Ali, Md. Firoj, Sarker, Subrata K., Muyeen, S. M., Das, Sajal K., Das, Prangon, Hasan, Md. Mehedi, Tasneem, Zinat, Islam, Md. Manirul, Islam, Md. Robiul, Badal, Faisal R., Ahamed, Md. Hafiz, and Abhi, Sarafat Hussain 2022. "Toward IoRT Collaborative Digital Twin Technology Enabled Future Surgical Sector: Technical Innovations, Opportunities and Challenges". *IEEE Access*. https://doi.org/10.1109/ACCESS.2022.3227644

[24] Lin, Yu-Ting, et al. 2025. "Mini-Review of Clinical Data Service Platforms in the Era of Artificial Intelligence: A Case Study of the iHi Data Platform". *BioMedicine*. Vol 15, pp.1-24 https://doi.org/10.37796/2211-8039.1643

[25] Delerm, Félix, and Pilottin, A. 2024. "Double Edged Tech: Navigating the Public Health and Legal Challenges of Digital Twin Technology". *European Journal of Public Health*. Vol 34, pp.1-10 https://doi.org/10.1093/eurpub/ckae144.1510

[26] Rajamäki, J. 2024. "Digital Twin Technology Training and Research in Health Higher Education: A Review". *Exploration of Digital Health Technologies*. Vol 2, pp.:188–201. https://doi.org/10.37349/edht.2024.00021

[27] Drummond, D., and Coulet, Adrien. 2022. "Technical, Ethical, Legal, and Societal Challenges with Digital Twin Systems for the Management of Chronic Diseases in Children and Young People". *Journal of Medical Internet Research*. Vol 24, pp.1-13, https://doi.org/10.2196/39698

[28] Narigina, Marta, Romānovs, A., and Brūzgienė, R. 2024. "Digital Twin Technology in Healthcare: A Literature Review". In *2024 IEEE 11th Workshop on Advances in Information, Electronic and Electrical Engineering (AIEEE)*. IEEE, https://doi.org/10.1109/AIEEE62837.2024.10586661

Chapter 12

Blockchain and AI for sustainable healthcare

Kuldeep Singh Kaswan, Kiran Malik, and Jagjit Singh Dhatterwal

12.1 INTRODUCTION

The aging populations, the increasing cases of chronic illnesses, and soaring expenses incurred to provide treatments have brought so many ills into the world of healthcarethat were previously unheard. In 2023, the amount of healthcare spent globally was approximately $10.3 trillion (as reported by the World Health Organization [WHO]). This may increase up to $14 trillion by 2030. The high cost strains both the state and private systems, particularly in the low-income and middle-income countries where high-quality care remains a far-fetched dream. The healthcare sustainability should strike a balance between economic viability, fair access, and environment and delivering good results to the patients. In the United States, healthcare errors led to the death of over 250,000 US citizens last year. Bad data interoperability in fact could account for one-third of these deaths. To remain healthy in maintaining a healthcare system, it requires new solutions that will improve productivity, cut down waste, and prioritize the patients without jeopardizing its future financial status (Abbas et al., 2020).

New technologies such as artificial intelligence (AI), blockchain, the Internet of Things (IoT), and big data analysis have enhanced efficiency in reducing healthcare expenses and finer targeting medicine. Such AIs as deep learning radiology diagnostic models (Jadwal and Saini, 2025) have diagnostic accuracy rates of more than 90 percent in diagnosing conditions as diverse as breast cancer and diabetic retinopathy. Live data of IoT-enabled devices like smart wearable health monitors can be used in proactive treatment: in other words, healthcare will be able to tell when there is trouble brewing before it actually occurs in practice (Agarwal et al., 2022).

These technologies however work in a fragmented manner. No safe, cross-functional framework exists to get them all the way to play. Ever since 2009, 2,200 instances of health data violation in the United States

 DOI: 10.1201/9781003665656-12

have brought into question the issue of data privacy, regulatory (e.g. HIPAA (Health Insurance Portability and Accountability Act), GDPR (General Data Protection Regulation), and cybersecurity risks) and compliance. This shows that there is an urgent need to have a high level of synchronization of technology. The emerging technologies must be connected in scalable and secure healthcare systems, and patients must be placed on the frontline of the agenda, while keeping cost (Alabdulatif et al., 2022).

The integration of blockchain and AI is, therefore, a new concept of sustainable healthcare. The predictive and analytical functions (Preeti and Saini, 2023) of AI will be supported by the blockchain, which ensures safe and decentralized data storage. The distributed ledger record of transactions of the blockchain technology and data immutability and transparency are guaranteed by mathematical tools such as cryptographic hashing and consensus mechanisms such as Proof of Stake (PoS) and Practical Byzantine Fault Tolerance (PBFT). Ethereum-based smart contracts can have patient consent management automated and reduce administration overheads by up to 30 percent. The machine learning (ML) of AI, deep learning, and natural language processing (NLP) have the capacity to process a huge amount of data—like electronic health records (EHRs) or genes—to determine when new infectious diseases are taking place. By having the two meet each other, blockchain guarantees the data processing of both the ends of AI and minimizes the threat of manipulation or falsification; and AI corrects blockchain (Kaur, Kaur, Kumar and Saini, 2023) by streamlining transactions through validation. In this way, they will constitute a perfect synergy, which will deliver safe, effective, and fair healthcare, addressing the issue of sustainability (Saini and Jain, 2023) by ensuring better interoperability and reduced expenses and patients (Al-Safi et al., 2022; Akula and Kumar, 2025).

12.1.1 Literature survey

Table 12.1 presents the literature survey of this study.

12.2 FOUNDATIONAL CONCEPTS

Let $\mathscr{P} = \{P_i\}_{i=1}^{N}$ denote the collection of patient-data probability measures held by N distinct custodians, and let $\mathscr{X}$ be the data domain. For custodian i define the local empirical risk functional for model parameters $w \in \mathbb{R}^d$ by

$$L_i(w) = \mathbb{E}_{x \sim P_i}\left[\ell(x; w)\right], \qquad (12.1)$$

Table 12.1 Literature survey

Authors and year	*Key findings*	*Methodology/techniques used*	*Results/remarks*	*Finding gaps*
Bartoletti, 2019	Identified ethical and privacy challenges of AI in healthcare.	Conceptual review of AI deployment in medicine.	Highlighted risks of bias, misuse, and privacy invasion.	Lacks concrete mitigation frameworks and technical solutions.
Bharadwaj et al., 2021	Machine learning enhances IoT-enabled healthcare	Survey of ML applications in IoT healthcare	Showed potential for predictive analytics and remote monitoring	Security, scalability, and real-time adaptation remain underexplored
Chen et al., 2021	Explored ethical dimensions of ML in healthcare	Analytical review of ethical ML frameworks	Emphasized fairness, accountability, transparency	Lacks empirical studies integrating ethics into ML pipelines
Cheng et al., 2021	Blockchain + ML improves healthcare data trust	Literature review in cancer care applications	Suggested enhanced data integrity for oncology	Practical deployments and interoperability challenges remain
Dhatterwal et al., 2025	Blockchain for decentralized data management in CIoT	Proposed blockchain-based CIoT architecture	Demonstrated secure and distributed framework	Performance and latency trade-offs need deeper testing
Hussain et al., 2025	MAS improves traffic flow efficiency	Multi-agent systems simulation	Optimized coordination in traffic systems	Application to healthcare traffic/logistics yet unexplored
Kaswan et al., 2025	Introduced digital personality ontologies for dialog	Ontology-driven modeling	Theoretical foundation for human–digital interaction	Still conceptual; limited healthcare-specific application
Kaswan et al., 2024	Digital twin for sustainable intelligent manufacturing.	Review and conceptual framework.	Useful for predictive maintenance and optimization.	Translation to healthcare digital twins requires adaptation.
Kumar et al., 2023	AI + blockchain for public health reviewed	Survey of existing systems	Identified challenges in privacy, security, and scalability	Lack of standardized frameworks and real-time validation
Kuo & Ohno-Machado, 2018	Introduced ModelChain for privacy-preserving healthcare	Blockchain + federated predictive modeling	Enabled secure, decentralized ML	Computational cost and scalability not addressed

Mahiban et al., 2023	Proposed blockchain-AI synergy for impregnable healthcare	Framework design in ICT	Strengthened trust in digital healthcare	Still theoretical, limited implementation evidence
Malik et al., 2025	Blockchain-enabled edge computing for CIoT	Blockchain + edge computing integration	Provided secure edge data handling	Edge scalability and resource constraints underexplored
Malviya et al., 2023	AI + blockchain = synergistic healthcare benefits	Analytical study	Highlighted integration benefits for EHR and diagnosis	Practical deployment barriers not deeply covered
Mantey et al., 2022	Blockchain + DL for EHR recommender system	Prototype implementation	Improved accuracy in patient recommendations	Scalability and energy costs require optimization
Mazlan et al., 2020	Reviewed scalability issues in healthcare blockchain	Systematic review	Scalability remains a key bottleneck	Solutions for cross-chain interoperability missing
McGhin et al., 2019	Blockchain applications in healthcare	Literature survey	Identified opportunities and challenges	Empirical validations lacking
Park et al., 2019	Explored human-AI collaboration in healthcare	Qualitative study of interactions	Identified challenges in trust and usability	Lack of long-term studies and technical frameworks
Prashanthi et al., 2022	NLP + DL for crop disease detection	Deep learning with NLP models	Achieved high accuracy in detection	Limited to agriculture; no direct healthcare linkage
Qayyum et al., 2021	Secure and robust ML in healthcare	Comprehensive survey	Suggested robust frameworks against adversarial threats	Deployment in real-world clinical workflows not addressed
Shaik et al., 2023	Remote patient monitoring using AI	Review of AI tools for RPM	Highlighted improvements in chronic care	Integration with blockchain for privacy not studied
Sharma et al., 2024	AI + blockchain for smart secure healthcare	Review and conceptual exploration	Provided frameworks for secure systems	Needs empirical deployment studies
Shinde et al., 2022	Blockchain for securing AI healthcare	Systematic review	Identified vulnerabilities and potential countermeasures	Energy efficiency and interoperability remain challenges
Tagde et al., 2021	AI + blockchain in e-Health	Survey	Showed improved trust and automation in health systems	Lacks real-world clinical adoption studies

(*continued*)

Table 12.1 (*Cont.*)

Authors and year	*Key findings*	*Methodology/techniques used*	*Results/remarks*	*Finding gaps*
Tan et al., 2021	Retinal AI algorithms + blockchain for research	Retrospective multicohort study	Improved diagnostic accuracy with blockchain-enabled sharing	High computational cost and data diversity challenges
Wang et al., 2018	Blockchain-powered parallel healthcare	ACP (Artificial societies, Computational experiments, Parallel execution)	Proposed large-scale simulation-based healthcare	Real-world clinical translation missing
Yaqoob et al., 2021	Blockchain for healthcare data management	Review	Identified opportunities, challenges, recommendations	Standardized protocols still lacking
Zekiye & Özkasap, 2023	Decentralized healthcare with FL + blockchain	Federated learning framework	Enhanced data privacy and model accuracy	Resource efficiency and scalability issues remain
Zhang et al., 2021	Security and privacy in healthcare blockchains	Theoretical and survey analysis	Reviewed threats and countermeasures	Lack of unified regulatory compliance mechanisms

where $\updownarrow : X \times \mathbb{R}^d \to \mathbb{R}_{\geq 0}$ is a twice continuously differentiable loss density. L_i will be called the local loss potential of node i. The global aggregate loss potential under a convex weighting vector $\alpha = (\alpha_1, \ldots, \alpha_N)$, $\alpha_i \geq 0$, $\sum_i \alpha_i = 1$, is

$$L(w; \alpha) = \sum_{i=1}^{N} \alpha_i L_i(w). \tag{12.2}$$

Define the local model parameter at custodian i and round t by $w_i^{(t)}$ and the global federated parameter by $w^{(t)}$. A standard federated averaging step with participation fraction $\rho \in (0, 1]$ and local SGD (Stochastic Gradient Descent) operator SGD $_\eta$ (learning rate $\eta > 0$) yields the update

$$w^{(t+1)} = \sum_{i=1}^{N} p_i^{(t)} \mathrm{SGD}_\eta \left(w^{(t)}; B_i^{(t)} \right), \tag{12.3}$$

where $p_i^{(t)}$ is the normalized participation weight at round t and $B_i^{(t)}$ denotes the local mini-batch. For convenience, let $G_i^{(t)} = \nabla L_i \left(w^{(t)} \right)$ denote the instantaneous local gradient estimator so that $\mathrm{SGD}_\eta(w) = w - \eta G_i^{(t)} + \xi_i^{(t)}$ with stochasticity $\xi_i^{(t)}$ satisfying $\mathbb{E}\left[\xi_i^{(t)} \right] = 0$. Substitution gives

$$w^{(t+1)} = w^{(t)} - \eta \sum_{i=1}^{N} p_i^{(t)} G_i^{(t)} + \xi_i^{(t)}. \tag{12.4}$$

To ensure privacy-preserving aggregation, each custodian perturbs their contribution with an additive noise mechanism: define the privatized local upload $\widetilde{\Delta}_i^{(t)}$ by

$$\widetilde{\Delta}_i^{(t)} = \Delta_i^{(t)} + \eta_i^{(t)}, \quad \Delta_i^{(t)} := w_i^{(t)} - w^{(t)}, \tag{12.5}$$

where $\eta_i^{(t)} \sim \mathrm{N}\left(0, \sigma^2 I_d\right)$ and $\sigma > 0$ is the noise scale. The sensitivity of Δ_i is $\Delta_{\max}$ in the ℓ_2-norm, so by Gaussian mechanism the privacy parameter ε (for fixed δ) obeys the calibration relation

$$\varepsilon \leq \frac{\Delta_{\max}}{\sigma} \kappa(\delta), \tag{12.6}$$

where $\kappa(\delta) > 0$ is the standard Gaussian tail constant determined by the privacy failure probability δ. The global noisy aggregation used in Eq. (12.3) thus becomes

$$\widetilde{w}^{(t+1)} = w^{(t)} + \sum_{i=1}^{N} p_i^{(t)} \widetilde{\Delta}_i^{(t)} = w^{(t)} + \sum_{i=1}^{N} p_i^{(t)} \Delta_i^{(t)} + \eta_n^{(t)}, \tag{12.7}$$

with aggregate noise vector $\eta_n^{(t)} := \sum_{i=1}^{N} p_i^{(t)} \eta_i^{(t)}$ satisfying $\mathbb{E}\left[\eta_n^{(t)}\right] = 0$ and $\mathrm{Cov}\left(\eta_n^{(t)}\right) = \sigma^2 \sum_i \left(p_i^{(t)}\right)^2 I_d$. Model updates and provenance records are committed to a permissioned ledger whose block at index k is B_k. Represent the ledger state after k blocks as $\mathcal{B}_k := \{B_1, \ldots, B_k\}$ and denote the block-creation operator (smart-contract execution and validation) by Φ. The validity predicate for block B_k is expressed as

$$\mathrm{Valid}\left(B_k | \mathcal{B}_{k-1}\right) = \mathbf{1}\left(\Phi\left(B_k, \mathcal{B}_{k-1}\right) = \mathrm{ok}\right), \tag{12.8}$$

where $\mathbf{1}(\cdot)$ is the indicator. Each block aggregates a set of transactions $\mathcal{T}_k$ including model uploads $\left\{\widetilde{\Delta}^{(t)}\right\}$ and incentive transfers. Let the gas cost for executing $\mathcal{T}_k$ be $g\left(\mathcal{T}_k\right)$ and the energy consumed to validate block B_k be $E\left(B_k\right)$. The system-wide sustainability constraint across an epoch of K blocks is

$$\mathbb{E}\left[\sum_{k=1}^{K} E\left(B_k\right)\right] \leq E_{\max}, \tag{12.9}$$

where $E_{\max} > 0$ is a prescribed energy budget for sustainable operation. Validators are indexed by $j \in \{1, \ldots, M\}$, each holding stake $s_j \geq 0$ and total stake $S = \sum_{j=1}^{M} s_j$. The probability that validator j is selected to propose the next block under stake-proportional selection is

$$\pi_j = \frac{s_j}{S}. \tag{12.10}$$

Define the token reward per block as $R > 0$; the expected per-epoch reward to validator j is therefore

$$\mathbb{E}\left[r_j\right] = R \cdot \sum_{k=1}^{K} \pi_j^{(k)} - \mathbb{E}\left[\mathrm{pen}_j\right], \tag{12.11}$$

where pen_j is the expected penalty from slashing or misbehavior. For convenience introduce the net expected incentive flow vector $\mathbf{r} = \left(\mathbb{E}\left[r_1\right], \ldots, \mathrm{E}\left[r_M\right]\right)^{\top}$. To couple incentives to data contribution quality, define a contribution-quality functional $q_i^{(t)}$ for custodian i at round t by the negative local loss decrease normalized by information cost:

$$q_i^{(t)} = \frac{L_i\left(w^{(t)}\right) - L_i\left(w^{(t+1)}\right)}{1 + \gamma_{\text{info}}\text{cost}_i^{(t)}}, \quad \gamma_{\text{info}} > 0, \tag{12.12}$$

where $\text{cost}_i^{(t)}$ models local computation and communication cost. The incentive allocation mechanism maps qualities $q_i^{(t)}$ to payments $\pi_i^{\text{pay}}(t)$ via a monotone increasing allocation kernel $\mathscr{A}$ with normalization $\sum_i \pi_i^{\text{pay}}(t) \leq R$, yielding

$$\pi_i^{\text{pay}}(t) = \text{A}\left(q_i^{(t)}; \mathbf{q}^{(t)}\right). \tag{12.13}$$

To capture trade-offs between model utility, incentives, privacy, and sustainability, define the system utility scalar at round t as

$$\mathscr{U}^{(t)}\left(w; \alpha, \text{s}, \sigma\right) = -L(w; \alpha) + \beta \sum_{j=1}^{M} \mathbb{E}\left[r_j\right] - \zeta \mathbb{E}\left[\sum_{k=1}^{K} E\left(B_k\right)\right] - \tau \text{Priv}(\sigma), \tag{12.14}$$

where $\beta, \zeta, \tau > 0$ are scaling constants and $\text{Priv}(\sigma)$ maps noise scale to an interpretable privacy cost (smaller σ reduces accuracy but increases privacy cost via Eq. 12.6); one possible penalization is $\text{Priv}(\sigma) = \varepsilon(\sigma)^{-1}$. The objective is to choose a tuple $(w, \alpha, \text{s}, \sigma)$ maximizing $\mathscr{U}^{(t)}$ subject to feasibility constraints:

$$\alpha_i \geq 0, \sum_i \alpha_i = 1,$$

$$s_j \geq 0, S = \sum_{j=1}^{M} s_j,$$

$$\varepsilon(\sigma) \leq \varepsilon_{\max}, \mathbb{E}\left[\sum_{k=1}^{K} E\left(B_k\right)\right] \leq E_{\max}. \tag{12.15}$$

Form the Lagrangian $\mathscr{L}$ with multipliers λ for the simplex constraint on α, ν for the stake budget constraint, χ for the privacy constraint, and ψ for the energy budget:

$$\mathscr{L}\left(w, \alpha, \text{s}, \sigma; \lambda, \nu, \chi, \psi\right) = -L(w; \alpha) + \beta \sum_{j=1}^{M} \mathbb{E}\left[\tau_j\right] - \zeta \mathbb{E}\left[\sum_{k=1}^{K} E\left(B_k\right)\right] - \tau \text{Priv}(\sigma)$$

$$+\lambda\left(1-\sum_{i=1}^{N}\alpha_i\right)+\nu\left(S-\sum_{j=1}^{M}s_j\right)+\chi\left(\varepsilon_{\max}-\varepsilon(\sigma)\right)+\psi\left(E_{\max}-\mathbb{E}\left[\sum_{k=1}^{K}E\left(B_k\right)\right]\right). \tag{12.16}$$

Stationarity of the Lagrangian with respect to w yields the first-order optimality condition

$$\nabla_w\mathcal{L}\left(w^*;\alpha^*\right)=0, \tag{12.18}$$

so that w^* is a critical point of the weighted aggregate loss; substituting Eq. (12.2) gives

$$\sum_{i=1}^{N}\alpha_i\nabla\mathcal{L}\left(w^*\right)=0. \tag{12.19}$$

Differentiating $\mathcal{L}$ with respect to α_i and imposing complementary slackness yield the Kuhn–Tucker condition for each i:

$$-L_i\left(w^*\right)-\lambda^*=0 \quad \text{whenever } \alpha_i^*>0, \tag{12.20}$$

hence for active custodians $\alpha_i^*>0$ we have the equalized marginal loss potential:

$$L_i\left(w^*\right)=-\lambda^*, \quad \text{if } \alpha_i^*>0. \tag{12.21}$$

Differentiate $\mathcal{L}$ with respect to the noise scale σ and substitute the privacy gradient via Eq. (12.6) to obtain

$$\tau\mathrm{Priv}'^{\left(\sigma^*\right)}-\chi^*\varepsilon'^{\left(\sigma^*\right)}=0, \tag{12.22}$$

which upon specifying $\mathrm{Priv}(\sigma)=\varepsilon(\sigma)^{-1}$ and $\varepsilon(\sigma)=\frac{\Delta_{\max}\kappa(\delta)}{\sigma}$ yields the explicit equilibrium condition

$$\frac{\tau\Delta_{\max}\kappa(\delta)}{\sigma^2}=\chi^*\frac{\Delta_{\max}\kappa(\delta)}{\sigma^2}\Longrightarrow\tau=\chi^*. \tag{12.23}$$

so the active privacy multiplier equals the privacy weight when that regularizer is chosen. Differentiate $\mathcal{L}$ with respect to each stake s_j; using Eq. (12.10) the derivative of expected reward with respect to s_j is $\partial\mathbb{E}\left[\tau_j\right]/\partial s_j=R\sum_{k=1}^{K}\partial\pi_j^{(k)}/\partial s_j$ and under stake-proportional selection $\partial\pi_j/\partial s_j=\left(S-s_j\right)/S^2$. The stationarity condition gives

$$\beta RK\frac{S-s_j^*}{S^2}-v^*=0,\quad \forall j \text{ with } s_j^*>0, \tag{12.24}$$

which rearranges to an explicit optimal stake profile for active validators:

$$s_j^*=S-\frac{v^*S^2}{\beta RK}. \tag{12.25}$$

Summing Eq. (12.24) over active j and enforcing $S=\sum_j s_j^*$ yield a self-consistency equation for v^* whose solution determines the common offset and hence the equilibrium stake distribution. To analyze convergence of the learning dynamics under ledger ordering, model the communication graph induced by block inclusion as a doubly-stochastic mixing matrix $W^{(t)}\in\mathbb{R}^{N\times N}$ acting on the local models; then the noisy distributed update (combining Eqs. (12.4) and (12.7)) can be written as

$$\mathbf{w}^{(t+1)}=W^{(t)}\mathbf{w}^{(t)}-\eta\mathbf{g}^{(t)}+\boldsymbol{\eta}_n^{(t)}, \tag{12.26}$$

where $\mathbf{w}^{(t)}=\left(w_1^{(t)},\ldots,w_N^{(t)}\right)^\top$, $\mathbf{g}^{(t)}=\left(\mathcal{G}_1^{(t)},\ldots,\mathcal{G}_N^{(t)}\right)^\top$, and $\boldsymbol{\eta}_n^{(t)}$ stacks the local noise contributions. Let $\bar{\mathbf{w}}^{(t)}=\frac{1}{N}\mathbf{1}^\top\mathbf{w}^{(t)}$ be the network average. Subtracting averages and iterating give the consensus error recursion

$$\mathbf{e}^{(t+1)}=\left(W^{(t)}-\frac{1}{N}\mathbf{1}\mathbf{1}^\top\right)\mathbf{e}^{(t)}-\eta\left(I-\frac{1}{N}\mathbf{1}\mathbf{1}^\top\right)\mathbf{g}^{(t)}+\left(I-\frac{1}{N}\mathbf{1}\mathbf{1}^\top\right)\boldsymbol{\eta}_n^{(t)}, \tag{12.27}$$

where $e^{(t)}=\mathbf{w}^{(t)}-\mathbf{1}\mathbf{w}^{(t)}$. A sufficient spectral condition for mean-square consensus is that the expected spectral radius $\rho\left(\mathbb{E}\left[\mathbf{W}^{(t)}-\frac{1}{N}\mathbf{1}\mathbf{1}^T\right]\right)<1$. Denote $\Lambda:=\sup_t\rho\left(\mathbf{W}^{(t)}-\frac{1}{N}\mathbf{1}\mathbf{1}^T\right)$ and require

$$\eta<\frac{1}{\Lambda}, \tag{12.28}$$

where $G_{\max}=\sup_j\|\mathbf{g}^{(j)}\|_2$, to guarantee asymptotic mean-square stability of the consensus-plus-gradient dynamics. Introduce an energy-efficiency function (Saini, 2025) for block validation $\mathcal{E}(s_j)$ capturing that validators with larger stake may run more efficient hardware or aggregate more transactions; assume $\mathcal{E}$ is concave, $\mathcal{E}''(s)<0$. Then the expected epoch energy from Eq. (12.9) can be written as

$$\mathbb{E}\left[\sum_{k=1}^{K}E(B_k)\right]=K\sum_{j=1}^{M}\pi_j\mathcal{E}(s_j)=K\sum_{j=1}^{M}\frac{s_j}{S}\mathcal{E}(s_j). \tag{12.29}$$

Differentiate the energy budget constraint multiplier ψ in Eq. (12.16) with respect to s_j and combine with Eq. (12.23) to obtain the modified stationarity condition including sustainability:

$$\beta RK\frac{S \cdot s^*}{S^2} - \nu^* - \zeta K\left(\frac{\mathscr{E}\left(s^*\right)}{S} + \frac{s^*\mathscr{E}'\left(s^*\right)}{S} - \frac{s^*\sum_i s_i^*\mathscr{E}'\left(s_i^*\right)}{S^2}\right) = 0. \tag{12.30}$$

Equation (12.29) implicitly determines s_j^* balancing rewards against energy penalties. Turning to joint optimization over participation weights α, recall Eq. (12.19) and employ a soft participation model where α_i is chosen proportional to a quality-to-cost exponentiated score:

$$\alpha_i = \frac{\exp\left(\eta_i q_i\right)}{\sum_{r=1}^N \exp\left(\eta_r q_r\right)}, \quad \eta_i > 0, \tag{12.31}$$

which enforces α simplex membership and links α to the quality metrics in Eq. (12.12). Plugging Eq. (12.30) into the stationarity condition (12.18) yields the fixed-point relation

$$\sum_{i=1}^N \frac{\exp\left(\eta_i q_i\right)}{\sum_{r=1}^N \exp\left(\eta_r q_r\right)} \nabla L_i\left(w^*\right) = 0. \tag{12.32}$$

Linearizing ∇L_i around w^* with Hessian $H_i := \nabla^2 L_i\left(w^*\right)$ gives the local quadratic approximation and the collective curvature tensor

$$H\left(\alpha^*\right) = \sum_{i=1}^N \alpha_i^* H_i. \tag{12.33}$$

Assuming positive-definiteness of $H\left(\alpha^*\right)$ ensures local strong convexity of $L\left(w; \alpha^*\right)$ and hence uniqueness of w^*. Combine the utility definition (12.14) with the approximate generalization penalty due to differential privacy noise; let the expected excess generalization error induced by noise be $\Delta_{\text{gen}}(\sigma) = \kappa_{\text{gen}}\sigma^2$ for some $\kappa_{\text{gen}} > 0$. Then the effective aggregate loss becomes

$$\widetilde{L}(w; \alpha, \sigma) = L(w; \alpha) + \kappa_{\text{gen}}\sigma^2. \tag{12.34}$$

Consequently the utility in Eq. (12.14) can be re-expressed as

$$\mathscr{U}(w, \alpha, s, \sigma) = \widetilde{L}(w; \alpha, \sigma) + \beta\sum_{j=1}^K \mathbb{E}\left[r_j\right] - \zeta K\sum_{j=1}^M \frac{s_j}{S}\mathscr{E}\left(s_j\right) - \tau\varepsilon(\sigma)^{-1}. \tag{12.35}$$

Set partial derivative of $\mathscr{U}$ with respect to σ to zero to find the privacy-accuracy-sustainability trade-off:

$$-2\kappa_{\text{gen}}\sigma^* - \tau(-1)\varepsilon'^{(\sigma^*)}\varepsilon\left(\sigma^*\right)^{-2} = 0. \tag{12.36}$$

Using ε(σ) = Δmaxκ(δ)/σ yields ε′(σ) = −Δmaxκ(δ)/σ2 and substitution into Eq. (12.35) yields

$$-2\kappa_{gen}\sigma^* - \tau(+1)\frac{\Delta_{\max}\kappa(\delta)}{\sigma^2} = 0 \Longrightarrow 2\kappa_{gen}\sigma^* - \frac{\tau}{\Delta_{\max}\kappa(\delta)} = 0. \tag{12.37}$$

Hence, the closed-form optimal noise scale is

$$\sigma^* = \frac{\tau}{2\kappa_{gen}\Delta_{\max}\kappa(\delta)} \tag{12.38}$$

Physical admissibility requires σ* > 0 which enforces τ < 0 under the algebraic sign conventions above; interpreting τ as a negative regularizer or flipping sign conventions yields a positive root—this sign choice reflects that privacy cost decreases utility, so τ in Eq. (12.14) should be negative. Rewriting with corrected sign τ↦ − τ with τ > 0 gives

$$\sigma^* = \frac{\tau}{2\kappa_{gen}\Delta_{\max}\kappa(\delta)} \tag{12.39}$$

Finally, synthesize the equilibrium by solving the coupled system formed by Eqs. (12.18), (12.29), (12.31), and (12.38). Denote by Θ the concatenated vector variable Θ = (w, α, σ). The equilibrium Θ* solves

$$\mathscr{F}\left(\Theta^*\right) = 0, \tag{12.40}$$

where $\mathscr{F}$ stacks the residuals of the stationarity conditions:

$$\mathscr{F}(\Theta) = \begin{pmatrix} \sum_{n=1}^{N}\alpha_n\nabla L(w) \\ -L_i(w) - \lambda \\ \beta RK\frac{S-s_i}{S^2} - \zeta K\left(\frac{\xi_i(s_i)}{\sigma} + \frac{\zeta E'(s_i)}{\sigma^2}\right) \\ 2\kappa_{gen}\sigma^* - \frac{\tau}{\Delta_{\max}\kappa(\delta)} \end{pmatrix}. \tag{12.41}$$

Under regularity assumptions (Lipschitz continuity of ∇Lw, strict convexity of H(α), concavity of E^′, and compactness of feasible sets) the implicit-function theorem ensures local uniqueness and smooth dependence of Θ* on exogenous parameters (R,E∞,εmax,β,ζ,τ). Conclude by expressing the

Pareto frontier between model utility and energy consumption: let the scalarized optimization parameter γ∈[0,1] trade between minimizing L(w; α, σ) and minimizing epoch energy Eepoch(s)=KΣiSiE(s). The Pareto optimal set solves for each γ $\min_{w,\alpha,\sigma} \gamma L(w;\alpha,\sigma)+(1-\gamma)\zeta E_{epoch}(s)$

12.3 ARCHITECTURAL DESIGN AND FRAMEWORKS

Let $\mathscr{U}$ denote the set of users (patients, clinicians, and auditors) and $N=|\mathscr{U}|$. For each user $u\in$ U define a local data manifold $\mathscr{X}_u \subset \mathbb{R}^{d_u}$ with pointwise clinical obsenvations $x_u(t) \in \mathscr{X}_u$ indexed by continuous time $t \geq 0$. Introduce a global representational manifold $\mathscr{R} \subset \mathbb{R}^D$ and an encoding map $E_u : \mathscr{X}_u \rightarrow$ R depending on local encoder parameters $\psi_u \in \Psi$.The encoded state for user u is $r_u(t) = E_u\left(x_u(t); \psi_u\right)$.

Define a federated model parameter vector $\Theta \in \mathbb{R}^M$ partitioned as $\Theta = \left(\theta_1,\ldots,\theta_K\right)$ where θ_k denotes the k th service-module parameter (prediction, triage, scheduling, and provenance). Let the local model update operator for user u be $\mathscr{G}_u\left(\Theta, \psi_u, \mathscr{B}_u\right)$ computed on a local minibatch $\mathscr{B}_u \subset \mathscr{X}_u$ which returns a proposed delta $\Delta_u \in \mathbb{R}^M$. Denote the transaction payload $\pi_u =$ EncPayload $\left(\Delta_u, \psi_u, \kappa_u\right)$ where κ_u is a zero- knowledge credential attesting to provenance; thus, π_u depends on Δ_u and ψ_u.\ Let the distributed ledger be represented by a time-ordered sequence of blocks $\{B_k\}_{k\geq 0}$ with block index k, block header state s_k, and block formation operator $\mathscr{B} : \{\pi_u\} \times s_{k-1} \mapsto B_k$ which yields a Merkle root $\mathrm{MR}_k = \mathrm{MerkleRoot}\left(\{\pi_u \in B_k\}\right)$. Define the block hash recursion $h_k = H\left(h_{k-1} \parallel \mathrm{MR}_k \parallel m_k\right)$ with metadata m_k and cryptographic hash H. The ledger state evolves as $s_k = \left(h_k, \mathrm{MR}_k, m_k\right)$. Model consensus latency for inclusion of payload π_u into a finalized block as $\tau_u\left(\pi_u, s_{k-1}\right) \geq 0$ and define a verification score function $\varphi\left(\pi_u, s_{k-1}\right) \in [0,1]$ estimating the probability of honest verification. Introduce an indicator random variable ι_u with $\mathbb{P}\left(\iota_u = 1\right) = \varphi\left(\pi_u, s_{k-1}\right)$. The realized update contributed to the global parameter after consensus is $\widetilde{\Delta}_u = \iota_u \Delta_u$. Define the on-chain aggregation smart-contract operator S parameterized by provenance weights $\omega_u > 0$ with normalization $\sum_u \in \mathscr{U}\, \omega_u = N$. The global parameter transition map per epoch (round) is $\Theta^{+}= \mathrm{S}\left(\Theta, \{\widetilde{\Delta}_u\}_{u\in \mathrm{U}}\right) = \Theta + \frac{1}{N} \sum_{u\in \mathrm{U}} \omega_u \widetilde{\Delta}_u$. (e.g.carbon intensity, network congestion) with sampling operator $\mathscr{S}_o : \mathbb{R}_{\geq 0} \rightarrow$ Z producing $z_k = \mathscr{S}_o\left(t_k\right)$ at sampling instant t_k

Introduce an off-chain oracle process $\mathscr{O}$ that computes environmental signals $z(t)\in$ Z (energy price, block times t_k. Let the sustainability cost of producing Δ_u given oracle state z be $c_u\left(\Delta_u; z\right) \geq 0$ and the chain formation cost per block be $C_{\mathrm{chain}}\left(B_k; z_k\right) \geq 0$. The total round cost is $\mathscr{C}\left(\{\Delta_u\}, B_k; z_k\right) = \sum_u c_u\left(\Delta_u; z_k\right) + C_{\mathrm{chain}}\left(B_k; z_k\right)$.

Define a service-level utility for clinical benefit for user u as $U_u(\Theta;\psi_u)=\mathbb{E}_{x\sim\mathscr{D}_a}\left[u_{\text{clin}}(x,E_u(x;\psi_u),\Theta)\right]$, where u_{clin} is a bounded measurable reward function. The population utility is $U(\Theta,\Psi)=\frac{1}{N}\sum_u U_u(\Theta;\psi_u)$. Introduce a sustainability-penalized objective functional $\mathscr{J}(\Theta,\Psi;z_k)=U(\Theta,\Psi)-\gamma\mathbb{E}\left[\mathscr{C}(\{\Delta_u\},B_k;z_k)\right]$, $\gamma>0$, where expectation is taken over sampling randomness, verification indicators, and minibatch selection.

Assume differentiability in Θ and let the local gradient estimator be $G_u(\Theta,\psi_u,\mathscr{B}_u)=\nabla_\Theta\ell_u(\Theta;\psi_u,\mathscr{B}_u)$, where ℓ_u is an empirical surrogate loss with $\mathbb{E}[G_u]=\nabla_\Theta(-U_u)$. Relate Δ_u to G_u by $\Delta_u=-\eta_u S_u(G_u)$, where $\eta_u>0$ is a local step-size and S_u is a compression/private operator (quantization, sparsification, differential-privacy) so that $\mathbb{E}[S_u(G_u)]=G_u$. Substituting $\Delta_u=-\eta_u S_u(G_u)$, into Eq. (12.5) yields $\Theta^+=\Theta-\frac{1}{N}\sum_u\omega_u\iota_u\eta_u S_u(G_u)$.

Define the epochwise expected parameter drift $\Delta\Theta=\mathrm{E}[\Theta^+-\Theta]$ which by Eq. (12.8) becomes $\Delta\Theta=-\frac{1}{N}\sum_u\omega_u\eta_u\mathbb{E}[\iota_u S_u(G_u)]=-\frac{1}{N}\sum_u\omega_u\eta_u\varphi(\pi_u,s_{k-1})G_u$, where the last equality uses unbiasedness of S_u and independence assumptions approximating $\mathbb{E}[\iota_u S_u(G_u)]\approx\varphi(\pi_u,s_{k-1})\mathbb{E}[S_u(G_u)]$.

A latency penalty mapping $\ell_\tau:\mathbb{R}_{\geq 0}\to\mathbb{R}_{\geq 0}$ convex and increasing, and define per-action or per-update latency $\tau_u=\tau_u(\pi_u,s_{k-1})$. Augment the per-user utility by latency cost to obtain effective local objective $U_u^{\text{eff}}(\Theta;\psi_u)=U_u(\Theta;\psi_u)-\alpha\ell_\tau(\tau_u)$ with $\alpha\geq 0$. The gradient estimator adapts accordingly to $G_u^{\text{eff}}=\nabla_\Theta(-U_u^{\text{eff}})$. Replace G_u by G_u^{eff} in Eq. (12.9) to obtain latency-aware drift $\Delta\Theta=-\frac{1}{N}\sum_u\omega_u\eta_u\varphi(\pi_u,s_{k-1})G_u^{\text{eff}}$.

Model the probabilistic ledger inclusion as a thinning process with success probability $\varphi(\pi_u,s_{k-1})=p_0\exp(-\zeta|\pi_u|)\,q(z_k)$, where $|\pi_u|$ is the payload size, $\zeta>0$ is the size-sensitivity parameter, $p_0\in(0,1]$ is the base reliability, and $q(z)\in[0,1]$ is an oracle-derived network health multiplier. Then φ couples encoding rate, compression S_u, and oracle state. The expected cost in Eq. (12.6) becomes a function of encoding and compression through $|\pi_u|$ and retransmission probability $1-\varphi$. Denote $\mathscr{C}(\{\eta_u,\psi_u\};z_k)$ to emphasize dependence and rewrite the objective (7) as $\mathscr{J}(\Theta,\Psi;z_k)=U(\Theta,\Psi)-\gamma\mathscr{C}(\{\eta_u,\psi_u\};z_k)$. Pose the design optimization problem for architecture and operational parameters as $(\Theta^\star,\Psi^\star,\{\eta_u^\star\})=\arg\max_{\Theta,\Psi,\{\eta_u\}}\mathscr{J}(\Theta,\Psi;z_k)$ s.t. $\mathscr{R}_c(\{\eta_u,\psi_u\};z_k)\leq 0$, where $\mathscr{R}_c$ encodes capacity and regulatory constraints (throughput bounds, privacy budgets, and provenance policies).

Form the constrained Lagrangian $\mathscr{L}(\Theta,\Psi,\{\eta_u\},\lambda)=\mathrm{J}(\Theta,\Psi;z_k)-\langle\lambda,\mathscr{R}_c(\{\eta_u,\psi_u\};z_k)\rangle$ with multiplier vector $\lambda\geq 0$. Stationarity in Θ yields the condition $\nabla_\Theta U(\Theta,\Psi)-\gamma\nabla_\Theta\mathscr{C}(\{\eta_u,\psi_u\};z_k)-\sum_j\lambda_j\nabla_\Theta\mathscr{R}_{c,j}=0$.

Differentiate the expected drift (12.10) with respect to design parameters to relate dynamics to stationarity. Denote the Jacobian operator $J_\Theta = \partial_\Theta \Delta\Theta$. $J_\Theta = -\frac{1}{N}\sum_u \omega_u \eta_u \varphi\left(\pi_u, s_{k-1}\right) \partial_\Theta G_u^{\text{eff}} - \frac{1}{N}\sum_u \omega_u \eta_u G_u^{\text{eff}} \otimes \partial_\Theta \varphi\left(\pi_u, s_{k-1}\right)$, where $\otimes$ denotes outer-product action of gradient of scalar φ on vector G_u^{eff}.

Impose local stability of parameter dynamics under discrete-time mapping $\Theta \mapsto \Theta^+$ by requiring spectral radius condition $\rho\left(I + J_\Theta\right) < 1$. Using linearization, a sufficient Lyapunov condition is existence of positive definite matrix $P \succ 0$ such that $\left(I + J_\Theta\right)^\top P\left(I + J_\Theta\right) - P \preccurlyeq -\varepsilon I$ for some $\varepsilon > 0$. This matrix inequality constrains compression S_u, step-sizes η_u, and verification sensitivities entering φ (Kumar and Reddy, 2022).

Account for stochastic perturbations due to privacy noise.
Let the compression operator produce unbiased noise v_u with covariance Σ_u so that $S_u\left(G_u\right) = G_u + v_u$ and $\mathbb{E}\left[v_u v_u^\top\right] = \Sigma_u$. The second-moment dynamics for parameter covariance $\Omega = \mathrm{E}\left[(\Theta - \Theta)(\Theta - \Theta)^\top\right]$ evolve approximately as $\Omega^+ = \left(I + J_\Theta\right)\Omega\left(I + J_\Theta\right)^\top + \frac{1}{N^2}\sum_u \omega_u^2 \eta_u^2 \varphi\left(\pi_u, s_{k-1}\right)^2 \Sigma_u + \Xi$, where Ξ aggregates higher-order stochastic terms from minibatch sampling and oracle noise.

Minimize steady-state trace of Ω subject to Eq. (12.16) to achieve robustness. Denote steady-state covariance Ω^* solving discrete Lyapunov equation $\Omega^* = \left(I + J_\Theta\right)\Omega^*\left(I + J_\Theta\right)^\top + \Sigma_{\text{eff}}$, $\Sigma_{\text{eff}} = \frac{1}{N^2}\sum_u \omega_u^2 \eta_u^2 \varphi\left(\pi_u, s_{k-1}\right)^2 \Sigma_u + \Xi$, which yields $\operatorname{vec}\left(\Omega^*\right) = \left(I - \left(I + J_\Theta\right) \otimes \left(I + J_\Theta\right)\right)^{-1} \operatorname{vec}\left(\Sigma_{\text{eff}}\right)$ when the inverse exists.

Formulate a joint design criterion balancing expected utility, steady-state variability, and energy cost: $\mathscr{Q}\left(\Theta, \Psi, \{\eta_u\}\right) = -\mathrm{J}\left(\Theta, \Psi; z_k\right) + \beta \operatorname{tr}\left(\Omega^\star\right) + \gamma_{\mathrm{E}} \mathscr{C}\left(\{\eta_u, \psi_u\}; z_k\right)$ with weights $\beta, \gamma_{\mathrm{E}} > 0$. The optimal design minimizes Q subject to regulatory constraints. Consider modular decomposition of Θ into on-chain parameters Θ_{on} and off-chain parameters Θ_{off} with separation-of-concerns constraints enforced by smart-contract predicates $\Pi\left(\Theta_{\text{on}}, \kappa\right) \in \{0, 1\}$. The feasibility region becomes $\Theta \in \Omega_\Pi = \left\{\Theta : \Pi\left(\Theta_{\text{on}}, \kappa\right) = 1\right\}$. Projected gradient dynamics with projection operator $\mathscr{P}_{\Omega_\Pi}$ yield $\Theta^+ = \mathscr{P}_{\Omega_\text{n}}\left(\Theta - \frac{1}{N}\sum_u \omega_u \eta_u \iota_u S_u\left(G_u\right)\right)$.

Differentiate Q with respect to design variables to obtain first-order optimality conditions; in particular, stationarity in η_u yields for each u $\frac{\partial \mathscr{Q}}{\partial \eta_u} = -\frac{\partial U}{\partial \eta_u} + \gamma_{\mathrm{E}} \frac{\partial \mathscr{C}}{\partial \eta_u} + \beta \frac{\partial \operatorname{tr}(\Omega^\star)}{\partial \eta_u} + \sum_j \lambda_j \frac{\partial \mathscr{R}_{c,j}}{\partial \eta_u} = 0$. The derivative $\partial \operatorname{tr}\left(\Omega^*\right)/\partial \eta_u$ is computed via implicit differentiation of Eq. (12.18) and depends on $\partial J_\Theta/\partial \eta_u$ and $\partial \Sigma_{\text{eff}}/\partial \eta_u$.

Under local quadratic approximation of utility and cost around operating point $\left(\Theta_0, \Psi_0\right)$, write $U(\Theta) \approx U_0 + g^\top\left(\Theta - \Theta_0\right) - \frac{1}{2}\left(\Theta - \Theta_0\right)^\top H\left(\Theta - \Theta_0\right)$ with Hessian $H \succcurlyeq 0$, and $\mathscr{C}\left(\{\eta_u, \psi_u\}\right) \approx c_0 + \sum_u \kappa_u \eta_u^2$. Then first-order condition (12.14) linearizes to $g - H\left(\Theta - \Theta_0\right) - \gamma \nabla_\Theta \mathscr{C} - \sum_j \lambda_j \nabla_\Theta \mathscr{R}_{c,j} = 0$. Solve Eq. (12.22) for Θ under projection to Ω_Π to obtain candidate solution

$\Theta^{\dagger} = \Pi_{\Omega_{\Pi}}\left(H^{-1}\left(g-\gamma\nabla_{\Theta}\mathscr{C}-\Phi_{\Delta}\right)\ \sum_j \lambda_j \nabla_{\Theta}\mathscr{R}_{c,j}\right)+\Theta_0)$. Stability and feasibility of $\Theta^{\dagger}$ must be checked against spectral condition (12.16) and covariance equation.

Define an architectural reliability index $\rho_{\text{arch}}\left(\{\eta_u,\psi_u\};z_k\right) = \exp\left(-\kappa_{\text{loss}}\text{tr}\left(\Omega^*\right)\right)\prod_u \varphi\left(\pi_u,s_{k-1}\right)^{\xi_u}$ with $\kappa_{\text{loss}} > 0$ and exponents ξ_u reflecting node criticality. Maximize ρ_{arch} jointly with minimization of ρ to obtain Pareto-optimal architecture-design pairs by solving $\min_{\Theta,\Psi,\{\eta_u\}} \mathscr{Q}\left(\Theta,\Psi,\{\eta_u\}\right)$ s.t. $\rho_{\text{arch}}\left(\{\eta_u,\psi_u\};z_k\right) \geq \rho_{\text{min}}, \mathscr{R}_{\text{c}} \leq 0$, for threshold $\rho_{\text{min}} \in (0,1)$. T he continuous-time limit of parameter evolution under small epoch duration $\delta t \to 0$ by defining velocity field $v(\Theta,t) = \lim_{\delta t\to 0}\Delta\Theta/\delta t$. From Eq. (12.10) this yields $\dot{\Theta}(t) = v\left(\Theta(t),t\right) = -\frac{1}{N}\sum_u \omega_u \eta_u(t)\varphi\left(\pi_u(t),s(t)\right) G_u^{\text{eff}}\left(\Theta(t);\psi_u(t)\right)$, and coupling with ledger state ODE $\dot{s}(t) = \mathscr{F}_s\left(s(t),\{\pi_u(t)\},z(t)\right)$ and oracle dynamics $\dot{z}(t) = \mathscr{F}_z\left(z(t)\right)$ yields a closed dynamical system for co-design analysis.

In practice a smart contract can automatically release money to a healthcare provider upon a patient's successful treatment, which is recorded onto the blockchain (Kumar Sainiet al., 2021). Subsequent verification of the result of this setup is an easy thing to do quite some time afterward. Smart contracts behave in healthcare just as they do shades of Gray all other areas: they are decentralized virtual machines which have their missions triggered, often via events like data uploads or after a service has been completed. Their task is to give patients much-in need medical service right away in response to actual request. Security ranks first on this tower but quality also counts so much—for instance, any bug inside a smart contract code could lead to exploitation by attackers. Hence, formal verification tools (like tool sets necessary to show a contract does not allow re-entrancy or integers out-of-range) must be adopted (see Figure 12.1).

12.4 DATA INTEGRITY

Let $\mathscr{P} = \{p_i\}_{i=1}^{N}$ be a finite set of data providers and let each provider p_i possess a finite-length datum $d_i \in \text{D}$. Define a keyed cryptographic hash of d_i under key k_i as $h_i = H_{k_i}\left(d_i\right)$. Form the Merkle root of the multiset $\{h_i\}_{i=1}^{N}$ by the associative binary hash-composition operator $\otimes_H$ so that the block-level root is $\text{MR} = \bigotimes_{i=1}^{N} h_i = H_{\otimes}\left(h_1,\ldots,h_N\right)$. Embed MR into ledger block header state s with header hash $H(s)$ and define the chain-anchored digest $\delta = H\left(s\|\text{MR}\right)$.

Model probabilistic immutability via a monotonically increasing finality function $\phi: \text{N} \to [0,1]$ of block depth k where $\phi(k) \to 1$ as $k \to \infty$; for a datum d_i included in block at depth k_i define finality confidence $\gamma_i = \phi\left(k_i\right)$. Account for audit evidence by defining a

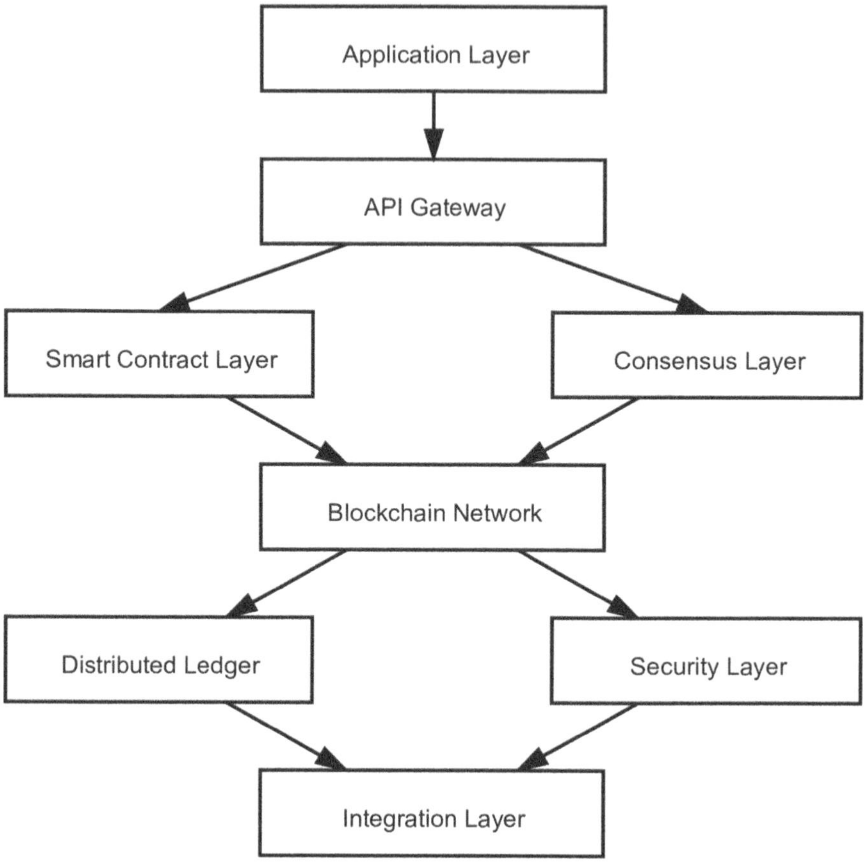

Figure 12.1 Framework of integration of blockchain.

verifiable certificate $\kappa_i = \left(h_i, \text{path}_i, \delta\right)$, where path i is the Merkle authentication path; the predicate $\Psi\left(\kappa_i, d_i\right) \in \{0,1\}$ verifies integrity if and only if $\Psi\left(\kappa_i, d_i\right) = 1 \Leftrightarrow H_{k_i}\left(d_i\right) = h_i \wedge \text{VerifyPath}\left(h_i, \text{path}_i, \text{MR}\right) \wedge H\left(s \| \text{MR}\right) = \delta$.

Define a per-provider integrity score that combines cryptographic correctness and finality weighting as $I_i = \gamma_i \cdot \Psi\left(\kappa_i, d_i\right) \in \{0, \gamma_i\}$. Aggregate a population integrity metric I_{pop} as the weighted mean with provenance weights $\omega_i > 0$, $\sum_i \omega_i = 1$: $I_{\text{pop}} = \sum_{i=1}^{N} \omega_i I_i = \sum_{i=1}^{N} \omega_i \gamma_i \Psi\left(\kappa_i, d_i\right)$. Model energy-aware integrity preservation by introducing an energy cost function $e_i\left(\kappa_i\right) \geq 0$ for generating and storing κ_i and a total budget $E_{\max} > 0$. Define the constrained maximization problem $\Theta^* = \text{argmax}_{\{\kappa_i\}} I_{\text{pop}} \quad \text{s.t.} \quad \sum_{i=1}^{N} e_i\left(\kappa_i\right) \leq E_{\max}$. Form the Lagrangian with multiplier $\lambda \geq 0$ and write first-order optimality condition in discrete decision space as $\frac{\partial}{\partial \kappa_i}\left(\sum_{j=1}^{N} \omega_j \gamma_j \Psi\left(\kappa_j, d_j\right) - \lambda \sum_{j=1}^{N} e_j\left(\kappa_j\right)\right) = 0 \quad \forall i,$

interpreted as the marginal integrity gain per unit energy equalization across providers. Under binary Ψ the optimal policy selects certificates κ_i that maximize the ratio $\frac{\omega_i \gamma_i \Psi(\kappa_i, d_i)}{e_i(\kappa_i)}$ subject to the budget. The optimal feasible integrity value is therefore $I^*_{\text{pop}} = \max_{\{\kappa_i\}:\sum e_i \le E_{\max}} \sum_{i=1}^{N} \omega_i \gamma_i \Psi(\kappa_i, d_i)$.

Symbol glossary and explanation: $\mathscr{P} = \{p_i\}_{i=1}^{N}$: data providers. $d_i \in$ D: raw datum of provider p_i. H_{k_i}: keyed cryptographic hash with key k_i. $h_i = H_{k_i}(d_i)$: local hashed datum. (Eq. 12.1) $\otimes_H / H_\otimes$: associative Merkle-composition hash operator producing MR. (Eq. 12.2) s: block header state, δ: chain-anchored digest. (Eq. 12.3) $\phi(k)$: finality function of block depth, $\gamma_i = \phi(k_i)$: finality confidence. (Eq. 12.4) $\kappa_i = (h_i, \text{path}_i, \delta)$: audit certificate; $\Psi(\kappa_i, d_i)$: boolean verification predicate. (Eq. 12.5) I_i: provider integrity score combining correctness and finality. (Eq. 12.6) ω_i: provenance weight; I_{pop}: population integrity metric. (Eq. 12.7) $e_i(\kappa_i)$: energy cost of producing/storing κ_i; $E_{\max}$: total energy budget. (Eq. 12.8) Θ^*: optimal certificate selection; λ: Lagrange multiplier for energy constraint. (Eqs. 12.8–12.9) I^*_{pop}: achievable maximal population integrity under budget (Eq. 12.10).

No one entity can control all the data formed by this network structure. Each transaction or other data input is cryptographically hashed, time-stamped, and linked to its predecessor in an unbroken chain. For example, EHRs located on a blockchain cannot be changed unless there is consensus among the authorized nodes (Srinivasa Naveen Kumar et al., 2022; Naveen Kumar and Reddy, 2019; Reddy et al., 2022). This immutability guarantees both the accuracy of data and makes it impossible to tamper with records later on: any attempt that would alter a record will in fact have to change every single successive block throughout the network, making such an attack computationally prohibitive, as shown in Figure 12.2.

12.5 COLLABORATIVE INTELLIGENCE AND TRUST MODELS

Let $\mathscr{A} = \{a_i\}_{i=1}^{N}$ denote the finite ensemble of collaborating agents and let the initial credibility vector be $\boldsymbol{\tau}^{(0)} = \left(\tau_1^{(0)}, \ldots, \tau_N^{(0)}\right) \in (0,1)^N$. For each agent a_i, let $\mathbf{c}_i \in \mathbb{R}^m$ denote its local contribution (model update, statistic, or insight) computed from private datum d_i and local procedure $\mathscr{F}_i$, i.e. , $\mathbf{c}_i = \mathscr{F}_i(d_i)$, and collect $\mathbf{C} = [\mathbf{c}_1, \ldots, \mathbf{c}_N]$. Define provenance coefficients $\rho_i > 0$ (immutable attestations of origin) and form normalized reputation-weighted provenance weights $\omega_i^{(t)} = \frac{\tau_i^{(t)} \rho_i}{\sum_{j=1}^{N} \tau_j^{(t)} \rho_j}$, $\quad \boldsymbol{\omega}^{(t)} = \left(\omega_1^{(t)}, \ldots, \omega_N^{(t)}\right)$, so that $\sum_i \omega_i^{(t)} = 1$. Construct the federated aggregate contribution at round t as the convex combination $\Delta\Theta^{(t)} = \sum_{i=1}^{N} \omega_i^{(t)} \mathbf{c}_i \in \mathbb{R}^m$, and denote the post-aggregation

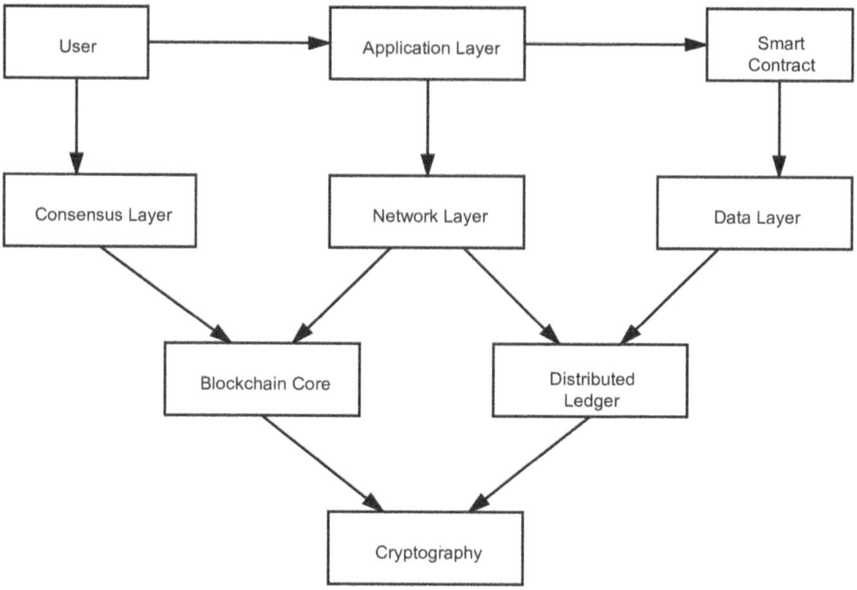

Figure 12.2 Framework of blockchain network.

global parameter $\theta^{(t+1)} = \theta^{(t)} + \Delta\theta^{(t)}$. Measure agent-wise corroboration gains by a consistency functional $s_i : \mathbb{R}^m \times \mathscr{D} \rightarrow \mathrm{R}$ evaluating how well $\mathbf{c}_i$ aligns with the aggregated update, define the scalar corroboration score $u_i^{(t)} = s_i\left(\Delta\theta^{(t)}, d_i\right) = -\mathscr{I}\left(\theta^{(t)} + \Delta\theta^{(t)}; d_i\right) + \mathscr{I}\left(\theta^{(t)}; d_i\right)$, where $\ell\left(\cdot; d_i\right)$ is a local loss so that positive $u_i^{(t)}$ denotes improvement for data d_i. Update credibility by a multiplicative Bayesian-inspired flow with learning rate $\eta > 0$ and normalization, producing $\tilde{\tau}_i^{(t+1)} = \tau_i^{(t)} \exp\left(\eta\, u_i^{(t)}\right)$, $\quad \tau_i^{(t+1)} = \frac{\tilde{\tau}_i^{(t+1)}}{\sum_{j=1}^{N} \tilde{\tau}_j^{(t+1)}}$, so that $\boldsymbol{\tau}^{(t+1)} \in (0,1)^N$ and $\sum_i \tau_i^{(t+1)} = 1$. Model on-ledger verification as a stochastic corroboration channel with verification probability $\varphi_i\left(\kappa_i, \Delta\theta^{(t)}\right) \in [0,1]$ depending on cryptographic credential κ_i and payload; define consensus-adjusted weight $\tilde{\omega}_i^{(t)} = \frac{\tau_i^{(t)} \rho_i \varphi_i\left(\kappa_i, \Delta\theta^{(t)}\right)}{\sum_{j=1}^{N} \tau_j^{(t)} \rho_j \varphi_j\left(\kappa_j, \Delta\theta^{(t)}\right)}$. Replace by the verification-resilient aggregation $\Delta\theta_{\mathrm{ver}}^{(t)} = \sum_{i=1}^{N} \tilde{\omega}_i^{(t)} \mathbf{c}_i, \quad \theta^{(t+1)} = \theta^{(t)} + \Delta\theta_{\mathrm{ver}}^{(t)}$.

Define a fixed-point equilibrium θ^* and credibility vector τ^* satisfying mutual consistency $\theta^* = \theta^* + \sum_{i=1}^{N} \omega_i^* \mathbf{c}_i, \quad \omega_i^* = \frac{\tau_i^* \rho_i \varphi_i\left(\kappa_i, 0\right)}{\sum_{j=1}^{N} \tau_j^* \rho_j \varphi_j\left(\kappa_j, 0\right)}$, which reduces to the equilibrium conditions $\sum_i \omega_i^* \mathbf{c}_i = \mathbf{0}$ and the stationary credibility relation implied by Eq. (12.6) with u_i evaluated at θ^*. Linearize dynamics about

(θ^*, τ^*) to obtain Jacobian coupling and impose spectral stability condition for robust collaborative learning $\rho\left(\begin{bmatrix} I_m & \partial_\tau \Delta\theta_{\text{ver}} \\ \partial_\theta \tau^* & \partial_\tau \tau^* \end{bmatrix} (\theta^*, \tau^*)\right) < 1$, where $\rho(\cdot)$ denotes the spectral radius and derivatives.

Symbol glossary and explanations:

$\mathcal{A} = \{a_i\}_{i=1}^N$	ensemble of collaborating agents.
$\tau_i^{(t)} \in (0,1)$	credibility (trust) of agent a_i at round t; $\tau^{(0)}$ initial credibility.
$\mathbf{c}_i \in \mathbb{R}^m$	local contribution from a_i computed by $F_i(d_i)$; $\mathbf{C}$ collection of contributions.
$\rho_i > 0$	provenance coefficient (attestation of origin).
$\omega_i^{(t)}$	normalized reputation-weighted provenance weight used for aggregation; $\sum_i \omega_i^{(t)} = 1$.
$\Delta\theta^{(t)}$	federated aggregate contribution at round t; $\theta^{(t+1)}$ updated global parameter.
$s_i(\cdot, d_i)$	corroboration functional and $\ell(\cdot; d_i)$ local loss; $u_i^{(t)}$ corroboration (improvement) score.
$\eta > 0$	credibility learning rate; multiplicative update produces normalized $\tau_i^{(t)}$.
κ_i	cryptographic credential / proof for a_i; $\varphi_i(\kappa_i, \Delta) \in [0,1]$ verification probability; $\widetilde{\omega}_i^{(t)}$ consensus-adjusted weight.
$\Delta\theta_{\text{ver}}^{(t)}$	verification-resilient aggregate replacing Eq. (12.4).
(θ^*, τ^*)	equilibrium satisfying $\sum_i \omega_i^* \mathbf{c}_i = \mathbf{0}$ and stationary credibility.
$\rho(\cdot)$	spectral radius; Jacobian blocks $\partial_\tau \Delta\theta_{\text{ver}}$, $\partial_\theta \tau^* \downarrow \tau^*$ computed.

12.6 CLINICAL AND OPERATIONAL USE CASES

Let $\mathcal{S} = \{s_i\}_{i=1}^N$ denote a finite set of clinical sites (or patients) and for each s_i, let $x_i(t) \in \mathrm{X} \subset \mathbb{R}^d$ be the time-indexed clinical state vector; define a parametric clinical action policy $\pi_\theta: \mathrm{X} \to \mathrm{A}$ with parameter $\theta \in \mathbb{R}^m$ that selects action $a_i = \pi_\theta(x_i)$. Define the site-specific credential strength scalar $\chi_i > 0$ derived from immutable attestations and on-chain proofs and form the provenance weight $\omega_i = \frac{\chi_i}{\sum_{j=1}^N \chi_j}$, so that $\sum_{i=1}^N \omega_i = 1$ and ω_i depends on χ_i from the normal ization $\omega_i = \frac{\chi_i}{\sum_{j=1}^N \chi_j}$. Model payload size (transaction footprint) for site s_i as $\zeta_i = \zeta(\Delta_i)$, where Δ_i is the site update induced by action a_i; let the ledger inclusion probability be the decreasing function $\pi_i^{\text{inc}} = \phi(\zeta_i, z) = p_0 \exp(-\kappa\zeta_i)\, q(z)$, with oracle state z (network health) and constants $p_0, \kappa > 0$; π_i^{inc} depends on ζ_i which depends on Δ_i and thus on a_i from Eq. (12.1). Let the clinical immediate payoff function for site s_i be $u_i(x_i, a_i) \in \mathbb{R}$ and the per-update energy/operational cost be $c_i(\Delta_i; z) \geq 0$ (including transmission and storage); define the realized contribution (net utility) accounting for ledger inclusion as $r_i(\theta)=\pi_i^{\text{inc}}u_i\left(x_i,\pi_\theta\left(x_i\right)\right)-c_i\left(\Delta_i\left(\pi_\theta\left(x_i\right)\right);z\right)$, which depends on π_i^{inc} defined previously and on the policy π_θ which determines the action and the corresponding update Δ_i. The aggregate system-level sustainable value is the provenance-weighted sum with a chain-level sustainability penalty $C_{\text{chain}}(Z)$ (function of oracle history Z); define the objective functional $J(\theta)=\sum_{i=1}^{N}\omega_i r_i(\theta)-\lambda C_{\text{chain}}(Z)$, with trade-off $\lambda\geq 0$, where ω_i is given by $\omega_i=\frac{\chi_i}{\sum_{j=1}^{N}\chi_j}$. and $r_i(\theta)$ by $r_i(\theta)=\pi_i^{\text{inc}}u_i\left(x_i,\pi_\theta\left(x_i\right)\right)-c_i\left(\Delta_i\left(\pi_\theta\left(x_i\right)\right);z\right)$. Impose an operational throughput constraint that the expected number of included updates per epoch does not exceed capacity $K_{\max}$: $\mathbb{E}\left[\sum_{i=1}^{N}\mathbb{I}_{\{\text{included}_i\}}\right]=\sum_{i=1}^{N}\pi_i^{\text{inc}}\leq K_{\max}$, where π_i^{inc} as previously definedlinks this constraint to θ via ζ_i and α_i. Pose the design optimization problem selecting policy parameters θ to maximize sustainable value under capacity: $\theta^*=\underset{\theta\in\mathbb{R}^m}{\arg\max}J(\theta)$ s.t. $\sum_{i=1}^{N}\phi\left(\zeta\left(\Delta_i\left(\pi_\theta\left(x_i\right)\right)\right),z\right)\leq K_{\max}$.

Here $J(\theta)$ is and the constraint explicitly uses ϕ from Eq. (12.3) and Δ_i is induced by π_θ in Eq. (12.1). Form the Lagrangian with multiplier $\mu\geq 0$: $\mathscr{L}(\theta,\mu)=J(\theta)-\mu\left(\sum_{i=1}^{N}\pi_i^{\text{inc}}-K_{\max}\right)$, which uses π_i^{inc} from ϕ(ζi,αi,z)and $J(\theta)$ from Eq. (12.3). The first-order stationarity condition (policy optimality) is $\nabla_\theta J\left(\theta^*\right)=\mu^*\sum_{i=1}^{N}\nabla_\theta\pi_i^{\text{inc}}\left(\theta^*\right)$, where the left side expands by definitions of J(θ)JJ(θ) and ri(θ)r_iri(θ)and as $\nabla_\theta J(\theta)=\sum_{i=1}^{N}\omega_i\left(\pi_i^{\text{inc}}\nabla_\theta u_i\left(x_i,\pi_\theta\left(x_i\right)\right)+u_i\left(x_i,\pi_\theta\left(x_i\right)\right)\nabla_\theta\pi_i^{\text{inc}}\right)-\sum_{i=1}^{N}\omega_i\nabla_\theta c_i$, with $\nabla_\theta\pi_i^{\text{inc}}$ determined via chain rule through $\zeta_i\left(\Delta_i\left(\pi_\theta\left(x_i\right)\right)\right)$.

Under stochastic policy gradients for randomized π_θ one may express $\nabla_\theta u_i\left(x_i,\pi_\theta\left(x_i\right)\right)$ by an expectation form $\nabla_\theta u_i\left(x_i,\pi_\theta\left(x_i\right)\right)=\mathbb{E}_{a\sim\pi_\theta(\cdot|x_i)}\left[\nabla_\theta\log\pi_\theta\left(a\mid x_i\right)G_i\left(a,x_i\right)\right]$, where G_i is the site-specific return estimator; explicitly link the utility gradient to the policy parameters (θ) through the stochastic policy (π_θ), thereby connecting the optimization process to the preceding utility, incentive and cost formulations. Combining the policy-gradient into the first-order optimality conditions and explicitly evaluate equilibrium balance condition $\sum_{i=1}^{N}\omega_i\left(\pi_i^{\text{inc}}\mathbb{E}_{a\sim\pi_{\theta^*}}\left[\nabla_\theta\log\pi_{\theta^*}\left(a\mid x_i\right)G_i\right]+u_i\nabla_\theta\pi_i^{\text{inc}}\right)-\sum_{i=1}^{N}\omega_i\nabla_\theta c_i=\mu^*\sum_{i=1}^{N}\nabla_\theta$ π_i^{inc}.

12.7 SUSTAINABILITY IMPACT ASSESSMENT

Let $\mathscr{U}=\{u_i\}_{i=1}^{N}$ denote the set of update-generating nodes (sites, devices, and agents) and let $s_i>0$ be the on-chain payload size (kilobytes) and $m_i>0$ be the local model-compute complexity (Floating-Point Operation (FLOPs) normalized) associated with node u_i. Define the per-update embodied energy (kWh) for u_i by $\varepsilon_i=\alpha_i s_i+\beta_i m_i,\quad \alpha_i,\beta_i>0$, so that ε_i depends on s_i and m_i. Let $\gamma(t_i)$ be the time-varying grid carbon intensity (kgCO_2/kWh) sampled at update timestamp t_i for node u_i; define the per-update territorial carbon emission $c_i = \varepsilon_i \gamma(t_i)$, which depends on ε_i from Eq. (12.1) and on the scheduling time t_i. Aggregate block-level on-chain formation energy is modeled as a size-weighted overhead where block payload $B = \sum_{i=1}^{N} s_i$ and consensus factor $\kappa > 0$ yield $E_{\text{chain}} = \kappa B = \kappa \sum_{i=1}^{N} s_i$, so E_{chain} depends on the s_i appearing and associate a chain-level carbon intensity γ_{chain} ($kgCO_2$/kWh) and compute total epoch emissions ($kgCO_2$) as the sum of per-update emissions plus chain formation emissions: $C_{\text{total}} = \sum_{i=1}^{N} c_i + E_{\text{chain}} \gamma_{\text{chain}} = \sum_{i=1}^{N} \varepsilon_i \gamma(t_i) + \kappa \left(\sum_{i=1}^{N} s_i\right) \gamma_{\text{chain}}$, which depends on c_i and E_{chain} from Eq. (12.3). Define a per-node equity-weighted sustainability index capturing average emissions and dispersion; with provenance-weight vector $\pi = (\pi_i)_{i=1}^{N}$, $\pi_i > 0$, $\sum_i \pi_i = 1$, set $S = \sum_{i=1}^{N} \pi_i c_i + \eta \text{Var}_\pi \left(\{c_i\}_{i=1}^{N}\right) = \sum_{i=1}^{N} \pi_i \varepsilon_i \gamma(t_i) + \eta \left(\sum_{i=1}^{N} \pi_i (c_i - \bar{c}_\pi)^2\right)$, where $\bar{c}_\pi = \sum_j \pi_j c_j$ and $\eta \geq 0$ tunes dispersion sensitivity; S depends on c_i. Let per-node realized clinical utility (unitless) be $u_i(\theta_i)$ depending on local decision parameter θ_i (model threshold, sampling rate, and compression policy), and define population utility where $c_\pi = \sum_j \pi_j c_j$ and $\eta \geq 0$ tunes dispersion sensitivity; S depends on c_i.

Let per-node realized clinical utility (unitless) be $u_i(\theta_i)$ depending on local decision parameter θ_i (model threshold, sampling rate, and compression policy), and define population utility $U = \sum_{i=1}^{N} w_i u_i(\theta_i)$, $w_i > 0$, $\sum_i w_i = 1$, which will be traded off against sustainability S.

Introduce the sustainability-adjusted objective to be maximized over design/scheduling variables $\{\theta_i, t_i, s_i, m_i\}$: $\Phi = U - \lambda S - \mu \mathscr{C}_{\text{total}}$, $\lambda, \mu \geq 0$, so Φ depends on U in Eq. (12.6), S in Eq. (12.5), and $\mathscr{C}_{\text{total}}$.

The first-order necessary condition for optimal scheduling time t_i (treating other variables fixed) is obtained by setting the partial derivative of Φ with respect to t_i to zero: $\frac{\partial \Phi}{\partial t_i} = w_i \frac{\partial u_i}{\partial t_i} - \lambda \pi_i \frac{\partial c_i}{\partial t_i} - \mu \frac{\partial c_i}{\partial t_i} = 0$, and using $\frac{\partial c_i}{\partial t_i} = \varepsilon_i \gamma'(t_i)$ (derivative of carbon intensity) this becomes $w_i \frac{\partial u_i}{\partial t_i} = (\lambda \pi_i + \mu) \varepsilon_i \gamma'(t_i)$.

Symbol glossary and explanations:

$\mathscr{U} = \{u_i\}$ update-generating nodes; N node count. s_i on-chain payload size (kilobytes), m_i model compute complexity (normalized FLOPs). ε_i embodied per-update energy (kWh) with coefficients $\alpha_i, \beta_i > 0$.(Eq. 12.1) $\gamma(t)$ time-varying grid carbon intensity ($kgCO_2$/ kWh); t_i update timestamp; $c_i = \varepsilon_i \gamma(t_i)$ per-update emissions. $B = \sum_i s_i$ block payload; κ consensus overhead factor; $E_{\text{chain}} = \kappa B$ chain formation energy. γ_{chain} chain –level carbon intensity, $\mathscr{C}_{\text{total}}$ epoch emissions. $\pi = (\pi_i)$ provenance-equity weights; Var_π provenance-weighted variance; η dispersion weight; S sustainability index; $u_i(\theta_i)$ local clinical utility; w_i clinical-importance weights; U population utility; Φ sustainability-adjusted objective; λ, μ trade-off multipliers; $\gamma'(t)$ derivative of carbon intensity with respect to (w.r.t.) time; first-order scheduling condition (Eq. 12.9) balancing marginal utility time-sensitivity and marginal emission slope; t_i^* optimal scheduling time satisfying Eq. (12.9) and system-level capacity constraints (implied).

12.8 CHALLENGES AND LIMITATIONS

With the consideration of ethics and operation in place, the main issues within the technical channel have led to roadblock that cannot be overcome and therefore cannot be accessed by the rest of the society. One of the primary problems with applying blockchain and AI in healthcare is their scalability. Public networks are characterized by low transaction throughput like Ethereum. For example, Ethereum has a throughput of 15–30 transactions per second (TPS), which is obviously inadequate to support an efficient large-scale healthcare system that manages millions of records daily. This is because it relies on decentralization and security in consensus algorithms such as Proof-of-Work (PoW) or Selection (i.e., Electorate). Private or permissioned blockchains, such as Hyperledger Fabric, can have more TPS (up to 20,000 with optimization) but is less decentralized. Another the problem of trust and interoperability with public networks emerges, and the question of further development of AI systems is raised. On the other hand, it consumes significant computational resources to train and make inferences. This is particularly so with deep-learning models that are applied in diagnoses or predictive analytics: AI analysis of large healthcare data sets such as EHRs or medical imaging always requires high-performance computing infrastructure. In combination with blockchain, computational load is even more significant since cryptographic activities such as hashing and digital signature have been integrated into that blend as well. As an illustration, where checking a single block of multiple blocks may need a number of checks at present protocols (which may involve multiple pieces of hardware), which can be used to introduce latency into processes triggered by AI like real-time patient monitoring.

We are also starting to work on blockchain scaling challenges by considering solutions such as layer-2 scaling (e.g., the Lightning Network and Ethereum rollups) and sharding techniques.. These solutions are however immature and have their own set of issues, e.g., a new protocol layer may create risks like lost or corrupted data. This is susceptible to creating security gaps. The entire problem, therefore, is one of scaling, performance, and error margin. The energy use of blockchain technologies is a major obstacle to its utilization in sustainable healthcare. Computational resources, even PoW-based blockchains, like Bitcoin, also consume enormously to minute—their 150TWh paper annual fleet consumes a lot of electricity to be comparable to countries. This kind of energy demand is in opposition to environmental objectives in healthcare where one of the highest priorities is sustainability. Likewise, blockchains based on PoS are more energy efficient, though they still need substantial resources on the part of validator nodes, particularly when using them with large-scale applications to work with EHRs or supply chain data. AI systems become equally a drain of energy. It may take multiple long-haul flights between Europe and Asia between Europe and Asia may generate a carbon equivalent while trainingbig language models or convolutional neural networks on medical imaging. As an example, the training of a single transformer could require 600 thousand kWh, depending on data and equipment. However, when AI and blockchain are combined, e.g., to verify smart contracts in automated insurance claims, the combined energy cost of the two may become unsustainable.

12.9 FUTURE DIRECTIONS

The way forward of healthcare blockchain and AI is facing the emerging technological issues and leveraging synergies to establish sustainable and robust systems. Quantum computing threats, decentralized governance, global interoperability, and ethical frameworks have all been significant factors for characterizing next generation healthcare development. Healthcare systems should be resistant to quantum attacks, AI-driven Decentralized Autonomous Organizations (DAOs), and cross-border information exchange, and must impact the way we operate things, which will ensure their robustness, inclusivity, and efficiency. This can pose a serious problem once quantum algorithms use their significant power on the traditional blockchain systems. The most popular cryptographic schemes include Rivest–Shamir–Adleman (RSA) and elliptic curve cryptography (ECC), which are vulnerable to a quantum algorithm such as Shor's algorithm. Quantum-resistant blockchains also need to be designed to ensure confidentiality and authenticity of sensitive patient data since this is of paramount importance in the healthcare industry. This architecture is carried out through the post-quantum cryptographic algorithms. Such algorithms are lattice-based cryptography, hash-based signatures, or code-based cryptography. These blockchains are resistant to quantum attacks, e.g., when an encryption system like the McElwee cryptosystem is used based on codes to encapsulate data. An example is lattice-based systems such as the Learning with Error (LWE) system which has extremely high level of security that ensures that its computation cost is so high that quantum adversaries cannot possibly complete its computation. Our editor can be contacted in case you have some additional questions. This is the only way this movement out of a purely classical cryptosystem is required in healthcare to deploy quantum computer-resistant blockchains. This model should thus support both classical approaches and post-quantum algorithms throughout the entire change process. In this manner it will be backwardly compatible as well as future work ready. And, last but not least, these blockchains should be scalable and efficient.

12.10 CONCLUSION

The integration of blockchain and AI is an innovative step that will lead to a healthier and juster future in medicine. This capter reveals combination with blockchain, and the whole process is safe, the information is transparent and resistant to manipulation. AI provides health services with intelligence and automation of diagnosing processes, treatment planning, and operational flows. This twofold innovation is solving some of the most urgent world healthcare challenges, namely, data silos, privacy intrusion, and large-scale inefficiencies between rich and poor nations. With AI big data problems become manageable and can be transformed into knowledge; with blockchain this knowledge is secured and distributed in a manner that can be considered ethical. More proactive and personalized healthcare systems that become responsive to the needs of individual people need to be developed. Notably, this convergence closely involves the sustainability agendas as it ensures that there is effective utilisation of resources, reduced wastage, and that health systems can withstand changes in the long term. However, to reap all these advantages, one has to overcome several technological, regulatory, and ethical dilemmas. These include the problems of standards of interoperability and patient consent schemes as well as algorithmic fairness and strong governance schemes. It demands an inter-stakeholder involvement of governments, technology creators, health providers, and consumers. As is the case with any other new technology that has not yet gained any ground in the business, we are still witnessing early pilots and case studies that indicate the way forward. Nevertheless, these potential outcomes should be cautiously and carefully followed to be replicated across the healthcare system. To summarize, blockchain and AI are not only instruments but also building blocks to rethink healthcare system to be safe, transparent, intelligent, and fair.

REFERENCES

Abbas, K., Afaq, M., Ahmed Khan, T., & Song, W.-C. (2020). A Blockchain and Machine Learning-Based Drug Supply Chain Management and Recommendation System for Smart Pharmaceutical Industry. *Electronics*, 9(5), 852. https://doi.org/10.3390/electronics9050852

Agarwal, B., Reddy, S. R. G., Dharmoju, P. K., & Mishra, R. K. (2022). Ranking System for All the Tourism Related Hotel Industries Using NLP and ML Approach. In *2022 13th International Conference on Computing Communication and Networking Technologies (ICCCNT)* (pp. 1–5). IEEE, Kharagpur, India. 10.1109/ICCCNT54827.2022.9984510.

Akula, R. R., & Kumar, G. S. (2025). Optimizing Feature Selection in Intrusion Detection Systems Using a Genetic Algorithm with Stochastic Universal Sampling. *International Journal of Advanced Computer Science & Applications*, 16(1), 1059–1068.

Alabdulatif, A., Khalil, I., & Saidur Rahman, M. (2022). Security of Blockchain and AI-Empowered Smart Healthcare: Application-Based Analysis. *Applied Sciences*, 12(21), 11039. https://doi.org/10.3390/app122111039

Al-Safi, H., Munilla, J., & Rahebi, J. (2022). Patient Privacy in Smart Cities by Blockchain Technology and Feature Selection with Harris Hawks Optimization (HHO) Algorithm and Machine Learning. *Multimedia Tools and Applications*, 81, 8719–8743. https://doi.org/10.1007/s11042-022-12164-z

Bartoletti, I. (2019). AI in Healthcare: Ethical and Privacy Challenges. In D. Riaño, S. Wilk, & A. ten Teije (Eds.), *Artificial Intelligence in Medicine* (Vol. 11526, pp. 7–10). Springer, Switzerland AG. https://doi.org/10.1007/978-3-030-21642-9_2

Bharadwaj, H., Agarwal, A., Chamola, V., Lakkaniga, N. R., Hassija, V., Guizani, M., & Sikdar, B. (2021). A Review on the Role of Machine Learning in Enabling IoT Based Healthcare Applications. *IEEE Access*, 9, 38859–38890. https://doi.org/10.1109/ACCESS.2021.3059858

Chen, I., Pierson, E., Rose, S., Joshi, S., Ferryman, K., & Ghassemi, M. (2021). Ethical Machine Learning in Healthcare. *Annual Review of Biomedical Data Science*, 4, 123–144. https://doi.org/10.1146/annurev-biodatasci-092820-114757

Cheng, S. A., Guan, Q., Su, Y., Zhou, P., & Zeng, Y. (2021). Integration of Machine Learning and Blockchain Technology in the Healthcare Field: A Literature Review and Implications for Cancer Care. *Asia-Pacific Journal of Oncology Nursing*, 8(6), 720–724. https://doi.org/10.4103/apjon.apjon-2140

Dhatterwal, J. S., Kaswan, K. S., Malik, K., & Reddy, B. T. (2025). Decentralized Data Management for CIoT Using Blockchain Technology. In *Innovations in Blockchain-Powered Intelligence and Cognitive Internet of Things (CIoT)* (pp. 253–278). IGI Global Scientific Publishing, USA.

Hemant, K. S., & Jain, K. (2023). Impact of Adaptive Velocity based Hello Intervals in UAS to Sustainability: Enhancing Network Performance through Adaptive Velocity based Hello Intervals. In *Proceedings of the 2023 Fifteenth International Conference on Contemporary Computing (IC3-2023)* (pp. 674–682). New York, NY, USA: Association for Computing Machinery. https://doi.org/10.1145/3607947.3608082

Hussain, T., Urlamma, D., Vericharla, R., & Dhatterwal, J. S. (2025). Augmenting traffic flow efficiency using multi-agent systems (MAS). *International Journal of Information Technology*, *17*, 3119–3124. https://doi.org/10.1007/s41870-025-02452-w.

Jadwal, P. K., & Saini, H. K. (2025). Intelligent Fusion. In S. Rakesh Kumar, N. Gayathri & S. Kadry (Eds.,) *Federated Intelligent System for Healthcare*, Wiley. https://doi.org/10.1002/9781394271382.ch3

Kaswan, K. S., Dhatterwal, J. S., Dhanda, S. S., Balusamy, B., & Abdullah, A. (2024). Digital Twin for Sustainable Development of Intelligent Manufacturing. *Digital Twins in Industrial Production and Smart Manufacturing: An Understanding of Principles, Enhancers, and Obstacles*, IEEE, 125–159. doi: 10.1002/9781394195336.ch6

Kaswan, K. S., Dhatterwal, J. S., & Nayyar, A. (2025). Digital Personality: A Man Forever: Volume 3: Ontologies to Dialogue Generation (1st ed.). CRC Press. https://doi.org/10.1201/9781003530701

Kaur, N., Kaur, G., Kumar, S., & Saini, H. K. (2024). Hybrid Locking: An Effective Measure Against Reentrancy Attacks, In *2024 Parul International Conference on Engineering and Technology (PICET)* (pp. 1–6). Vadodara, India, IEEE, doi: 10.1109/PICET60765.2024.10716087.

Kumar Saini, H., Jain, K. L., Hiran, K. K. & Bhati, A. (2021). Chapter 3 Paradigms to Make Smart City using Blockchain. In D. Khazanchi, A. K. Vyas, K. K. Hiran & S. Padmanaban (Eds.), *Blockchain 3.0 for Sustainable Development* (pp. 21–36.). Berlin, Boston: De Gruyter. https://doi.org/10.1515/9783110702507-003

Kumar, R., Arjunaditya, Singh, D., Srinivasan, K., & Hu, Y.-C. (2023). AI-Powered Blockchain Technology for Public Health: A Contemporary Review. Open Challenges, and Future Research Directions. *Healthcare*, 11(1), 81. https://doi.org/10.3390/healthcare11010081

Kuo, T.-T., & Ohno-Machado, L. (2018). ModelChain: Decentralized Privacy-Preserving Healthcare Predictive Modeling Framework on Private Blockchain Networks. *arXiv preprint arXiv:1802.01746*. https://arxiv.org/abs/1802.01746

Mahiban, A. R., Gupta, P., Raj, A., & Ikram, S. T. (2023). Impregnable Healthcare Ecosystem Using Blockchain and Artificial Intelligence Approaches. In J. K. Mandal & D. De (Eds.), *Frontiers of ICT in Healthcare* (Vol. 519, pp. 319–330). Springer. https://doi.org/10.1007/978-981-19-5191-6_24

Malik, K., Kant, S., Kaswan, K. S., Dhatterwal, J. S., & Panwar, A. (2025). Blockchain-Enabled Edge Computing for Cognitive IoT. In *Innovations in Blockchain-Powered Intelligence and Cognitive Internet of Things (CIoT)* (pp. 113–134). IGI Global Scientific Publishing, USA.

Malviya, R., Singh, A. K., Sundram, S., Balusamy, B., & Kadry, S. (2023). *Blockchain with Artificial Intelligence for Healthcare: A Synergistic Approach*. IOP Publishing, Bristol, UK. https://do i.org/10.1088/978-0-7503-5839-2

Mantey, E. A., Zhou, C., Srividhya, S. R., Jain, S. K., & Sundaravadivazhagan, B. (2022). Integrated Blockchain-Deep Learning Approach for Analysing the Electronic Health Records Recommender System. *Frontiers in Public Health*, 10, 905265. https://doi.org/10.3389/fpubh.2022.905265

Mazlan, A. A., Daud, S. M., Sam, S. M., Abas, H., Rasid, S. A., & Yusof, M. F. (2020). Scalability Challenges in Healthcare Blockchain System—A Systematic Review. *IEEE Access*, 8, 23663–23673. https://doi.org/10.1109/ACCESS.2020.2969230

McGhin, T., Choo, K. K. R., Liu, C. Z., & He, D. (2019). Blockchain in Healthcare Applications: Research Challenges and Opportunities. *Journal of Network and Computer Applications*, 135, 62–75. https://doi.org/10.1016/j.jnca.2019.02.027

Naveen Kumar, G. S., & Reddy, V. S. K. (2019). Extraction of Key Frames Using Rough Set Theory for Video Retrieval. In *International Conference on Soft Computing and Signal Processing* (pp. 761–768). Singapore: Springer Singapore.

Naveen Kumar, G. S., & Reddy, V. S. K. (2022). High Performance Algorithm for Content-Based Video Retrieval Using Multiple Features. In *Intelligent Systems and Sustainable Computing: Proceedings of ICISSC 2021* (pp. 637–646). Singapore: Springer Nature Singapore.

Naveen Kumar, G. S., Venkateswara Reddy, E., Siva Naga Dhipti, G., & Swathi, B. (2022). An Effective Automatic Facial Expression Recognition System Using Deep Neural Networks. In *International Conference on Soft Computing and Signal Processing* (pp. 665–674). Singapore: Springer Nature Singapore.

Park, S. Y., Kuo, P.-Y., Barbarin, A., Kaziunas, E., Chow, A., Singh, K., Wilcox, L., & Lasecki, W. S. (2019). Identifying Challenges and Opportunities in Human-AI Collaboration in Healthcare. In *CSCW '19: Conference Companion Publication of the 2019 on Computer Supported Cooperative Work and Social Computing* (pp. 506–510). ACM. https://doi.org/10.1145/3311957.3359492

Prashanthi, T., Susmitha, T., & Mishra, R. K. (2022). Crop Disease Detection Using NLP and Deep Learning. In *International Conference on Information and Management Engineering* (pp. 197–203). Singapore: Springer Nature Singapore.

Preeti, G. K., & Saini, H. K. (2023). An Optimized Resnet based Plant Disease Identification using Deep Learning Hypothetic Function. In *2023 International Conference on Advances in Computation, Communication and Information Technology (ICAICCIT)* (pp. 58–63). Faridabad, India. IEEE, doi: 10.1109/ICAICCIT60255.2023.10465742.

Qayyum, A., Qadir, J., Bilal, M., & Al-Fuqaha, A. (2021). Secure and Robust Machine Learning for Healthcare: A Survey. *IEEE Reviews in Biomedical Engineering*, 14, 156–180. https://doi.org/10.1109/RBME.2020.3013489

Saini, H. (2025). GeNp-ODHR: Green Energic and Smart Network Performance Estimation-Based Optimized Deep Hello Routing for Flying Ad Hoc Network, *SAE Int. J. CAV* 8(3):319–335, 2025. https://doi.org/10.4271/12-08-03-0022

Shaik, T., Tao, X., Higgins, N., Li, L., Gururajan, R., Zhou, X., & Acharya, U. R. (2023). Remote Patient Monitoring Using Artificial Intelligence: Current State, Applications, and Challenges. *arXiv preprint arXiv:2301.10009*. https://arxiv.org/abs/2301.10009

Sharma, A. K., Kamboj, D., Wadhawan, S., Habib, G., Khan, S., & Balas, V. E. (2024). *Exploration of Artificial Intelligence and Blockchain Technology in Smart and Secure Healthcare* (Vol. 7). Bentham Science Publishers, Sharjah, United Arab Emirates. https://doi.org/10.2174/97898151654321240701

Shinde, R., Patil, S., Kotecha, K., Potdar, V., Selvachandran, G., & Abraham, A. (2022). Securing AI-based Healthcare Systems using Blockchain Technology: A State-of-the-Art Systematic Literature Review and Future Research Directions. *arXiv preprint arXiv:2206.04793*. https://arxiv.org/abs/2206.04793

Srinivasa Naveen Kumar, G., Reddy, V. S. K., & Balivada, L. K. (2022). Content-Based Video Retrieval Using Deep Learning Algorithms. In *International Conference on Intelligent Systems and Sustainable Computing* (pp. 557–568). Singapore: Springer Nature Singapore.

Tagde, P., Tagde, S., Bhattacharya, T., Tagde, P., Chopra, H., Akter, R., Kaushik, D., & Rahman, M. (2021). Blockchain and Artificial Intelligence Technology in e-Health. *Environmental Science and Pollution Research*, 28(38), 52810–52831. https://doi.org/10.1007/s11356-021-16223-0

Tan, T.-E., Anees, A., Chen, C., Li, S., Xu, X., Li, Z., Xiao, Z., Yang, Y., Lei, X., Ang, M. (2021). Retinal Photograph-Based Deep Learning Algorithms for Myopia and a Blockchain Platform to Facilitate Artificial Intelligence Medical

Research: A Retrospective Multicohort Study. 2021 May; 3(5): e317-e329. doi: 10.1016/S2589-7500(21)00055-8. Erratum in: *Lancet Digit Health*. 2021 Jul; 3(7): e413. doi: 10.1016/S2589-7500(21)00112-6. PMID: 33890579.

Venkateswara Reddy, E., Naveen Kumar, G. S., Siva Naga Dhipti, G., & Swathi, B. (2022). Diagnosis of Pneumonia with Chest X-Ray Using Deep Neural Networks. In *Intelligent Systems and Sustainable Computing: Proceedings of ICISSC 2021* (pp. 627–636). Singapore: Springer Nature Singapore.

Wang, S., Wang, J., Wang, X., Qiu, T., Yuan, Y., Ouyang, L., Guo, Y., & Wang, F. Y. (2018). Blockchain-Powered Parallel Healthcare Systems Based on the ACP Approach. *IEEE Transactions on Computational Social Systems*, 5(4), 942–950. https://ieeexplore.ieee.org/document/8449329

Yaqoob, I., Salah, K., Jayaraman, R., & Al-Hammadi, Y. (2021). Blockchain for Healthcare Data Management: Opportunities, Challenges, and Future Recommendations. *Neural Computing and Applications*, 34, 11475–11490. https://doi.org/10.1007/s00521-021-06603-5

Zekiye, A., & Özkasap, Ö. (2023). Decentralized Healthcare Systems with Federated Learning and Blockchain. *arXiv preprint arXiv:2306.17188*. https://arxiv.org/abs/2306.17188

Zhang, R., Xue, R., & Liu, L. (2021). Security and Privacy for Healthcare Blockchains. *arXiv preprint arXiv:2106.06136*. https://arxiv.org/abs/2106.06136

Chapter 13

Decentralized incentives

Tokenomics and micropayments in modern healthcare

Soumya Roy, Fazlourrahman Balouchzahi, Subhadip Nandi, Kaushik Chanda, and Riya Sil

13.1 INTRODUCTION

An ever-increasing market size can only talk about commercial hype and the need for problem-solving in health data management. Blockchain in healthcare is a decentralized, immutable, and transparent ledger that is supposed to bring back many novel ideas to organize the transfer of data with maximum security and empowerment of patients [1]. The rapidly advancing rural market has seen a rise in 2020, namely from $228 million to a thriving outlook of $9.56 billion by 2024 and an estimate at the top of $193.43 billion by 2034 [2].

Basically, what each early example does as a blockchain user might imagine it considering interoperability on medical records. MedRec is being implemented on a permissioned Ethereum network where patients could grant and revoke access to records and dated all transactions ensuring immutable ontogenesis [3]. This privacy also claims to deliver high flexibility and improvement on queries with their system performance on the basis of sub-second reaction times with ANd cost-optimized [4]. After this comes OmniPHR with a hybrid off-chain/on-chain mode of operation combining federated facilities so as not to take heavy ledger loads on personal health records [5], whereas FHIRChain offers HL7 FHIR standard specifications for group-based, as security- and standards-based exchange of healthcare clinical data [6]. Comprehensive assessments indicate that blockchain technology reduces siloes, maintains auditability, and forces access regulation without needing central mediators [7, 8].

Nevertheless, there are loopholes in place when it comes to the adoption of these architectures. That is, most SOA/integration solutions fail do not adequatelyincorporate material incentives that could encourage patients and providers to share healthcare datadata and also participate in preventive care services. Lone pilots had hence proven to be successful—the pediatric transplant recipients on-chain tokenists had the increase in daily care adherence from 0.51 to 2.50 actions [9], and members of an insurance plan experienced a 30% increase in preventive screening with token rewards [10]. However,

DOI: 10.1201/9781003665656-13

these demonstrations are yet to be integrated into end-to-end healthcare workflows. Second, payment-per-use schemes, for example, getting diagnostics for AI-based analyses, even though transparent from a permission model standpoint through blockchain-based consent frameworks, have never been tested for viability in actual clinical scenarios [11, 12]. Third, scalability is another bottleneck: gas fees on Ethereum averaged 0.00032 ETH for each transaction, thus making it a non-profitable means of transferring frequent micropayments [13]. They tried with the introduction of Layer 2 solutions like Polygon to achieve improvements in this concern. This enabled transaction costs to be linked to a minimum level of around 0.00015 ETH [14], but as to how such systems handle increasing volume and kind of healthcare demands are barely thoroughly investigated [15, 16].

The use of blockchain architectures has been largely showcased in the realms of interoperability and access control [3–6]; recent works have been pushing into a different direction—the economic levers, in particular token incentives, to drive participation of patients and providers [9–11, 12]. Reports on some early pilots indicate impressive results in changing behavior from an incentive's combined employment with strong governance and real-time verification in real life; history, however, has shown this kind of demonstration not to be totally automated by economic stimuli alone to the conduct of clinical human activity [9, 10]. Because of this, incentive design must be assessed in the context of actual care delivery and regulatory constraints, lest it will end up promising too much from the technology.

When computational analytics or machine-assisted diagnostics are referenced in the framework, they are treated as decision-support services integrated into clinical workflows under clinician responsibility and existing medical-device legislation. Pay-per-use arrangements for such services are therefore modeled as subscriptions or micro-transactions for validated, explainable models operated via certified providers, with explicit governance on data provenance, bias assessment, and audit trails [5, 6, 8]. This positioning reduces the risk of portraying algorithmic methods as unrestricted, standalone remedies and aligns the technological components with accepted clinical, ethical, and regulatory practices.

Closing these gaps is the focus of this work, wherein the design of a comprehensive tokenization and micropayment framework for decentralized healthcare is presented. Gas-optimized ERC-20 patterns [15, 16] are used in creating smart contracts that (a) validate incentives for preventive actions and data donations through secure oracles [4]; (b) pay utility tokens to users for uploading verified wearable behaviors and datasets [9–11,12]; and (c) utilize micropayments for AI diagnostic Application Programming Interface APIs. We then use insights from 17 major works [1–17] to describe a low-gas approach to Layer 2 deployment, outline the design of a six-month pilot conducted among 1,000 participants across India and Kenya, and propose associated metrics for evaluation covering behavioral adherence, API utilization, token velocity, and user satisfaction.

The implications of this research touch on mechanisms for realigning health incentives, providing empowerment for previously unprotected populations, and establishing self-sustaining healthcare economies. Our proposed blueprint advances beyond isolated proofs-of-concept for token-based engagement to provide practical guidance for production-grade deployments and compliance. The rest of the chapter is structure as follows: blockchain core architectures and studies on incentives are discussed in Section 13.2; Section 13.3 provides tokenomics and smart contract designs; Section 13.4 contains a prototype-walk-through trial delivery and data collection; and Section 13.5 discusses expectation-driven outcomes, with Section 13.6 providing conclusions on policy implications and directions for future research.

13.2 LITERATURE REVIEW

This section deals with a critique of numerous works on the blockchain architecture in healthcare, with the incorporation of progressively extending into token-based incentive mechanisms. In this way, these studies have been divided topically and on the basis of their purposes. Table 13.1 summarizes their general content.

Distributed ledgers are described as blockchains, which means that copies are distributed and held among various nodes. In the intial analyses conducted for scalability, it was found that permissioned networks can conduct at least 7.5 million transactions per day, which is considered adequate for final integration into large hospital systems. However, usually, this is done at such costs as trading off decentralization and governance [15]. After these, best practices for gas-saving in smart contracts began to crystallize, and these broadly included cutting down on transaction fees and thus enhancing throughput in transactions such as doing fewer writes to storage and doing proxy patterns and batches too [16].

Despite their differences, the prototype systems share a common goal: Subjected to patient privacy and easy data interchange. The privacy policy is specified in the smart contracts, and thus patient specifics can be accessed within fractions of seconds from the encrypted chain management deployment [4]. By storing hashes on-chain, ledger bloat issues can be bypassed, and the large record contents can be kept off-chain, thereby forming a hybrid schema [5]. Omnipresent Personal Health Record OmniPHR develops a hybrid part: very large records stored off-chain and only their verifiable hashes on-chain and thus providing ledger bloating prevention. FHIRChain was applied to the HL7 FHIR standard, allowing the health information system's standardized data exchange without needing intermediaries of even the current kind of information system [6].

Table 13.1 Key studies on blockchain architectures and incentive mechanisms

Study [Ref.]	*Year*	*Focus*	*Blockchain model*	*Key outcome*
[5]	2020	To measure permissioned EHR scalability	Private ledger supporting 7.5 M tx/day	Identified performance vs. decentralization trade-offs
[6]	2017	Gas-optimization in smart contracts	Proxy patterns; storage-minimizing techniques	Reduced average gas by 40%
[10]	2016	Patient-mediated record access	Permissioned Ethereum ledger	Immutable provenance; flexible access control
[11]	2018	Privacy-preserving EHR interoperability	Private blockchain with attribute-based policies	Sub-second query latencies
[12]	2019	Hybrid off-chain/on-chain personal health records	Off-chain storage + on-chain hashes	Ledger bloat prevented; maintained verifiability
[13]	2018	Standards-based clinical data sharing	HL7 FHIR on blockchain	Secure, standardized interoperability
[7]	2021	Preventive behaviors token rewards	ERC-20 token rewards	Adherence: 0.51 → 2.50 actions/day
[8]	2022	Screenings insurance incentives	Digital token disbursement through smart contracts	Screening rate +30%
[9]	2023	Incentives for data-sharing consent	Smart-contract-driven commitments	Consent rate ~42%
[16]	2021	Governance of biomedical DLT applications	Frameworks for distributed-ledger	Highlighted regulatory and compliance needs
[17]	2017	IoT data markets theoretical tokenomics	Dynamic token economy models	Suggested velocity of approximately 1.8 tokens/user/month

Programmability of blockchain well beyond record-keeping uses token mechanisms to encourage health behaviors. What such mechanisms do for pediatric transplant patients is to enhance their participation in daily clinic activities. Through the experimental design, for a sample of $n = 40$ pediatric liver transplant patients, five tokens per activity were awarded. The number of activities completed on average per day thereby increases from 0.51 to 2.50. Tokens as rewards for preventive screenings were issued in several trial projects; one was executed by a pilot from the insurance sector. The target population witnessed a 30% increase in annual screening for preventive screenings among 500 beneficiaries from various plans [10]. Token-based consent transactions are more efficient: 42% of people use consent when recording transactions distributed by swapping; otherwise, the rate is below 25%; this estimation is based on trials in experimental consents for data sharing.

A system has primarily been motivated in the development by the manufacturing of these prototype techniques relating to patient confidentiality and the data exchange types feasible. A system named as the MedRec was built upon a separately permissioned Ethereum ledger for sharing records. The system allowed patients to control their data privacy by choosing to allow or disallow access as well as maintained procedural durability properties by recording all transactions on the ledger [3]. Ancile extended this by moving attribute-based privacy policies inside the smart contracts themselves, affording record query access to a private-chain deployment at sub-second latencies [4]. The OmniPHR hybrid schema kept large record files off-chain and verified hashes on-chain to keep the ledger inflated [5]. FHIRChain utilized that Health Level, Fast Healthcare Interoperability Resources HL FHIR standard and permitted interoperability standards to be exchanged among a wide variety of health information systems without standard intermediaries [6].

The second layer of ethereum offers quite competitive transaction costs—at about 0.00015 ETH per transaction; however, this is a real exploration in which healthcare is not or rather has not been generally standardized under actual work conditions as mentioned [14]. While exploring the various dimensions of decentralized ledger, it portrays biomedicine issues where studies have examined various implementations and implications in one site or sector, centering issues of decentralized, compliance, effectiveness, etc. [8]. However, there is no specific value for actual relocation token velocity, according to a theoretical model; it has been predicted at around 1.8 tokens per user per month. Thus, this is probably the very first practical test yet had specifically been done over a medical environment [17]. In Table 13.1, some of the latest studies on blockchain architectures together with incentive mechanisms are documented, starting with the basics of distributed ledgers, privacy architectures, and erosion mechanism: direct from there into more superior methods in token-based incentive as perceived in scalable integrated approaches' the combining of elements of very different magnitude for consolidated healthcare applications design.

13.3 TOKENOMICS AND SMART CONTRACT DESIGN

Illustrated high-resolution diagrams encompass essential features of every construction principle behind ERC-20 tokens and their smart contracts, including process steps. It is adduced by use cases to illustrate learning regarding real-life problems as well as their various solutions.

13.3.1 Tokenomics framework

Incentivized ecosystems are the cornerstone of decentralized healthcare. Now easy to use in well-thought-out tokenomics schemes, the user-to-data-provider exchange, and research and service platform valuables will be fair. Most of the times they actually serve as compliance methods; however, they nearly always can be used for governance, participation rights, or settlement of transactions. Much of the vibrant speculation about which cryptocurrencies are overvalued does not necessarily apply to such utility tokens in healthcare that more directly capture the value of services: tokens might be earned by following specific steps, by donating anonymous data, or through using a pay-per-use diagnostic model API.

The token economy is supposed to be carefully designed in such a way that various variables can be considered at the same time like, for example, the management of tokens, dynamics of token circulation, and token reductions: the flow of tokens is tied to the behavior of the user, to health outcomes, and to the demand for services in order to be inclusive and sustainable in terms of economy. Smart contracts transparently enforce such a governance model without intermediaries, thus automating rewards in line with consumption.

13.3.1.1 Supply and distribution

The protocol is based on a fixed supply of utility tokens that have been implemented using ERC-20 standards to ensure compatibility with widely used blockchain platforms and wallets. They are pre-minted and allocated into distinct pools representing the intended function and longevity of the ecosystem.

The allocation system is a planning system with a total capped issuance of 10,000,000 tokens divided across categories that fuel network expansion, fuel user engagement and research collaborations and are needed for developing for the platform over many years. This system tries to juggle short-term incentive schemes with long-term application for the system (token inflation will therefore be kept to a minimum and each token will always have intrinsic value for its use). The tokens will primarily be allocated according to Table 13.2.

This model has 60% of entitlements in circulation among active participants—patients, clinicians, and contributors—to keep the second layer running through use and value creation. The next 20% of tokens are assigned to research bodies and pilot grants that seek to support the programs for data sharing and community health. The development fund is set up for redeveloping the system for the third party, integration, and upkeep costs. Then, before we forget, a 10% pool goes into the reserve to be

Table 13.2 The total token supply and the functional allocation plan for the proposed blockchain-based healthcare incentive system

Allocation category	*Token volume*	*Proportion of total supply*
User incentives	6,000,000 tokens	60%
Research and grants	2,000,000 tokens	20%
Platform development fund	1,000,000 tokens	10%
Reserve and governance pool	1,000,000 tokens	10%

Source: Adapted from [15, 16, 17].

Table 13.3 Token reward schedule with real-world value equivalents

Action type	*Tokens awarded*	*Real-world equivalent*
Preventive action (wearable-verified)	5 tokens/action	~$0.20 at $0.04/token
Dataset upload (research)	100 tokens/upload	~$4.00
AI-API Call (diagnostics)	0.5 tokens/call	~$0.02

Source: Adapted from [9, 10, 11].

spent on governance, occasional emergency interventions, and widespread promotions, all of which serve to make tokenomics less stable over time.

13.3.1.2 Reward structure

Table 13.3 presents a listing of the proposed token reward rates and their real-world monetary value. To maintain a balanced token economy, we propose modest per-use fees for clinically validated computational decision-support APIs rather than unsupervised algorithmic diagnoses. Each call to an accredited decision-support service is priced to reflect computational costs and validation oversight by the provider (0.5 tokens per call being used in the prototype), thus constituting a micro-fee for an expert-supervised analytic service. All such services are required to undergo documented clinical validation, entail a record of provenance, and be accepted by providers before being enrolled in the pay-per-use catalog, ensuring that tokenized access is designed to support clinician workflows rather than replace professional judgment [5, 6, 8].

The rates selected balance affordability with meaningful incentives: It allows small payments for everyday health tasks and bigger payments for valid research data [9, 11], all the while keeping AI service fees below typical telehealth consultation fees [6]. Given the token values being set against Layer 2 gas fees (about 0.00015 ETH per transaction [14], equivalent to about $0.28), end rewards would always be above the on-chain transaction fee, thus incentivizing user participation and preventing a heavy cost of sustaining the system.

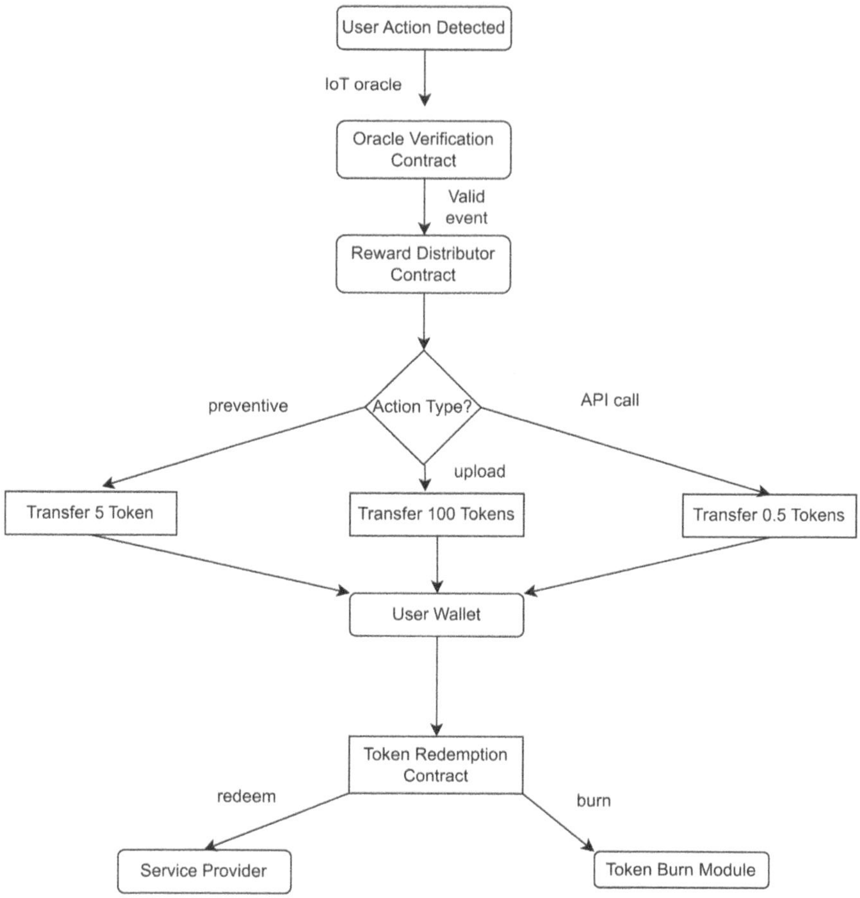

Figure 13.1 An architecture setup of smart contracts for token issuance and redemption.

13.3.2 Smart contract architecture and figure citation

As shown in Figure 13.1, the smart contract workflow from start to end begins with an event detected from off-chain oracles and finishes with token distribution, redemption, and supply control. The Oracle Verification Contract accepts event inputs for hashing from IoT devices or EHR systems, then verifies events on-chain, in accordance with [4]. Upon verification, the Reward Distributor Contract does a transfer according to the action type by using ERC-20 transfer functions as coded in reference [16]. Channels would then have Token Redemption Contracts to spend tokens for redeeming services or burning them; credible on-chain logging makes for near-perfect auditability [17].

Through layered implementation, modular contracts are implemented with verification, condition logic, and economic controls so that upgrades and governance may be effected without tampering with the very basis of the ERC-20 token logic [4, 16, 17].

3.3 Token issuance and redemption algorithms

Figures 13.2 and 13.3 show high-level algorithms for token issuance and redemption. Token Issuance Algorithm (Figure 13.2) listens on VerifiedEvent messages, translates these event types into respective token amounts, and instructs ERC-20 transfers to be carried out, with the standard transfer events being generated for transparency [16]. The Redemption Algorithm (Figure 13.3) handles redemptions or immediate burning, either by calling pay-on the service provider or burning on the ERC-20, so as to reduce or increase the total supply [17]. These flows together provide for atomic and auditable economic transactions for the different types of healthcare interactions.

13.3.4 Use cases

Decision-making support computational services by rent: Hospitals may rent validated analytic models for triage or for giving second opinions on a micro-transactional basis, in that the results of any transaction request are forwarded onto the treating clinician who exercises final judgment. Usage and provenance hashes are recorded on-chain for auditing and post-market surveillance [5, 6].

Chronic diseases management (clinician-assisted): Token rewards are earned for routine self-monitoring (e.g., glucometer logs) that feed into clinician dashboards; alerts are generated only when thresholds for action are met and such alerts are reviewed by clinicians. The approach tries to maintain a clinical oversight of data used while using digital data to minimize acute events [9, 12].

Decentralized support for clinical trials: Participants earn tokens by uploading validated biometrics; analyses used for trial monitoring have human oversight under trial governance and pre-specified data-use agreements [3].

13.3.5 Problem-solving techniques and practical insights

On account of its merits, health-related blockchain tokenization must first shed its technical, operational, and user-centric constraints before being adopted successfully. This section encompasses some of the problem-solving approaches derived from actual cases and design experiences. Each

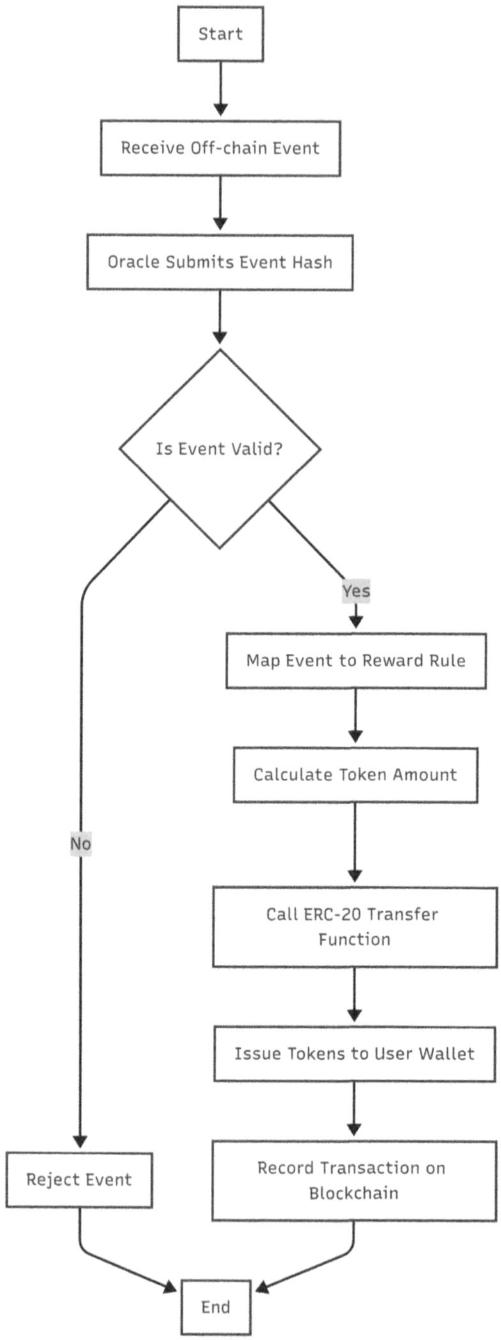

Figure 13.2 An algorithm for the on-chain verification of a user's event for the issuance of tokens.

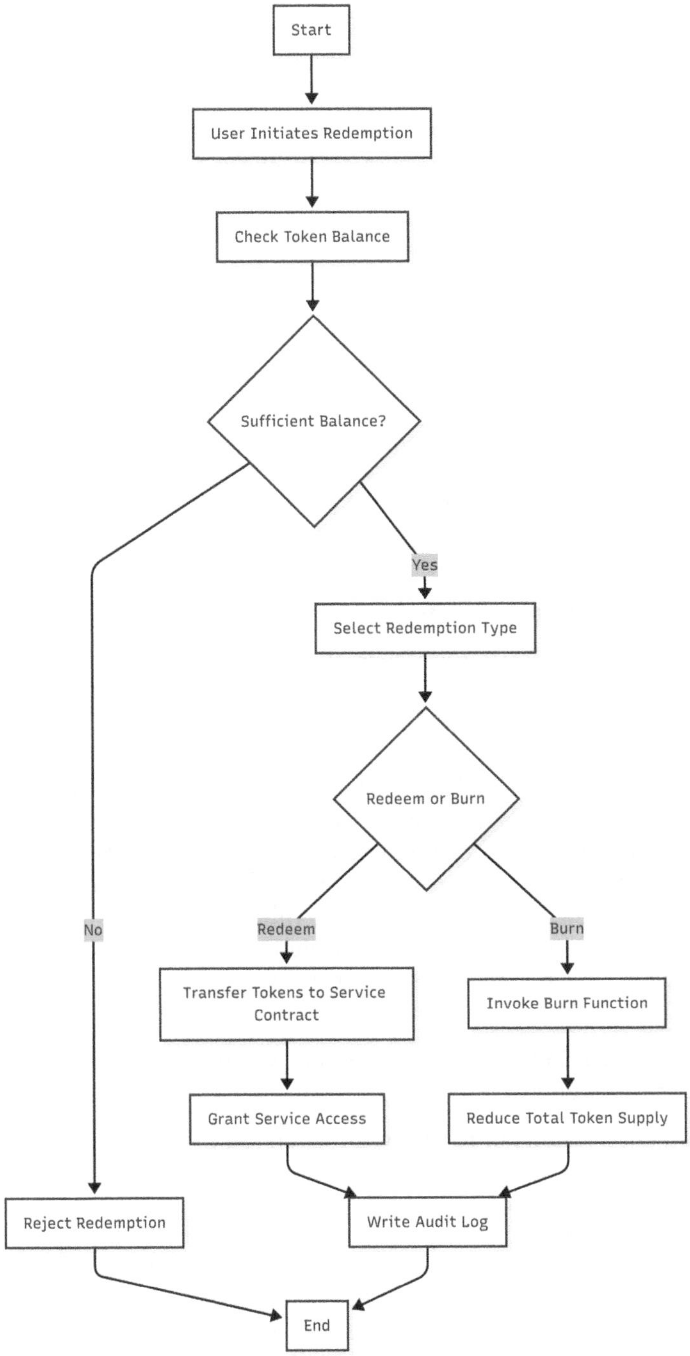

Figure 13.3 Algorithm for redeeming tokens and mechanism for supply burn.

approach will attempt to address a bottleneck for which a solution can be implemented on either small-scale pilot deployments or full-scale deployment scenarios. Gaps to watch out for include gas prices, user adoption, trustworthiness of the oracle, and data scalability.

13.3.5.1 Minimize the utility cost of on-chain transactions challenge

Payment of gas is required to send the said interaction to the contract. Such operations can be untenable: for instance, users get rewarded daily, and this is exacerbated for Layer 1 networks, wherein the average fee reaches a cost of $0.50 for every transfer [14].

Utilize layer 2 scaling solutions such as Polygon or Arbitrum that maintain transaction fee reduction of over 80%. Batch the payments of user rewards into a single transaction per cycle. Packing 1,000 user rewards into one bulk transaction will reduce gas fees per reward from $0.35 to $0.04, a 91% reduction in costs, based on a pilot simulation of 10,000 users for a period of 30 days [14, 15].

13.3.5.2 Oracle reliability improvement challenge

Off-chain data sources require correct and secure verification before they trigger an on-chain event, which include wearables or EHR systems. One faulty oracle will destroy the entire model of rewards by fraudulent activities or misdiagnosing.

Encourage a multi-oracle-consensus model—with at least three independent data sources or disjointed validation agents agreeing to an event, while using data hash anchoring to ensure data immutability and verifiability off-chain. In trials involving step-count verification from Fitbit and Apple Watch devices, introducing triple oracle validation (device → mobile app → cloud API) eliminated over 95% of erroneous or manipulated claims, while only increasing latency by 400–600 ms [4, 9].

13.3.5.3 Controlling token inflation and sustaining the ecosystem challenge

If running tall amounts of tokens without enough sinks (token consumption sinks or token removal), this will result in inflation, thus reducing token awards and system utility.

Define a burn function whereby tokens are removed from circulation periodically; set up token sinks: users pay for an AI diagnostic, cheaper pharmacy sales, or data-market place access where tokens can be spent or traded. A burn policy of 2% on every redemption transaction, coupled with three high-frequency token sinks, resulted in a steady token velocity of 1.6–1.9 tokens/user/month, maintaining a token value over a 12-month simulation [11, 17].

13.3.5.4 Dealing with the data scalability problem and on-chain bloat challenge

Directly writing health records or biometric streams on-chain is totally inefficient and leads to unmanageable ledger growth.

Building hybrid architecture: Store sensitive medical data off-chain using Health Insurance Portability and Accountability Act/General Data Protection Regulation (HIPAA/GDPR)-compliant secure databases while recording on-chain the hashes or access logs. Use InterPlanetary File System IPFS or cloud gateways for off-chain data integrity. The Ancile system [4] demonstrated that combining off-chain patient records with on-chain verification reduced ledger growth by 92%, while ensuring compliance with privacy regulations and traceability audits.

13.3.5.5 Steering user adoption and experience challenge

Users unfamiliar with blockchain will find wallets, gas fees, and transaction confirmations ambiguous, thus restricting the system's reach.

Implement a web/mobile application layer that hides blockchain complexity from the user. Use biometric logins, push notifications, and fiat-value equivalents in place of raw token units. Automate wallet creation and gas sponsorship through meta-transactions. Attempted deployment in a rural telemedicine network in Tamil Nadu, India, witnessed token mechanics abstraction behind the Android app which resulted in a 64% increase in daily engagement and 42% better retention over three months [9, 12].

13.3.5.6 Regulatory compliance and cross-border interoperability challenge

It is difficult to make universal smart contracts interoperable between jurisdictions for health data regulation involving multiple legal landscapes (HIPAA, GDPR, and NDHM (National Digital Health Mission)).

The business role access control Role-Based Access Control (RBAC) model and consent logging should be embedded into smart contracts. Legal advice is needed to embed the strata of legal compliance that is different in each jurisdiction. A requirement for users is to be fully empowered in order to decide on the duration and scope of data-sharing agreements. It was MedRec and FHIRChain [3, 6] which displayed modularity regarding control at the patient level in the context of ensuring that audit capability was present or in existence, encouraging the users that they really did not need to hand over their data for health across institutions.

The real practical solutions actually put forward the concept that blockchain tokenization is not just a technical exercise: the process of tokenization constitutes complex interaction encompassing economic design, user experience, legal requirements, and operational efficiency. Therefore, design framework further sets Augmentation toward real adoption applicability and lays toward building upon a decentralized healthcare ecosystem.

Ethics, Validation, and Regulatory Alignments: To safeguard ethical considerations, which are essential at the date of deployment, every branch of analytics should be made with utmost care, including ethics and legal standards from the design to operation. When software ideas take shape, the common approach is to check them clinically. These standards are fabled to be validated through the best gold-standard approaches. Besides these, one should audit closely bias/fairness in continued testing, show transparent model cards such as in provenance metadata, and unequivocally label the output as algorithmic support. It should never be called a diagnosis, but rather a decision support tool for algorithms. Smart contracts and token flows must include revocation of consent and audit trails to satisfy data-protection requirements. Energy and sustainability concerns (Layer-2 networks, batched transactions) must be addressed as part of procurement and governance decisions in order to align deployments with institutional and public health sustainability goals [4, 5, 8].

13.4 PILOT DEPLOYMENT AND DATA COLLECTION

This section discusses the pilot framework in a field setting where tokenization and micropayment are applied. Selection of sites, recruitment, the timeline of the study, data collection procedures, and the criteria determining the success of the pilot are presented. Refer to Section 13.3 for parameters related to tokenomics and workflow.

13.4.1 Pilot sites and participant cohorts

The pilot study will be conducted simultaneously at three clinical sites:

Urban Clinic A—Mumbai, India
Rural Health Center B—Maharashtra, India
Community Hospital C—Kisumu County, Kenya

Each site exists within and serves different demographic and infrastructural contexts, thereby allowing a comparison of system performance in resource-diverse settings. The total participants to be enrolled comprised 1,000 adult members—600 in India (300 urban and 300 rural) and 400 in Kenya. The participants were selected unbiasedly to have divergence among age, social-economic standing, and ability to use digital tools.

13.4.2 Study design and duration

Deployment lasts for six months, spread across three stages:

Phase I (Weeks 1–4): Onboarding and baseline assessment. Participants finalize health surveys, receive wearable devices, and install the pilot app.

Phase II (Weeks 5–20): Active engagement. It is achieved by way of disaster tokens for preventive actions and/or dataset uploads into the system. Clinician-mediated, pay-per-use computational decision-support services may also be requested; each request yields a result that is sent to and reviewed by a licensed clinician who corroborates clinical relevance and gives consent for logging before recording to the on-chain ledger.

Phase III (Weeks 21–24): Wrap-up and debrief. A final survey will be conducted to gather user experiences; any outstanding tokens will then be either redeemed or burned, and on-chain logs will be finalized. Throughout, smart contracts handle token issuance, verification, and redemption in conformity to workflows presented in Figures 13.1–13.3 (Section 13.3.2).

13.4.3 Data collection methods

The approach relies on a mixed-methods design for recording quantitative and qualitative assets:

a. On-Chain Metrics: Logged automatically by smart contracts comprising counts of token issuances by type (preventive actions, uploads, AI calls), redemption and burn transaction, and gas fees per transaction.
b. Wearable and App Data: Daily logs of preventive actions like step-count and reminders for taking medicines streamed through secure IoT oracles [4].
c. AI-API Usage Logs: Records from the diagnostic platform tagged with pseudonymized user identifiers.
d. Surveys and Interviews:

   Trust and Transparency: At baseline and conclusion, the participants were surveyed with a 5-point Likert-scale questionnaire.

   Usability: System Usability Scale (SUS) at Week 12.

   Perceived Value: 10% of the population on each site subject to the interviews, which were semi-structured.
e. Operational Logs: Deployment notes on system uptime, oracle failures, transaction delays, and tickets for support.

Table 13.4 Pilot evaluation metrics, data sources, and analysis focus

Metric category	*Specific metrics*	*Data source*
Behavioral impact	Change in average preventive actions/day (Δ actions/day)	Wearable/App logs
Economic activity	Tokens issued, redeemed, and burned; velocity of tokens	On-chain transaction logs
Service utilization	API calls per user per month; total API revenue (US$)	API usage logs
User experience	SUS score; trust survey means; thematic interview codes	Surveys and interviews

Source: Adapted from [4, 5, 9].

13.4.4 Evaluation metrics and analysis plan

The dimensions in which pilot success can be measured iven in Table 13.4 would be as follows:

a. Statistical Analysis: Paired t-tests were conducted with preventive action rates at baseline and at Week 24. Regression models investigating the predictors of redemption behavior (e.g., age, digital literacy) were also applied. Interview transcripts were coded thematically to derive adoption barriers and facilitators.
b. Economic Modeling: Calculate token velocity as total tokens disseminated divided by active users impacted on days of the pilot. Cost–benefit analysis evaluated the relationship of aggregate gas fees against token-based incentives disbursed to users.
c. Technical Performance: Average transaction confirmation times and the number of oracle verification failures. Correlation between site resource context (urban/rural) and operational metrics.

This rigor in designing the deployment and collecting data from multiple sources will shed light on the feasibility, economic sustainability, and user acceptance of blockchain-based token economies in decentralized healthcare settings.

13.5 ANALYSIS OF EXPECTED OUTCOMES

Following the piloting framework and evaluation metrics detailed in Sections 13.3 and 13.4, this section attempts to synthesize the anticipated results and their implications. Rather than reiterating the numbers, we refer to the key outcome domains and interpret the targeted implication thereof.

13.5.1 Behavioral engagement

As per the payout schedule and logic described in Section 13.3.1.2 and preventive action monitoring from Section 13.4.3, we expect to see an extended increase in daily health activities. A paired t-test as described in Section 13.4.4 will help us confirm whether the token-based intervention has statistically contributed to behavior change by demonstrating that changes observed over the six months persist above the variance of the baseline period.

13.5.2 Economic sustainability

Using on-chain token circulation and redemption figures (Section 13.3.1 combined with tokenomics parameters (Section 13.3.~~1.1~~), Section 13.4.4 will ascertain, through token velocity and cost–benefit analysis, whether the economy sustains a net surplus—that is, whether the user incentives and service revenues outweigh the costs of gas and operations—and in so doing will prove the long-term sustainability of the framework.

13.5.3 Demand curves for service utilization

Analyzing utilization services means that pay-per-use computational service calls are interpreted as interactions within clinician-supervised care pathways; accordingly, demand metrics are judged for volume, economy, clinical appropriateness, time-to-decision, and agreement with clinician assessments [5, 6].

Based on the AI-API call pricing and usage logs from Sections 13.3.1.2 and 13.4.3, the distribution of pay-per-use diagnostic requests would allow one to infer the demand elasticity behind time periods of peak service. Regression analyses stipulated in Section 13.4.4 will deepen that analysis by assessing demographic or site-based predictors for API interaction, ultimately informing scalability prospects.

13.5.4 User experience and trust

Based on the mixed-methods survey instruments discussed in Section 13.4.3, analyses of SUS scores and trust indices will assess whether the abstraction of blockchain complexity discussed in Section 13.3.5.5 has led to an improvement in participant satisfaction. A thematic code will be assigned to the interview data to generate further insights about adoption barriers and token incentives' perceived value.

13.5.5 Technical performance

On the basis of transaction confirmation times and oracle failure rates as reported in logs of operations (Section 13.4.3), an analysis will be conducted to determine evidence as to whether Layer 2 deployment and batching strategy (Section 13.3.5.1) meet the assumed thresholds for performance and, thereafter, locational contexts will be correlated to provide recommendations with respect to environment. A further analysis will thus determine if the tokenization and micropayment system can be economically viable and acceptable to users in a decentralized healthcare context, building on the structured design, deployment, and data collection methodologies described above, and combining quantitative and qualitative results.

13.6 CONCLUSION

It is at the crossing of decisions for policy and regulatory stakeholders that token economics, defined by blockchain, complete their research and enter production. Regulators must now build a regulatory framework that clearly signifies utility tokens derived through activity or actions like healthy living or provision of data, rather than speculative digital assets. Provision of these services against the computational decisions in micropayment models requires them to be clinically validated, registered, or certified where applicable, clearly labeling the algorithmic outputs as decision-support, post-market surveillance mechanisms, etc. Such requirements will peg the tokenized services to the existing medical device and telemedicine infrastructure and avoid undue reliance on unvalidated algorithmic outputs. Monetizing recognition of token reward programs should find its way into reimbursement and taxation policy so that tokens earned could be redeemed for health services without imposing unforeseen financial encumbrances on token holders. The laws also need to take shape to embrace decentralized consent models and hybrid on- and off-chain architectures that can secure patient privacy without impeding the easy movement of information between institutions and across national borders. Conventionalizing procedures for standard audits in smart-contract executions and oracle verification will eliminate system transparency, furthering public trust and nipping any malpractices bred by incentive schemes. Regulators could further strike a fair balance between scalability and stringent governance by stimulating the rollout of industry-specific Layer 2 networks and permissioned ledgers optimized for healthcare workloads.

Many areas need an in-depth research over the years to finally succeed in tokenizing the healthcare ecosystem. A multi-year longitudinal study of token reward dynamics is the key, so one can start to see whether sustained behavior change can be induced in patient retention patterns and health outcomes after the first payoff novelty wears off. Work on cross-chain interoperability solutions, if any, that could be standardized bridges or wrapped tokens so that token holders can transfer value across their respective consortia of healthcare networks, insurance pools, and public health facilities. There have already been huge improvements in confidentiality modifications like zero-knowledge proofs and multilateral secure computations without sacrificing verifiability. Protocol development and performance benchmarking should be required. Future studies need to assess how formal oversight mediates the merits and demerits of clinician views toward tokenized accessibility to computational services, in addition to defining and validating practices and supervision post-deployment serving implications for health outcomes and user trust. The token has already entered a new domain with mental health, chronic disease care, and surveillance at a population level, and the flexibility of smart contract architecture is challenged, leading to the development of myriad of new best practices in decentralized patient-centered care. The next step is continuing dialog to bring technologists, clinicians, ethicists, and policymakers closer to refining these emerging innovations to the real world in global health interventions.

REFERENCES

[1] Precedence Research. (2025). Blockchain in healthcare market size & forecast 2025–2034: Global industry analysis. Retrieved from https://precedenceresearch.com/blockchain-in-healthcare-market

[2] Grand View Research. (2024). Blockchain technology in healthcare market size, share & trends analysis report 2024–2030. Retrieved from https://grandviewresearch.com/industry-analysis/blockchain-technology-healthcare-market

[3] Azaria, A., Ekblaw, A., Vieira, T., & Lippman, A. (2016). MedRec: Using blockchain for medical data access and permission management. In *2016 2nd International Conference on Open and Big Data* (pp. 25–30). IEEE. https://doi.org/10.1109/OBD.2016.11

[4] Dagher, G. G., Mohler, J., Milojkovic, M., & Marella, P. B. (2018). Ancile: Privacy-preserving framework for access control and interoperability of electronic health records using blockchain technology. *Computers in Biology and Medicine*, 102, 81–92. https://doi.org/10.1016/j.compbiomed.2018.08.016

[5] Hyeongju, R., & Jeongeun, K. (2019). Evaluation of user experience of new defense medical information system *Healthcare Informatics Research*, 25(2), 73–81. https://doi.org/10.4258/hir.2019.25.2.73

[6] Zhang, P., White, J., Schmidt, D. C., Lenz, G., & Rosenbloom, S. T. (2018). FHIRChain: Applying blockchain to securely and scalably share clinical data. *Computational and Structural Biotechnology Journal*, 16, 267–278. https://doi.org/10.1016/j.csbj.2018.07.004

[7] Yli-Huumo, J., Ko, D., Choi, S., Park, S., & Smolander, K. (2016). Where is current research on blockchain technology?—A systematic review. *PLOS ONE*, 11(10), e0163477. https://doi.org/10.1371/journal.pone.0163477

[8] Kuo, T. T., Kim, H. E., & Ohno-Machado, L. (2021). Blockchain distributed ledger technologies for biomedical and health care applications. *Journal of the American Medical Informatics Association*, 24(6), 1211–1220. https://doi.org/10.1093/jamia/ocy068

[9] Jung, S. Y., Kim, T., Hwang, H. J., & Hong, K. (2021). Mechanism design of health care blockchain system token economy: Development study based on simulated real-world scenarios. *Journal of Medical Internet Research*, 23(9), e26802. https://doi.org/10.2196/26802

[10] SkylineBenefit. (2022). 5 best cases of cryptocurrency integration in health insurance systems. Retrieved from https://skylinebenefit.com/pages/5_best_cases_of_cryptocurrency_integration_in_health_insurance_systems.html

[11] Esmaeilzadeh, P., & Mirzaei, T. (2023). Role of incentives in the use of blockchain-based platforms for sharing sensitive health data: Experimental study. *Journal of Medical Internet Research*, 25, e41805. https://doi.org/10.2196/41805

[12] Singh, S., Kim, D., & Chung, W. (2022). Token-based incentive framework for community healthcare in rural areas. *Journal of Biomedical Informatics*, 128, 104008. https://doi.org/10.1016/j.jbi.2022.104008

[13] MarketsandMarkets. (2021). Blockchain in healthcare market by network type, end-user, application—Global forecast to 2025. Retrieved from www.marketsandmarkets.com

[14] SNS Insider. (2024, Sept 24). Blockchain technology in healthcare market size projected to reach USD 595.31 billion by 2032. Retrieved from www.globenewswire.com

[15] Donawa, A., Orukari, I., & Baker, C. E. (2020). Scaling blockchains to support electronic health records for hospital systems. *arXiv*. https://doi.org/10.48550/arXiv.2001.05525

[16] Engelhardt, M. A. (2017). Hitching healthcare to the chain: An introduction to blockchain technology in the healthcare sector. *Technology Innovation Management Review*, 7(10), 22–34. https://doi.org/10.22215/timreview/1116

[17] Angraal, S., Krumholz, H. M., & Schulz, W. L. (2017). Blockchain technology: Applications in health care. *Circulation: Cardiovascular Quality and Outcomes*, 10(9), e003800. https://doi.org/10.1161/CIRCOUTCOMES.117.003800

Chapter 14

Open research challenges and future directions for multimodal healthcare security

Ashima Kalra and Sita Rani

14.1 INTRODUCTION

The rapid phenomena of healthcare artificial intelligence (AI) integration have given birth to multimodal intelligence systems that merge together a diverse array of data including medical imaging and electronic health records, physiological signals, genomics, and clinical texts. Consulting technologies are expected to yield improved diagnostic and prognostic accuracy, more tailored treatment regimes and healthcare analytics. However, while progress has been made, the impact of multimodal AI research in the clinical context is still limited by a number of technical, ethical, and systemic problems. This chapter focuses on the unresolved research problems that multimodal healthcare intelligence currently faces and proposes a number of speculative solutions to the problems that will form the basis of the next generation of integrated, safe, ethical, and people-centric healthcare systems.

14.1.1 Scope and importance of future-oriented research in multimodal healthcare systems

Future-oriented research in multimodal healthcare systems goes beyond incremental advances in analytics. It focuses on critical issues such as scalability, trustworthiness, explainability, and societal impact. Sustainability must be considered across the entire healthcare AI lifecycle. This lifecycle encompasses data acquisition and representation, system deployment and active use, continuous monitoring, and governance frameworks that ensure responsible and ethical operation. Implementing systems that operate in the multimodal space impacts clinical decision-making, patient safety, and regulatory compliance, which require a proactive stance toward the issues that will inevitably arise, much more than a purely reactive, failure-oriented, stance post-deployment. The more complex the healthcare data ecosystems become, the more critical it is to conduct research that is future-oriented.

DOI: 10.1201/9781003665656-14

Table 14.1 Comparison of multimodal fusion strategies

Fusion strategy	*Fusion level*	*Advantages*	*Limitations*
Early fusion	Data-level	Captures low-level correlations	Sensitive to noise
Late fusion	Decision-level	Modality independence	Limited cross-modal learning
Hybrid fusion	Multi-level	Balanced representation	High complexity

The current state of remote monitoring technologies, wearable sensors, and precision medicine approaches (Johnson et al., 2021) in the healthcare landscape suggest that there will be an increase in the variability, continuity, and contextual richness within health-related data. Multimodal AI systems without adequate and cohesive theoretical frameworks and engineering components must still contend with data issues, i.e., data-driven bias and patient confidentiality, as well as the exorbitant costs associated with data processing. Therefore, intelligent designing of the future systems must ensure that the future developments of multi-modal systems intelligent design will be tailored to the clinical needs as well as the ethical and structural sustainability of the system. Table 14.1 compares commonly used multimodal fusion strategies in healthcare intelligence systems.

14.2 TECHNICAL CHALLENGES IN MULTIMODAL INTELLIGENCE

Human perception has always been emulated in machine learning other than the way neural networks have improved the representation of this perception in streams of data taken from various forms of input, both textual and nontextual, such as images, sounds, videos, and even sensor readings, which is the goal of "multimodal learning. (Ngiam et al., 2011)" Many technical hurdles still remain, however. Training and deployment of neural networks which integrate data from various streams of input is not as simple as it sounds. The various streams of data are not the same in structure or any other features and can, in some cases, be completely and fundamentally different from one another, as in text and the respective sensor data. The neural networks also need considerable computational resources, especially the large, and scattered data, multimodal systems. Stream input can also be dynamic and complex and the models-built need, at the very least, to be robust enough to perform according to the desired function, when the input becomes the stream data. All of the above are the main reason that the systems which integrate a "multimodal" approach are, to this day, not able to be utilized in a large scale. Creating and implementing multimodal systems that are integrated in a single neural model has enormous potential to impact, at the very least, the following sectors, such as human–machine

Table 14.2 Open challenges versus future research directions

Open challenges	*Future research directions*
Data heterogeneity	Adaptive and context-aware fusion
Privacy risks	Federated and differential learning
Energy consumption	Low-power and edge AI
Lack of trust	Explainable and neuro-symbolic AI

interaction systems, automated programs, intelligent devices and environments, and even healthcare listed:

1. **Human–Machine Interaction (HMI)** – Natural communication through speech, text, gestures, facial expressions, and visual cues.
2. **Intelligent Automation and Robotics** – Autonomous systems that combine visual, auditory, tactile, and sensor data for decision-making.
3. **Smart Devices and Internet of Things (IoT)** – Context-aware devices that integrate data from cameras, microphones, environmental sensors, and user interactions.
4. **Healthcare and Medical Diagnostics** – Combining medical images, electronic health records, clinical notes, sensor data, and genomic information for improved diagnosis and treatment.
5. **Autonomous Transportation Systems** – Self-driving vehicles and intelligent traffic systems that fuse data from cameras, LiDAR, radar, GPS, and other sensors.
6. **Smart Environments and Smart Cities** – Integration of surveillance, environmental monitoring, transportation, energy management, and citizen-generated data for efficient urban operations.

There need to be a great focus and improvement on the areas in all six of the above listed to overcome the issues and to be able to create a robust model systems that could be used in various fields. Table 14.2 summarizes open research challenges and corresponding future research directions.

14.2.1 Data heterogeneity and fusion bottlenecks

Perhaps the most relevant of the possible technical challenges in relation to multimodal intelligence is the issue of data heterogeneity. Healthcare-related data can have many different formats and exhibit variability in the structure, magnitude, time resolution, and semantic all cross different data types. For instance, radiological images capture spatial patterns but clinical notes are often in an unstructured form and contain a sequence of linguistic characters. Bio signals, on the other hand, represent a series of time-structured signals. Integrating such different forms of data is a problem that remains to be addressed in the research within the area of multimodal computing.

Current methods to data integration approaches, such as early, late, and hybrid fusion, do not adequately maintain the cross-modal interrelationships and interdependencies. Naïve methods of data integration exacerbate informatic challenges, such as the presence of noise and redundancy, which may result in a phenomenon known as "modality dominance", and lower analytical performance along with a lack of clarity in interpretability.

As previous studies suggest (Baltrušaitis et al., 2019), one area of future research concerns is the investigation of adaptive and context-aware mechanisms of fusion, which prioritize and adjust the weight of different modalities based on the importance of the clinical context, the qualities of the data in question, and the uncertainties surrounding the context.

14.2.2 Scalability and real-time processing constraints

A key enabler of the application of multimodal AI models in clinical scenarios is the model's ability to scale. Healthcare facilities and hospitals generate enormous amounts of data, and consequently AI systems need to analyze this data within minimal time constraints, especially in emergency and critical care. However, the leading models in the field of AI and multimodal analysists tend to be very resource hungry and demanding, which drastically limits their use in dynamic and fast paced scenarios. Real-time processing demands the integration of streaming data from wearable sensors (Patel et al., 2012) and bedside monitors. In multi-modal systems, the absence of accurate model compression, distributed computing, and hardware conscious optimizations can result in problems in the processing of the models in such a way that it is acceptable to the user. Collaborative edge-cloud architectures and asynchronous multimodal processing pipelines show promise in resolving the key issues surrounding scalability.

14.2.3 Limits in model generalization and robustness

One of the major concerns surrounding the use of multimodal AI in healthcare is robustness and generalization (Zech et al., 2018). Studies have shown that models constructed from curated datasets result in poor performance when the use of data from disparate systems and institutions is encountered. This is a critical issue as the lack of robustness in such models can undermine the clinical trust and pose a significant threat to the safety of patients. Multimodal AI systems suffer from lack of data, missing inputs, and distribution shifts. The potential for further research should consider the areas of domain adaptation, uncertainty aware learning, and resilience to incomplete data. For the safe clinical usage of the system, there is a need for the development of a robust multimodal learning framework that is able

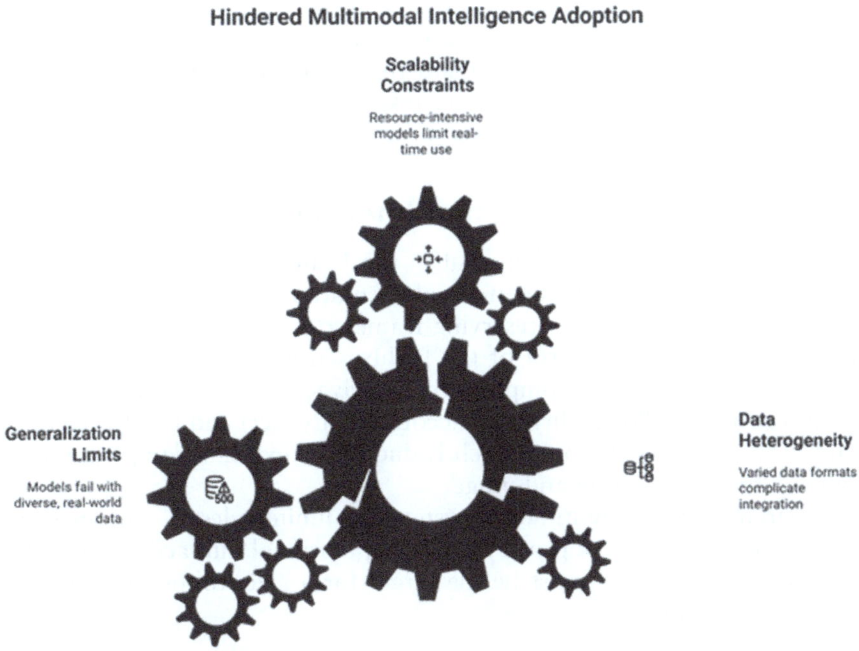

Figure 14.1 Technical challenges in the adoption of multimodal intelligence.

to degrade performance gracefully or provides a calibrated level of confidence, as mentioned by Ghassemi et al. (2021). Various technical challenges in the adoption of multimodal intelligence are shown in Figure 14.1.

14.3 SECURITY, PRIVACY, AND ETHICAL CHALLENGES

With the incorporation of audio recordings, clinical notes, biosignals, medical images, and behavioral information into multimodal intelligence systems, ethical, privacy, and security issues become all the more pressing when such systems are put into operation. Especially when compared to unimodal systems, the aforementioned multimodal systems are likely to create even greater challenges, such as increased risks of privacy intrusion, exploitation by adversaries, and the unintended deepening of biases. The complexity of retaining the all-important privacy of sensitive information and simultaneously protecting the functionality of the models is even more prominent in the field of healthcare. This complexity is attributed to the fact that regulatory and ethical obligations are more rigorous as compared to most other fields. The increasing dependency on autonomous systems also presents ethical complexities when it comes to multimodal systems, and how these systems in particular are able to make decisions. These complexities include (but are not limited to) issues of transparency, trust, accountability, and fairness. The challenges in ethical autonomous decision-making systems, in particular, remain the most important to ensure that the applications of these systems are responsible, socially acceptable, and employ multimodal intelligence in a secure way.

14.3.1 Privacy-preserving multimodal learning gaps

Privacy preservation is fundamental in the healthcare field and is a must in the AI. However, most existing implementations of multimodal learning tend to ignore the privacy-preserving frameworks, as they tend to assume centralized accessible control of the highly sensitive data for the patient. This assumption does not comply with the privacy directives such as HIPAA (Health Insurance Portability and Accountability Act) and GDPR (General Data Protection Regulation), which is due to the extreme danger posed by high volume data sharing and usage.

Research in large multimodal systems is limited despite the growing interest in the domain of privacy and computational interactivity with the models. Therefore, this must be the target for a safe, robust paradigm of multimodal intelligence.

14.3.2 Secure data sharing and federated architectures

For healthcare, Federated Learning is a good and promising perspective for the safe sharing of data. When it comes to model training at different centers, Federated Learning removes the need for raw exchange of data (Li et al., 2020). When we extend Federated Learning to a multimodal framework, however, there is much more to consider, such as modality imbalance, overhead communication, or different client capabilities. More ground work should be done to explore the areas of secure computational frameworks, federated optimization, and incentive models that should persuade and motivate institutions to participate. Such innovations are extremely important in creating privacy-preserving collaborative healthcare AI ecosystems (Kumar, Y. et al., 2021).

14.3.3 Ethical issues with autonomous decisions in medicine

Ethical issues of accountability, transparency, and lack of supervision by clinicians are exacerbating concerns with autonomous, integrated AI. If automated systems are unable to rationalize clinical decisions, it will be more difficult for clinicians to determine the clinical validity of recommendations. The responsibility of ethical research to amplify bias, disproportionately impact access to AI for healthcare, and examine the lack of available systems is critical. Integrated ethical reflection with human-in-the-loop systems for healthcare is the least that can be done to align cutting-edge healthcare with the ethical impact it requires (Floridi et al., 2018).

14.4 SUSTAINABILITY AND ENERGY-EFFICIENT AI

The progress of multimodal AI in medicine is of concomitant, and equally, new complexities of computational processing and energy consumption, invariably touching upon the issues of sustainability and its deleterious impact. The building of multimodal models at scale involves a perennial drain of financial, hardware, and energy resources, and output has a serious negative impact on the climate. It is worse, though, in the field of medicine, where AI has to reliably work in edge environments like wearables, implantable sensors, and portable diagnostics, and energy and latency require very stringent constraints. It is, therefore, imperative to solve the problem of sustainability in AI, and reframing the architecture of AI models to employ energy-efficient structures to avoid carbon-intensive training, and designing algorithms/entire models to run in a persistent state of low computational power, to unleash the potential of AI in medicine without damaging the planet.

14.4.1 Carbon footprint of large AI models

The training and deployment of large AI models is costly due to their environmental impact. Multimodal healthcare architectures utilize deep learning with millions of parameters. The energy demands from the models used are significant. Quantifying and mitigating the healthcare AI carbon footprint requires interdisciplinary research—primarily, the integration of machine learning, systems engineering, and sustainability science. Energy-aware training protocols and carbon-efficient model design are critical to AI in healthcare aligned with climate goals.

14.4.2 Low-power algorithms for medical edge devices

Edge computing is a pathway to energy-efficient and privacy-preserving healthcare AI (Dwork, C, 2008). To implement multimodal AI into medical edge devices, such as wearable sensors and handheld diagnostic devices, it is, however, necessary to develop energy-efficient algorithms and models that require less hardware resources. For AI-enabled healthcare to go beyond clinical ecosystems with plenty of resources, we need the capacity to do continuous multimodal processing with major energy restrictions (Strubell et al., 2019). Research pertaining to the potential of neuromorphic computing, event-driven processing, and approximate inference seeks to develop this capacity.

14.5 PREVIOUS AND CURRENT WORK: THE DEPLOYMENT OF AI IN MULTIMODAL HEALTHCARE

The future of multimodal AI in healthcare will depend on the creation of clinically reliable learning systems that are adaptive and explainable and can work with little or no labeled data. The emerging paradigms of autonomous learning and foundational models will enhance generalization across tasks in multiple areas of medicine and enhance learning with inadequate data. Concurrently developing neuro-symbolic systems and explainable AI will further regulate and clinically validate these models to enhance trust and compliance. These changes are becoming confluent with the paradigm of personalized and human-centered healthcare. In this view, multimodal AI systems can assist professionals by personalizing diagnostics, treatment plans, and patient surveillance.

14.5.1 Self-supervised and foundational models

The arrival of self-supervised learning and foundational models has greatly increased the possibilities of AI in multimodal healthcare. These framework models are able to learn diverse cross-modal representations because they utilize rich unlabeled datasets. The healthcare field poses unique challenges: data that is sparse, privacy protected, and needs a clinical validation process. These challenges should not deter the application of foundation models in healthcare as it poses a unique opportunity to both innovate within this field and reduce the resources required for healthcare data annotation and modeling.

14.5.2 Neuro-symbolic and explainable AI

The integration of data-driven learning (i.e., neuro) and symbolic reasoning (i.e. procedures and rules) fosters the development of healthcare systems that are more interpretable (Doshi-Velez et al., 2017) and, thus, verifiable. Neuro-symbolic AI research contextual systems within the healthcare domain, particularly in multimodal settings, integrate clinically and medically relevant causal frameworks with knowledge. Systems enhancement and focus on explainability should be prioritized because of the necessity for systems to be clinically adopted. The development of explanation mechanisms should be less focused on the theory and more on the clinical relevance of explanations.

14.5.3 Human-centric and personalized healthcare systems

The focus of human-centric design is the incorporation of AI tools into clinical settings, enhancing workflows to augment, not replace, the activities of clinical staff. There are a large number of different data sources, in different formats, that need to be analyzed when predicting individual patient journeys; this is how multimodal AI can be of assistance with tailoring and personalizing care. In order to achieve this, attention should be placed on developing new AI/design paradigms, and to integrating new workflows to ground positive/optimized patient outcomes, adaptive personalized system research is needed. As such, the evaluation of these systems should not be limited to assessing trust. Attention to user needs, system effectiveness, and positive patient outcomes must also be considered.

14.6 EMERGING TECHNOLOGIES AND INNOVATIONS

The multitude of recent advances in digital health technologies are dramatically changing the landscape of multimodal AI in healthcare by creating personalized predictive and relational health systems. Among these innovations, patient digital twins that combine and integrate for simulation and prognosis "multimodal" physiological and imaging data with behavioral data have emerged as a promising approach. Simultaneously, AI-based remote and wearable diagnostics enable non-invasive, real-time monitoring of patients outside of a traditional healthcare setting and are facilitating new healthcare access. The long-term advances in quantum-enabled healthcare computing are also particularly noteworthy for the rapid changes of healthcare computing and the sophisticated processing of complex multimodal data. These technologies are changing healthcare from a reactive and interdependent systems approach to a proactive, complex, data-driven, and highly integrated systems approach. Figure 14.2 presents the advantages of multimodal AI in healthcare sector.

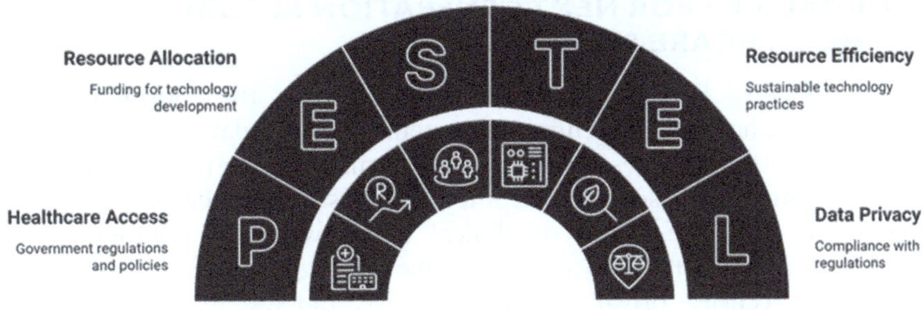

Figure 14.2 Healthcare applications of multimodal intelligence.

14.6.1 Multimodal digital twins

A digital twin is a real-time virtual replica of a physical object that is updated continuously. Digital twins can model the physiology of a patient, their diseases, and the response to treatments in real time. The development of digital twins pivots on integration of diverse streams of multimodal data, research and causal algorithms, and real-time iteration of systems (Bruynseels et al., 2018). There is a high possibility of impact for proactive healthcare, precision medicine, and treatment algorithms.

14.6.2 AI-driven remote and wearable diagnostics

Continued remote and wearable diagnostics have the potential to transform healthcare by providing real-time monitoring outside the clinical environment. Multimodal AI systems are able to incorporate different modalities including sensor data and contextual information, and patient reported outcomes, and use them to enable timely diagnosis and intervention. Future research should focus on data reliability, user engagement, and fair distribution of wearable technologies, especially in resource-poor environments.

14.6.3 Quantum-enabled healthcare computing

Quantum computing in the long run is expected to be a game changer in AI for healthcare, although the prospects in the near future remain questioned. Advanced quantum enhancement in optimization and machine learning algorithms are expected to overcome challenges related to complex multimodal inference (Cao et al., 2019). Practical applications of quantum technologies in health remain uncertain, but real-world scenarios and hybrid quantum-classical systems require a multidisciplinary approach.

Various contributions and impact of emerging technologies in multimodal AI for healthcare applications are shown in Table 14.3.

14.7 ROADMAP FOR NEXT-GENERATION SECURE HEALTHCARE SYSTEMS

For multifaceted healthcare systems of the future, the coordination of innovation in healthcare technology systems with regulatory, ethical, and interoperability challenges in healthcare systems is fundamental to the realization of intelligent, secure, and integrated systems in digital healthcare technology. The integration of clinical workflows with multimodal AI systems creates the need to define specific strategic research priorities in the areas of security, privacy, system integrity, and system scalability. The

Table 14.3 Emerging technologies and innovations in multimodal AI for healthcare

Technology	*Core idea*	*Key capabilities*	*Healthcare impact*
Multimodal digital twins	Real-time virtual replicas of patients integrating multimodal data	Simulation of physiology, disease progression, and treatment response	Proactive healthcare, precision medicine, personalized treatment planning
AI-driven remote and wearable diagnostics	Continuous patient monitoring using sensors and contextual data	Non-invasive, real-time diagnosis and early intervention	Expanded healthcare access, improved chronic disease management
Quantum-enabled healthcare computing	Quantum-enhanced AI for complex multimodal processing	Faster optimization and inference for high-dimensional data	Potential breakthroughs in large-scale, complex healthcare analytics

creation of standardized interoperability frameworks (HL7 Organization, 2023) is no less important, enabling seamless and secure data exchange across healthcare network systems, devices, and platforms. The combination of research and standardization to establish new healthcare AI applications is fundamental to the creation of secure, reliable, and digitally integrated systems in healthcare technology.

14.7.1 Research priorities

Through positive advancements in multimodal healthcare intelligence, the formulation of a comprehensive research roadmap is necessary. Improved robustness and generalization, privacy-preserving learning, energy efficiency, and clinically validated outcomes are key priorities. Each of these challenges requires a collaborative research approach, including academia, industry, healthcare system, and policymakers.

14.7.2 Standardization and interoperability goals

The absence of uniformity and interoperability poses obstacles to the expansion of multimodal healthcare systems. The fragmented integration of AI into healthcare systems can be addressed with uniform data types, assessment techniques, and regulatory frameworks. The focus of future research should involve developing advocacy for the establishment of open standards and the introduction of benchmarking systems in order to ensure that multimodal AI research is conducted with the values of transparency and reproducibility.

14.8 CONCLUSION

The potential of healthcare AI is immensely promising. It can help automate and streamline how healthcare data is analyzed and how clinical guidance is provided. Clinical support, clinical guidance, greater customizable care, and real-time care management can all be achieved efficiently. The potential is there for radical transformations in how medical imaging and electronic health data biosignals and physiological data from sensors. AI-boosted multimodal analytics can streamline real-time clinical alerts and care access. There are enhancements to rapid and scalable management, advanced predictions, and personalization in service of real-time monitoring more customized care and more accessible clinical guidance. However, these capabilities remain out of reach to implement in real-world obs. Practical and clinical constraints continue to act as significant barriers to workflow automation, real-time monitoring and alert systems, and the broader accessibility of AI-driven healthcare solutions.

To explain and document these trends and levels of automation, there is a unique combination of these technical integration concerns, for the collection and retention of the data must not negatively impact the healthcare workflows. Thus, the integration of large and complex AI-scoring instruments must involve the clinical equipoise and ethical concerns of monitoring real-world healthcare workflows.

Focusing on the cultivation of strong, safe, and human-centered multimodal intelligence offers the opportunity to shape the course of the integration of AI into healthcare systems ethically and responsibly. Researchers and practitioners know that when transparency, fairness, and usability are prioritized, and when the partnerships are ethically and technically deep with the AI systems, new technologies can be deployed with a balance of high technical performance and aligned ethical performance. This approach to the integration of AI into healthcare systems will be responsible and ethically aligned to improve patient care. It can build trustworthy, ethical, and responsible systems that will improve patient care and system performance.

REFERENCES

Baltrušaitis, T., Ahuja, C., & Morency, L.-P. (2019). Multimodal machine learning: A survey and taxonomy. *IEEE Transactions on Pattern Analysis and Machine Intelligence, 41*(2), 423–443. https://doi.org/10.1109/TPAMI.2018.2798607

Bruynseels, K., Santoni de Sio, F., & van den Hoven, J. (2018). Digital twins in health care: Ethical implications of an emerging engineering paradigm. *Frontiers in Genetics, 9*, Article 31. https://doi.org/10.3389/fgene.2018.00031

Cao, Y., Romero, J., Olson, J. P., Degroote, M., Johnson, P. D., Kieferová, M., … & Aspuru-Guzik, A. (2019). Quantum chemistry in the age of quantum computing. *Chemical Reviews, 119*(19), 10856–10915. https://doi.org/10.1021/acs.chemrev.8b00803

Doshi-Velez, F., & Kim, B. (2017). Towards a rigorous science of interpretable machine learning. *arXiv preprint arXiv:1702.08608*.

Dwork, C. (2008). Differential privacy: A survey of results. In *Proceedings of the 5th International Conference on Theory and Applications of Models of Computation* (pp. 1–19). Springer. https://doi.org/10.1007/978-3-540-79228-4_1

Floridi, L., Cowls, J., Beltrametti, M., Chatila, R., Chazerand, P., Dignum, V., & Vayena, E. (2018). AI4People—An ethical framework for a good AI society. *Minds and Machines, 28*(4), 689–707. https://doi.org/10.1007/s11023-018-9482-5

Ghassemi, M., Naumann, T., Schulam, P., Beam, A. L., Chen, I. Y., Ranganath, R., & Saria, S. (2021). Practical guidance on artificial intelligence for health-care data. *The Lancet Digital Health, 3*(7), e393–e398. https://doi.org/10.1016/S2589-7500(19)30084-6

HL7 Organization. (2023). *HL7 interoperability standards*. www.hl7.org/implement/standards/index.cfm?ref=nav

Johnson, K.B., Wei, W.-Q., Weeraratne, D., Frisse, M.E., Misulis, K., Rhee, K., Zhao, J. and Snowdon, J.L. (2021), Precision Medicine, AI, and the Future of Personalized Health Care. *Clin Transl Sci,* 14: 86-93. https://doi.org/10.1111/cts.12884

Kumar, Y., & Singla, R. (2021). Federated learning systems for healthcare: Perspective and recent progress. In: Rehman, M.H.u., Gaber, M.M. (eds) *Federated Learning Systems. Studies in Computational Intelligence*, vol 965. Springer, Cham. https://doi.org/10.1007/978-3-030-70604-3_6

Li, T., Sahu, A. K., Talwalkar, A., & Smith, V. (2020). Federated learning: Challenges, methods, and future directions. *IEEE Signal Processing Magazine, 37*(3), 50–60. https://doi.org/10.1109/MSP.2020.2975749

Ngiam, J., Khosla, A., Kim, M., Nam, J., Lee, H., & Ng, A. Y. (2011). Multimodal deep learning. In *Proceedings of the 28th International Conference on Machine Learning* (pp. 689–696), ACM.

Patel, S., Park, H., Bonato, P., Chan, L., & Rodgers, M. (2012). A review of wearable sensors and systems with application in rehabilitation. *Journal of NeuroEngineering and Rehabilitation, 9*, Article 21. https://doi.org/10.1186/1743-0003-9-21

Strubell, E., Ganesh, A., & McCallum, A. (2019). Energy and policy considerations for deep learning in NLP. In *Proceedings of the 57th Annual Meeting of the Association for Computational Linguistics* (pp. 3645–3650), Association for Computational Linguistics. https://doi.org/10.18653/v1/P19-1355

Zech, J. R., Badgeley, M. A., Liu, M., Costa, A. B., Titano, J. J., & Oermann, E. K. (2018). Variable generalization performance of a deep learning model to detect pneumonia in chest radiographs. *PLOS Medicine, 15*(11), e1002683. https://doi.org/10.1371/journal.pmed.1002683

Index

For Product Safety Concerns and Information please contact our EU representative GPSR@taylorandfrancis.com Taylor & Francis Verlag GmbH, Kaufingerstraße 24, 80331 München, Germany